Clinical Nuclear Medicine Neuroimaging

Dafang Wu

Clinical Nuclear Medicine Neuroimaging

An Instructional Casebook

Springer

Dafang Wu, MD, PhD
Department of Diagnostic Radiology & Molecular Imaging
Oakland University William Beaumont School of Medicine
Royal Oak, MI
USA

ISBN 978-3-030-40892-3 ISBN 978-3-030-40893-0 (eBook)
https://doi.org/10.1007/978-3-030-40893-0

This Springer imprint is published by the registered company Springer Nature Switzerland AG
The registered company address is: Gewerbestrasse 11, 6330 Cham, Switzerland

Preface

Clinical nuclear medicine neuroimaging studies (*e.g.*, brain FDG PET, brain perfusion SPECT, or CSF scintigraphy, just to name a few) are often difficult to interpret, mainly due to a variety of limiting factors. These include relatively low neuroimaging study volume in many of nuclear medicine clinics, the complex neuroanatomy, and lack of dedicated reference books in this important medical imaging field. As human life expectancy increases, neurological diseases, especially neurodegenerative dementias, have become a growing public health issue. Additionally, accurate and appropriate interpretation of clinical nuclear medicine neuroimaging studies is imperative not only for the aid of clinical diagnosis of neurological disorders but also for the implementation of effective pharmacotherapy, if available. Therefore, the main purpose of this casebook is to fill these unmet needs in nuclear medicine clinical practice.

This casebook consists of eight chapters, with the first 4 Chapters focusing on PET and SPECT in dementia and epilepsy, respectively, which are the mainstay of clinical functional neuroimaging studies. Chapter 5 includes cases to show the value and limitation of FDG PET imaging of brain tumors, although clinical significance of this application is still under debate. Chapter 6 focuses on dopamine transporter scan (often abbreviated as DaTscan), a relatively new neuroimaging modality approved by the FDA in 2011 to help differentiate essential tremor (ET) from tremor due to dopamine neurodegenerative diseases such as Parkinson's disease (PD). Chapter 7 describes cerebrospinal fluid (CSF) scintigraphic studies that are divided into three sections: CSF imaging in normal pressure hydrocephalus (NPH), CSF leak imaging, and CSF imaging of shunt patency. Cases presented in this Chapter show that CSF imaging plays an important role in initial diagnosis and subsequent follow-up of certain patients with NPH, or CSF leak, or CSF shunt misfaction, especially those with persistent/recurrent symptoms and/or equivocal anatomic imaging results. Chapter 8 comprises several brain perfusion SPECT studies in the evaluation of brain death and chronic Lyme encephalopathy, as well as three unique cases: the WADA test (also referred to as intracarotid amobarbital procedure [IAP]), an intracerebral steal phenomenon (ISP) on brain perfusion SPECT with acetazolamide (Diamox) challenge, and finally an FDG PET of possible Mycoplasma encephalitis. Attached to the end of this book are two appendices, Self-Assessment Quiz and Imaging Protocols, which are provided for those who wish to test their own ability in the interpretation of clinical nuclear medicine neuroimaging studies and/or to adopt the practical nuclear medicine neuroimaging protocols used in our institution on a daily basis.

It took me 1.5 years to complete this project. During the course of the writing, I found myself from time to time on a steep learning curve in many of the topics, although I have been practicing nuclear medicine for nearly two decades, in addition to my prior years in basic neuroscience research. Advances occur at a fast rate in many neurological fields including diagnosis and treatment of patients with neurodegenerative diseases, epilepsies, and other neurodisorders. Meanwhile, practitioners in clinical nuclear medicine neuroimaging, likely physicians working in other medical specialties or subspecialties, are increasingly required to work more efficiently, often with limited resources. In this book, each case presentation starts with a chief complaint, followed by pertinent clinical information, representative images with illustrations, key imaging findings, concise discussion/follow-up data, and concludes with a case summary. Readers will be able to quickly catch the main teaching points of each case in a few minutes through reviewing the chief complaint, figure(s) with key findings, and case summary, although the clinical information and discussion/follow-up data are very informative. In Chapters 1 and 2 (*e.g.*, PET and SPECT in dementias, respectively), a detailed instruction was provided in each of the first case discussion section (Case 1.1, and Case 2.1, respectively) regarding appropriate neuroimaging display (transaxial, sagittal, coronal, and their sequences), color selection, and image reorientation. In summary, this book was written by a physician for the physicians at any level of clinical training or in their busy daily practice in nuclear medicine and radiology, with the sole intention to improve patient care and to enhance medical education.

That having been said, I have to acknowledge that the data equality of many cases in this book varies despite extensive efforts to improve. This is inevitable given the complex referral base and variable patient and physician preferences in diagnosis, treatment, and follow-up of neurologic disorders. Also, since antemortem biopsy is required for definitive diagnosis of many neurological diseases, the majority of the cases in this book did not have a definite diagnosis, except for a few patients with intractable epilepsy (Chapters 3 and 4) or brain tumor (Chapter 5), who ultimately underwent biopsy or surgical resection. The words of "possible" or "probable" were used for likely or most likely diagnosis/impression in most cases indicating different levels of confidence. It is my hope that this casebook can be significantly improved in the future editions through incorporation of readers' feedback, updated follow-up data of existing cases, and addition of new cases.

Royal Oak, MI, USA Dafang Wu, MD, PhD

Acknowledgments

First and foremost, I sincerely thank the leadership at the Beaumont Health System in Michigan for their strong support of this project, with special thanks to Dr. Richard H. Kennedy, PhD; Dr. Ray O. Bahado-Singh, MD; Dr. Duane G. Mezwa, MD; and Dr. Richard Silbergleit, MD. I would also like to acknowledge that all cases presented in this book were from patients we have been privileged to serve in our Nuclear Medicine Clinics. This project would not have been possible without their contributions to medical science and education.

I would also like to thank my Nuclear Medicine colleagues, Dr. Darlene Fink-Bennett, MD; Dr. Helena R. Balon, MD; Dr. John N. Rydberg, MD; Dr. Jane C. Palka, MD; Dr. John P. Seitz, MD; and Dr. Feng Qing, MD, PhD, for sharing many of their interesting cases from our daily clinical service, which have greatly inspired the selection I have included in this book. I would like to especially thank Dr. Helena R. Balon and Dr. Feng Qing for their support and passion for this project.

I am deeply grateful to my entire family for their support and contribution to this project. I thank my son, Sherwin, and my daughter-in-law, Anji, for their encouragement, support, and invaluable suggestions. I would like to give special thanks to my daughter, Shirley, for meticulously editing the chapters, her suggestion for adding a Self-Assessment Quiz section to the book, and her passion and strong support throughout this project. Most of all, I wish to thank my wife, Xiaoping, from the bottom of my heart, for her understanding, encouragement, and support not only in this project but also in all of my life endeavors.

Finally, I would like to thank Eric Zhou, a medical student at the New York University School of Medicine, for carefully editing chapters and providing invaluable suggestions and clarifications throughout the writing process.

Contents

Positron Emission Tomography (PET) in Dementias

1

Case 1.1 Probable Normal Brain FDG PET Study

Clinical Information

Chief Complaint *Memory loss*

The patient is a 45-year-old male presenting with memory loss, worsening after exposure to industrial waste of unknown kind. He denies hallucinations and there is no tremor on exam.

Current medications include alprazolam 1 mg daily; bupropion 300 mg daily; folate 1 mg daily; omeprazole 20 mg daily, albuterol, two puffs daily; and quetiapine 200 mg daily.

Past medical history includes essential hypertension, hypercholesterolemia, seizure disorder, asthma, depression, bipolar disorder, and tobacco and alcohol dependence. He denies a history of drug abuse, however. There is no family history of dementia.

A recent MR imaging of the brain was normal. Laboratory tests showed TSH, folate, and vitamin B_{12} in normal ranges.

The patient's blood glucose level was 112 mg/dL prior to FDG administration for the PET study.

FDG PET Findings (Fig. 1.1)

The images show essentially symmetric brain hemispheres and no evidence of brain atrophy (Fig. 1.1a, the upper panel). FDG activity is highest in the basal ganglia (white arrow) and essentially symmetric, despite slight head-tilting. FDG activity in the cerebral cortex is largely symmetric (red triangles), with relatively higher activity in the primary visual cortices (green arrow) and lower activity in the temporal lobes (red arrows), especially in the medial, anterior, and inferior portions, when compared to the other cortical regions. FDG activity in bilateral posterior cingulate gyri/precuneus (PCG/PCUN, hatched red arrows) is higher than the anterior cingulate gyri (ACG). This finding is best appreciated on the sagittal view (Fig. 1.1a, the middle panel). The PCG/PCUNs are bilateral medial (vertical) parietal lobes separated by the posterior interhemispheric fissure, and they are located on the two adjacent slides in the central of symmetrically displayed sagittal images. FDG activity in the thalami is also symmetric, despite slight head-tilting. FDG activity in the cerebellum (hatched yellow arrows) is overall lower than the cerebral cortices. This is best appreciated on the coronal view (Fig. 1.1a, the lower panel).

Discussion and Follow-Up

Prior to imaging review, it is necessary to emphasize the importance of knowing the patient's current clinical presentation and pertinent medical history. Briefly, this is a middle-aged male with a chief complaint of memory loss and history of

D. Wu, *Clinical Nuclear Medicine Neuroimaging*, https://doi.org/10.1007/978-3-030-40893-0_1

mood disorders and tobacco/alcohol dependence. A recent brain MRI was normal. Therefore, the pretest likelihood of neurodegenerative disorders is low.

Imaging review of FDG PET brain scans usually starts with reorientation (Fig. 1.1b), as difficulty in positioning and head-tilting during imaging acquisition often occur. Using the provided crosshair as a reference, scroll the transaxial slices to the level of the basal ganglia and thalami, and make the horizontal line in the middle of the temporal lobes and in parallel with the tails of the putamens, the vertical line centering in the right brain hemisphere, and then adjust the image to make the vertical line in parallel to the interhemispheric fissure (white line). On the sagittal view, rotate the image to make the inferior right frontal lobe and the inferior right cerebellum (red line) in an approximately 30-degree angle, and on the coronal view, make the bilateral inferior poles of the temporal lobes (green line) at the same level and in parallel with the horizontal line of the provided crosshair.

Although FDG PET brain scan images could be displayed in dozens of different colors, I recommend to use the 10-step color spectrum, as subtle but important imaging findings only can be appreciated on this particular color display, relative to others. In other words, the use of 10-step color display for visual imaging review could increase/improve detection sensitivity. The 10-step color spectrum corresponds to FDG intensities from highest to lowest in the following order: red, red-orange, yellow, yellow-green, green, black-green, cyan, cyan blue (sky blue), blue, and dark blue (navy blue). Since the normal highest FDG activity is distributed in the basal ganglia, imaging color normalization requires to adjust each set of the images (transaxial, sagittal, or coronal) to show the basal ganglia in red.

After reorientation and color selection/normalization, the images of this particular case show an essentially normal pattern of FDG distribution: highest tracer activity in the basal ganglia (assumed 100%), followed by essentially symmetric activity in the cerebral cortex (approximately 75–90% of the basal ganglia), and lowest activity in the cerebellum (approximately 50–65% of the basal ganglia) [2, 6]. Note that there is some slight cortical asymmetry likely due to FDG heterogeneity and head-tilting. There is no global or regional glucose hypometabolism to suggest a neurodegenerative process. Therefore, this patient's symptom of memory loss is likely due to known mood disorders or transient alcoholic encephalopathy or both.

In the ensuring 3-year follow-up, the patient never had any recurrent memory issues, although he was admitted to our hospital several times due to intermittent, generalized abdominal pain. He was effectively treated for acute and chronic alcohol hepatitis and pancreatitis.

Case Summary

Brain FDG distribution in normal adult individuals is essentially and largely symmetric, with regional variations in the following order [2]:

- *Basal ganglia (highest) > cerebral cortices (intermediate) > cerebellar cortices (lowest)*

Among the cerebral cortices, normal FDG distribution varies in the following order:

- *Primary visual cortices > frontoparietal cortices > temporal cortices*

Within the temporal lobes, normal FDG distribution varies in the following order:

- *Lateral/superior > anterior > medial (mesial)/ inferior*

The essentially normal FDG distribution pattern, in conjunction with a low pretest likelihood for neurodegenerative disorder in this patient, is indicative of a probable normal brain metabolic study, which was confirmed by clinical follow-up data.

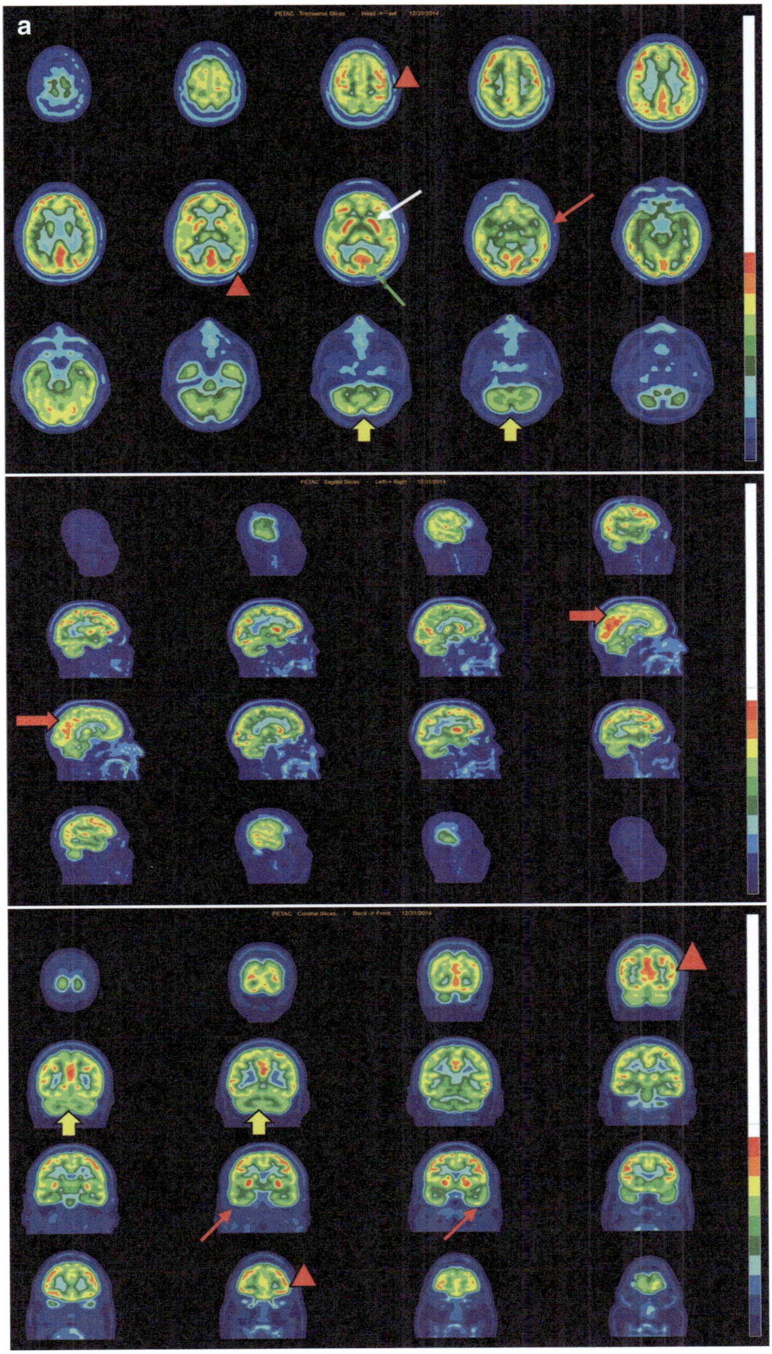

Fig. 1.1 (**a**) A 45-year-old male with probable normal brain FDG PET study. The brain FDG PET images are displayed in the following orders: *the upper panel* – transaxial view from superior to inferior or head to feet; *the middle panel* – sagittal view from left to right; *the lower panel* – coronal view from posterior to anterior, or back to front. (**b**) Image reorientation. On the transaxial view (the left), using the provided crosshair as a reference, scroll the slice to the level of the basal ganglia and thalami, and make the horizontal line of the red crosshair in the middle of the temporal lobes and in parallel with the tails of the putamens, the vertical line centering in the right brain hemisphere, and then adjust the image to make the vertical line in parallel to the interhemispheric fissure (white line). On the sagittal view (the middle), rotate the image to make the inferior surface of the right frontal lobe and the inferior surface of the right cerebellum (red line) in an approximately 30-degree angle. On the coronal view (the right), adjust the bilateral inferior poles of the temporal lobes (green line) at the same level and in parallel with the horizontal line of the provided crosshair

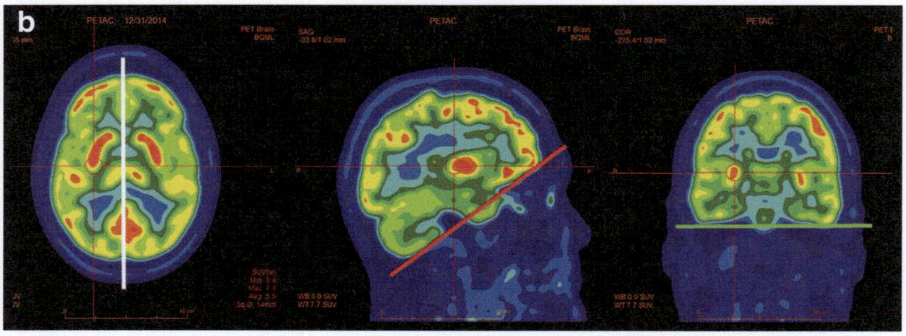

Fig. 1.1 (continued)

Case 1.2 Probable Normal Aging

Clinical Information

Chief Complaint *Memory loss for more than 1 year*

The patient is a 69-year-old male who is a current everyday smoker presenting with memory loss for more than 1 year, associated with malaise, fatigue, weight loss, and insomnia but no depression. He has had significant decline in his short-term memory, for which he has given up driving. He reports diminished appetite but denies any bowel issues.

Current medications include tadalafil 20 mg per day; clopidogrel 75 mg per day; albuterol inhaler, one puff every 6 hours; acetaminophen/oxycodone 325/10 mg, one tablet per day; isosorbide mononitrate 30 mg two tablets per day; metoprolol 25 mg twice a day; morphine 30 mg twice a day; nifedipine 60 mg per day; simvastatin 40 mg per night; and terazosin 1 mg per night.

Past medical history includes chronic low back pain, chronic hypertension, COPD (chronic obstructive pulmonary disease), dyslipidemia, and obesity.

Family history is positive for dementia of unspecified type.

Laboratory test showed TSH in a normal range.

The patient's blood glucose level was 95 mg/dL prior to FDG administration for the brain PET study.

FDG PET Findings (Fig. 1.2)

This study is technically limited due to difficult head positioning. As a result, the right cerebellum was not fully covered during the imaging acquisition (hatched yellow arrows).

The images show mildly prominent lateral ventricles, and separation of the deep brain structures (basal ganglia and thalami), suggestive of mild brain atrophy.

Mildly decreased FDG activity is noted in the bilateral medial forefrontal, superomedial parietal, and anteromedial temporal lobes (red arrows), right slightly more prominent than the left, whereas FDG activity in the bilateral PCG/PCUN (hatched red arrows) is well preserved.

Overall, FDG distribution still follows a normal order, *e.g.*, highest activity in the basal ganglia, intermediate in the remainder of the cerebral cortices, and lowest in the cerebellum. Note that FDG activity in the primary visual cortices is enhanced bilaterally (green arrow), likely due to physiological stimulation.

Discussion and Follow-Up

The imaging finding of minimal-to-mild brain atrophy in this 69-year-old male patient is likely age-appropriate. The mild cortical hypometabolism in the bilateral medial forefrontal, superomedial parietal, and anteromedial temporal lobes, despite slight asymmetry, is likely secondary to brain atrophy, given the locations and the pattern. The preserved glucose metabolic activity in the PCG/PCUN makes AD (Alzheimer's disease) less likely. There is normal FDG activity in the occipital lobes including enhanced activity in the primary visual cortices; therefore, DLB (dementia with Lewy bodies) is less likely. There is no evidence of cortical or lacunar infarct to suggest VD (vascular dementia), either. Finally, FTD (frontotemporal dementia) is less likely, given the mild hypometabolism confined to the medial forefrontal and anteromedial temporal lobes and the lack of behavioral or language issues in the clinical presentation.

During 1-year follow-up, the patient only had one family-doctor office visit for his chronic back pain and chronic hypertension, without memory issues. Later, he was diagnosed with lumbar radiculopathy, for which physical therapy was recommended in addition to prescribed pain medications.

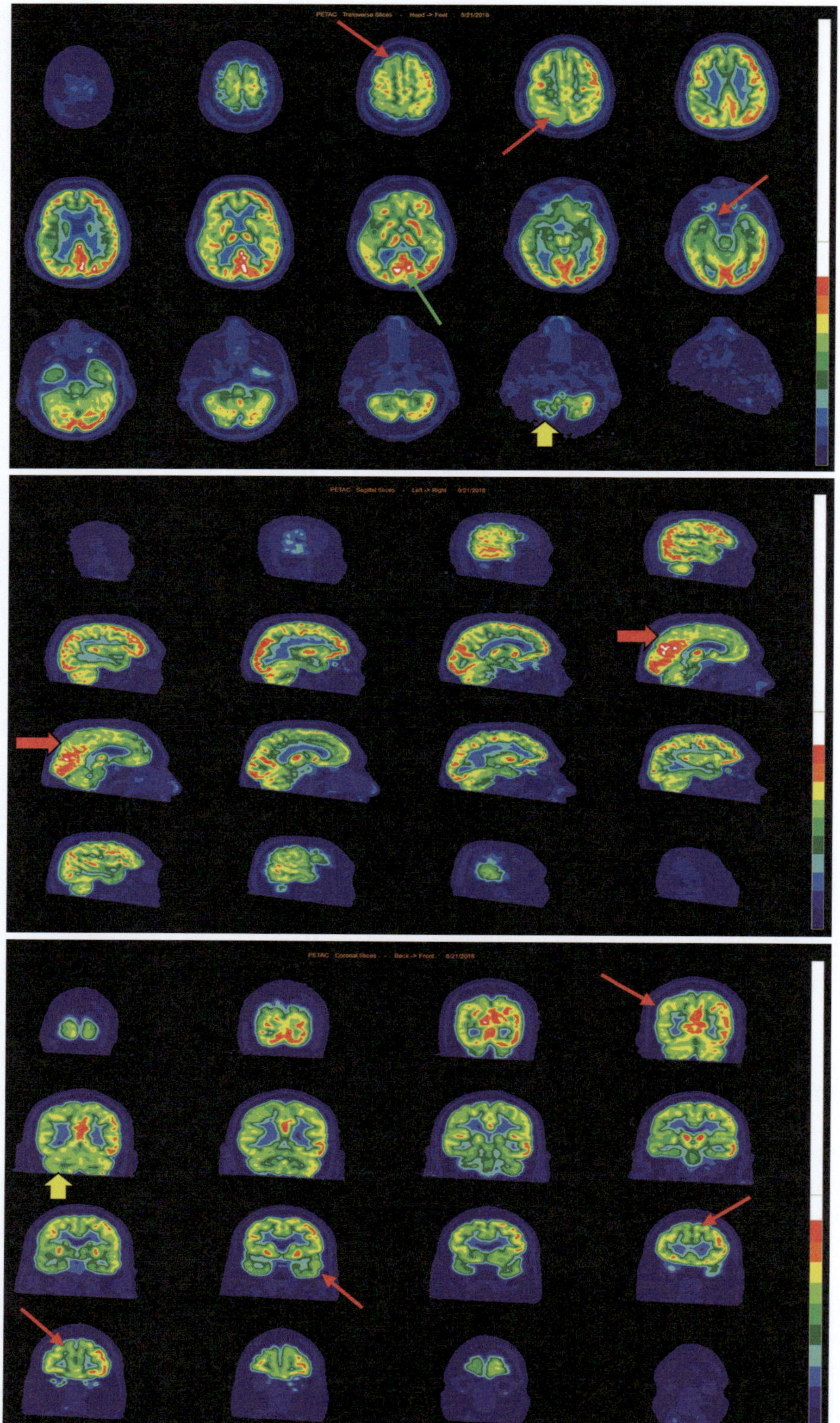

Fig. 1.2 A 69-year-old male with probable normal brain aging

Case Summary

Diagnosis of normal aging is often a judgment call after exclusion of commonly diagnosed neurodegenerative dementias, such as AD, FTD, DLB, or VD [12]. This 69-year-old male has minimal-to-mild brain atrophy as evidenced by prominent lateral ventricles and well-separated basal ganglia and thalami. The magnitude of cortical hypometabolism is minimal to mild, and the affected medial forefrontal, superomedial parietal, and anteromedial temporal lobes are common sites for brain atrophy. There is no typical pattern to suggest any commonly diagnosed neurodegenerative dementia. Therefore, the overall FDG PET findings, in conjunction with the clinical presentation and the follow-up data, are suggestive of mild brain atrophy, likely secondary to normal aging.

Case 1.3 Probable Mild Cognitive Impairment (MCI)

Clinical Information

Chief Complaint *Short-term memory loss and expressive difficulty for 2 years*

The patient is an 80-year-old right-handed male presenting with short-term memory loss that started approximately 2 years ago. He has difficulty in remembering what people have told him recently, sometimes forgetting where he put his things. In addition, he has difficulty in talking and expressing himself verbally. However, he is independent in his daily activities including driving a car. He is an attorney and still practices law. Neurological examination showed mild dysarthria and mild subcortical expressive aphasia. He scored 30/30 on the Mini-Mental State Examination (MMSE). The patient denies any history of head trauma, bleeding, infection, depression, hallucinations, or delusions.

Current medications include celecoxib 100 mg twice a day, amlodipine 10 mg daily, enalapril-hydrochlorothiazide 10/25 mg daily, atorvastatin 40 mg daily, and multivitamins.

Past medical history includes hypertension, hypercholesterolemia, prior stroke, smoking, back pain, osteoarthritis, and obstructive sleep apnea (OSA).

There is no family history of dementia.

Recent brain MRI revealed chronic ischemic changes, more prominent in the periventricular white matter, an old and stable lacunar infarction in the posterior left thalamus, and generalized brain atrophy with a greater central component.

Laboratory tests showed TSH, folate, and vitamin B_{12} in normal ranges.

The patient's blood glucose was 88 mg/dL prior to FDG administration for the brain PET study.

FDG PET Findings (Fig. 1.3)

Images show mildly dilated lateral ventricles, separated basal ganglia and thalami, and prominent sulci, in line with the MRI findings, consistent with generalized brain atrophy.

Mild-to-moderately decreased FDG activities are noted in the medial frontal lobes including the anterior cingulate gyri (the middle panel, white arrows) and bilateral temporal lobes (the upper and lower panels, white arrows). Mildly to moderately decreased FDG activity is seen in the left parietal and occipital lobes, when compared to the contralateral, but more prominent at the junction of the left parietal-temporal-occipital lobes (red arrows). The left thalamus is smaller (green arrow), with decreased FDG activity when compared to the right, likely due to known left posterior thalamic lacunar infarct. Although FDG activity in the posterior cingulate gyrus (PCG) is preserved, there is mild to moderately decreased activity in the bilateral precuneus (PCUN, hatched red arrows). FDG activities in the remainder of the cerebral cortices, bilateral basal ganglia, the right thalami, and cerebella are within normal limits.

Discussion and Follow-Up

This patient scored 30/30 on MMSE, although he reported short-term memory loss and difficulty in expressing for 2 years. Contrast to the subjective complaints, he is still able to maintain independent daily activities including practicing law.

On the brain FDG PET study, there is evidence of mild to moderate generalized brain atrophy. The dominant cortical hypometabolism is noted at the junction of the left parietal-temporal-occipital lobes, in line with a known prior lacunar infarction in the posterior left thalamus, suggestive of left-sided ischemic vascular disease instead of FTD. The preserved metabolic activity in PCG makes AD less likely. Since the metabolic activity in the majority of the occipital lobes is well preserved, dementia with Lewy bodies (DLB) is less likely. The cortical hypometabolism in bilateral precuneus (PCUN), however, is concerning for an early neurodegenerative process. Given all these considerations, the overall FDG PET findings are compatible with mild cognitive impairment (MCI), although an early neurodegenerative process cannot be excluded.

Nearly 4 years later, due to clinical concerns for normal pressure hydrocephalus (NPH), the

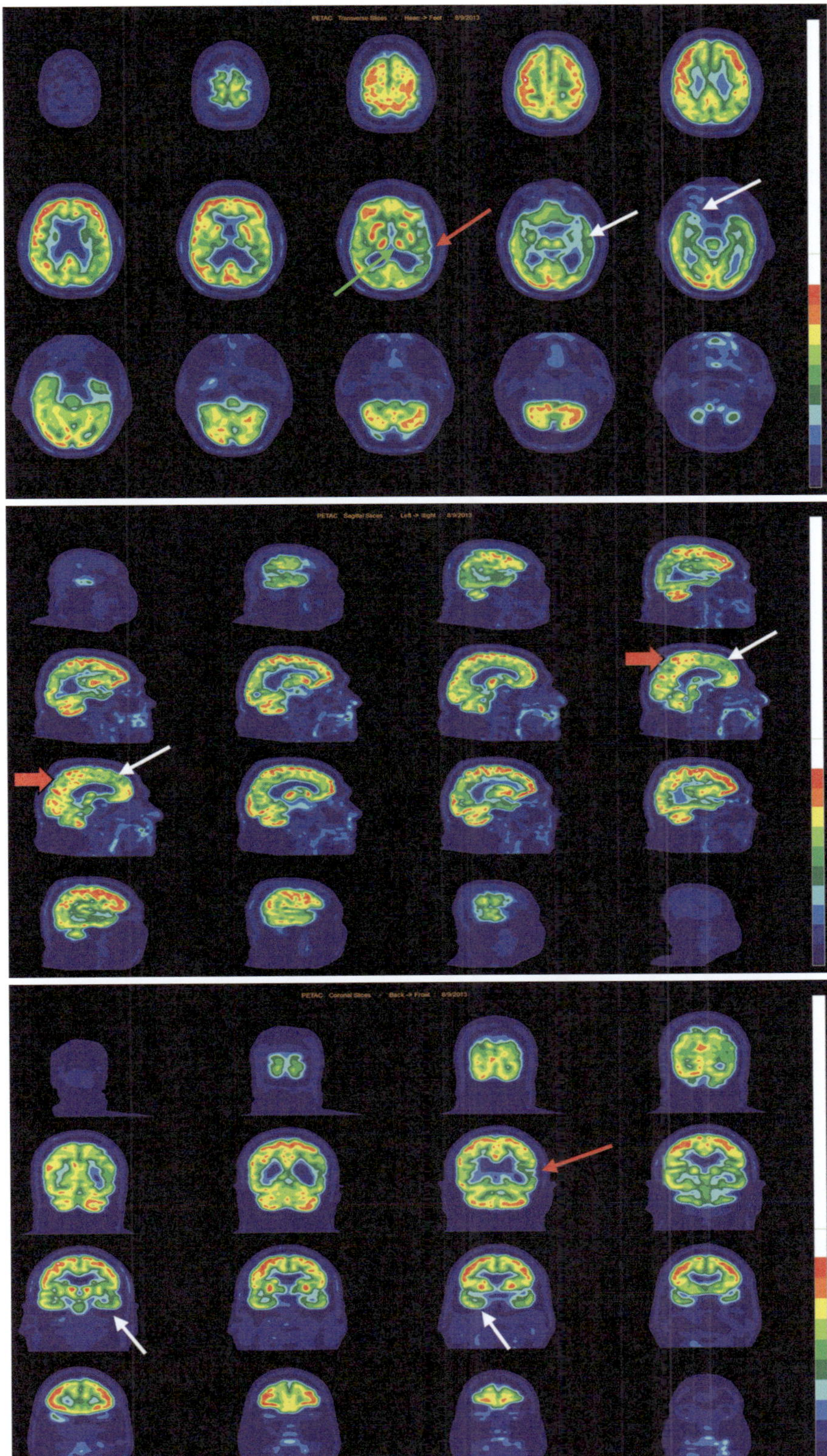

Fig. 1.3 An 80-year-old male with probable mild cognitive impairment (MCI)

patient underwent a nuclear medicine cisternogram, which was negative.

Follow-up brain MRI showed stable chronic ischemic changes. Brain MRA revealed no large vessel occlusion or aneurysm, except for stable basilar artery tortuosity and supraclinoid internal carotid artery ectasia.

Case Summary

MCI needs to be considered in patients with subjective complaint of memory loss but without evidence of dementia on neuropsychiatric examination [7, 15]. The FDG PET study showed no typical patterns to suggest commonly diagnosed neurodegenerative dementias, such as AD, FTD, DLB, or VD. However, cortical hypometabolism is identified in bilateral precuneus, for which an early neurodegenerative process cannot be excluded. Although there is evidence of left-sided ischemic vascular disease, the overall FDG PET findings, in conjunction with the clinical presentation, are compatible with MCI, which was further supported by follow-up imaging studies, including essentially normal cisternogram, MRI, and MRA.

Case 1.4 Probable Early-Onset Alzheimer's Disease (EOAD)

Clinical Information

Chief Complaint *Progressive short-term memory loss for 5–6 years*

The patient is a 51-year-old male presenting with progressive short-term memory loss that started 5–6 years ago. Although the patient believes he has been fairly stable, his wife has noticed a steady decline in his memory. He is a non-smoker and works as an insurance agent. He is frustrated with his loss of independence and particularly with difficulty in word finding. There is no history of drug or alcohol abuse. He denies history of stroke, head injury, or seizures.

Neurological examination reveals that his speech is fluent without any significant dysphasia or dysarthria. There is no tremor. Gait is steady and symmetric without any assistance.

Current medications include memantine 10 mg twice a day and sertraline 50 mg daily.

Past medical history is significant for depression and anxiety.

There is no family history of dementia.

Laboratory tests showed TSH and vitamin B_{12} in normal ranges.

A recent MR imaging of the brain at an outside institution was unremarkable, per report.

The patient's blood glucose level was 96 mg/dL prior to FDG administration for the brain PET study.

FDG PET Findings (Fig. 1.4)

Images show prominent sulci and enlarged lateral ventricles (green arrow), posterior horns > anterior horns, consistent with brain atrophy.

Global, mild to moderately decreased FDG activity indicating generalized hypometabolism is identified throughout the cerebral cortices, with relatively preserved activity only in the primary sensorimotor strips and the primary visual cortices. The most profound hypometabolism is noted in the bilateral parietal lobes (red arrows), with FDG activity being approximately 40–50% of the basal ganglia (normal 75–90%), right being more affected than left. This is followed, in a lesser degree, by hypometabolic involvement of the adjacent superior and lateral frontal lobes, the posterior and superior temporal lobes, and the superior lateral occipital lobes (white arrows). In contrast, FDG activity in the medial and inferior frontal lobes, anterior and medial temporal lobes, and medial and inferior occipital lobes is less affected. Severe cortical hypometabolism is also identified in the bilateral PCG/PCUN (hatched red arrows), whereas FDG activity in the anterior cingulate gyri (ACG) is relatively preserved.

FDG activity in bilateral basal ganglia, thalami, and cerebellum is essentially symmetric and appears within normal limits.

Discussion

In contrast to the reported "unremarkable" MRI study at an outside institution, brain FDG PET study is highly abnormal, with findings consistent with global and generalized brain atrophy that is age-disproportionate for this 51-year-old patient. In addition, the most profound cortical hypometabolism is identified in the bilateral parietal lobes including PCG/PCUN, which, in conjunction with the prominent posterior ventricular horns, is a classic functional neuroimaging biomarker for Alzheimer's disease (AD) – the most common type of neurodegenerative dementia [3, 14–16].

The less prominent cortical hypometabolism follows a spread pattern, mainly affecting the lateral superior occipital, and posterior lateral temporal lobes. In the frontal lobes, despite the preserved metabolism in the sensorimotor strips, cortical hypometabolism is more prominent in the superior and lateral regions when compared to the medial and inferior, which also supports a spread pattern from the dominantly affected parietal lobes.

Given the patient's symptoms started in his late 40s, well prior to the cutoff age of 65, this case is consistent with early-onset Alzheimer's disease (EOAD), a rare neurodegenerative disease affecting approximately 5.5% of the total AD patient population [17].

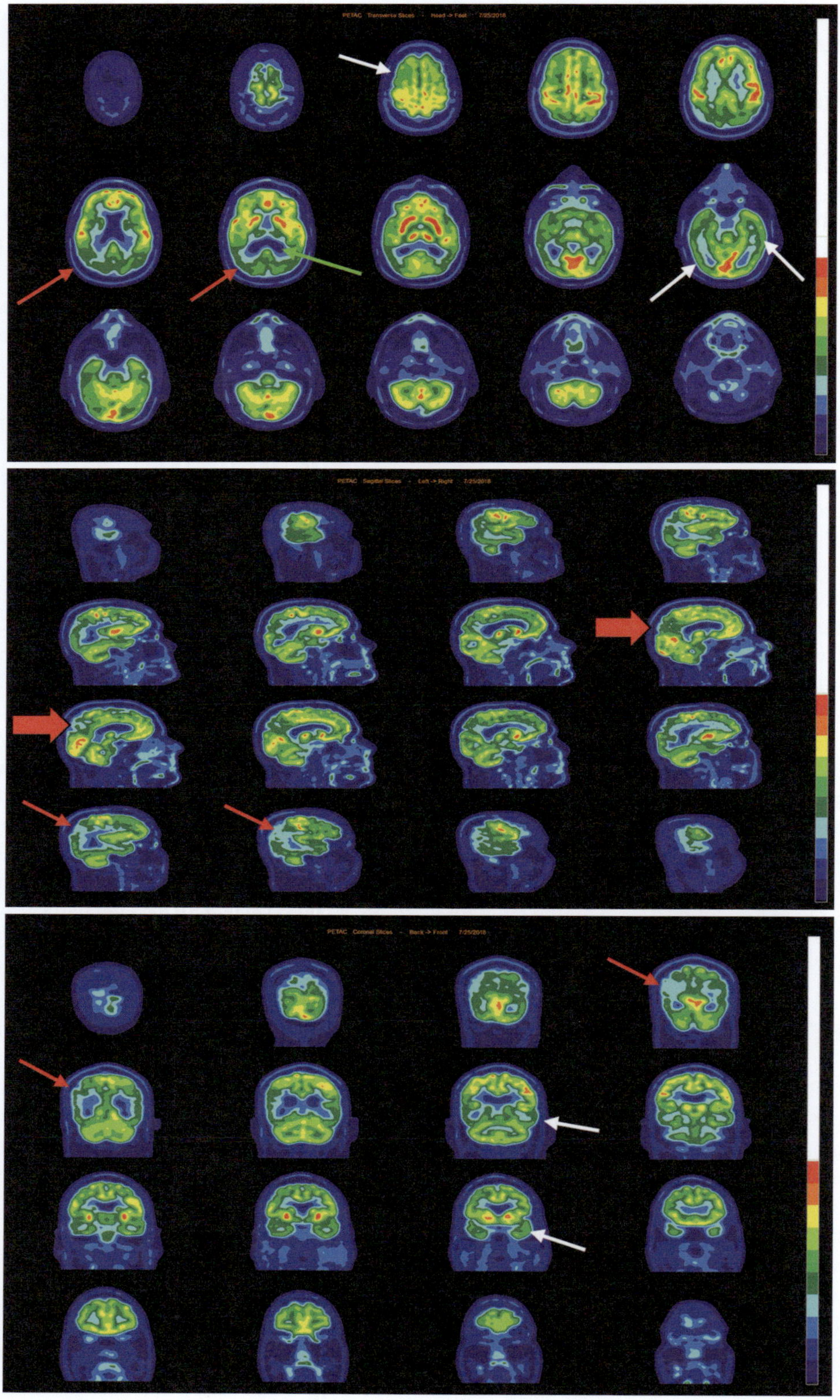

Fig. 1.4 A 51-year-old male with probable early-onset Alzheimer's disease (EOAD)

Case Summary

Progressive memory loss and functional decline in a 51-year-old businessman is suggestive of a neurodegenerative disorder. In contrast to the reported normal MR imaging, the FDG PET findings of age-disproportionate global brain atrophy and dominant cerebral cortical hypometabolism in the parietal lobes including PCG/PCUN, in conjunction with spread hypometabolism in the adjacent temporal, occipital and frontal lobes, are functional neuroimaging characteristics of probable AD. Since the patient's symptoms started in his late 40s, well prior to the cutoff age of 65, this case is consistent with early-onset AD (EOAD).

Case 1.5 Probable Late-Onset Alzheimer's Disease (LOAD)

Clinical Information

Chief Complaint *Progressive short-term memory loss*

The patient is a 69-year-old female presenting with progressive short-term memory loss for 13 months. On dementia screening interview, the patient had problems with judgment, demonstrated decreased interest in hobbies, and repeated the same things over and over. She had trouble learning and often forgot the date. She also had trouble remembering appointments and managing her personal finances.

Current medications include simvastatin 70 mg per day, sertraline 50 mg per day, and lisinopril 20 mg per day.

Past medical history includes hypertension, hyperlipidemia, depression, and overactive bladder. She is a former smoker but denies alcohol or drug abuse. She denies history of seizure, stroke, or head injury.

The patient does not have a family history of dementia.

Laboratory tests showed TSH, vitamin B_{12}, and folate in normal ranges.

Brain MRI was unremarkable except for an incidental finding of partial empty sella.

The patient's blood glucose level was 104 mg/dL prior to FDG administration for the PET study.

FDG PET Findings (Fig. 1.5)

Images show prominent sulci, wide separation of basal ganglia and thalami, and dilated lateral ventricles (green arrow), posterior horns > anterior horns, indicating global brain atrophy.

The most profound cortical hypometabolism is identified in the parietal lobes (red arrows), left > right (approximately 30–50% of the basal ganglia, normal 75–90%), including the PCG/PCUN (hatched red arrows). Mild to moderate cortical hypometabolism in a spread pattern is noted, more prominent in the adjacent posterior lateral temporal, superior lateral occipital, and superior lateral frontal lobes, again left > right (white arrows), although metabolism in bilateral sensorimotor strips and the primary visual cortices is relatively preserved or less affected.

Minimally decreased FDG activity is noted in the right cerebellum (hatched yellow arrows) relative to the left, suggestive of crossed cerebrocerebellar diaschisis.

Discussion and Follow-Up

The FDG PET shows global brain atrophy and dilated lateral ventricles, posterior horns > frontal horns. The most profound cortical hypometabolism is identified in the parietal lobes including PCG/PCUN. Mild to moderate hypometabolism, in a spread pattern, is noted in the adjacent posterior lateral portion of the temporal lobes, the superior lateral portion of the occipital lobes, and the superior lateral portion of the frontal lobes. These functional neuroimaging findings are characteristic of probable AD. The marked asymmetry, *e.g.,* left brain hemisphere being more severely affected than the right, raises the possibility of coexisting ischemic vascular disease of the left brain. However, the metabolism in the left basal ganglia and thalamus is preserved. There is no evidence of cortical infarcts or lacunar infarcts to suggest VD. Therefore, the left-sided dominant cortical hypometabolism is likely due to an asymmetric neurodegenerative process.

During the follow-up, the patient was treated with rivastigmine patch (a central acetylcholinesterase inhibitor), 4.6 mg/day, and memantine (a NMDA receptor antagonist), 10 mg, two tablets a day, with reported cognitive improvement.

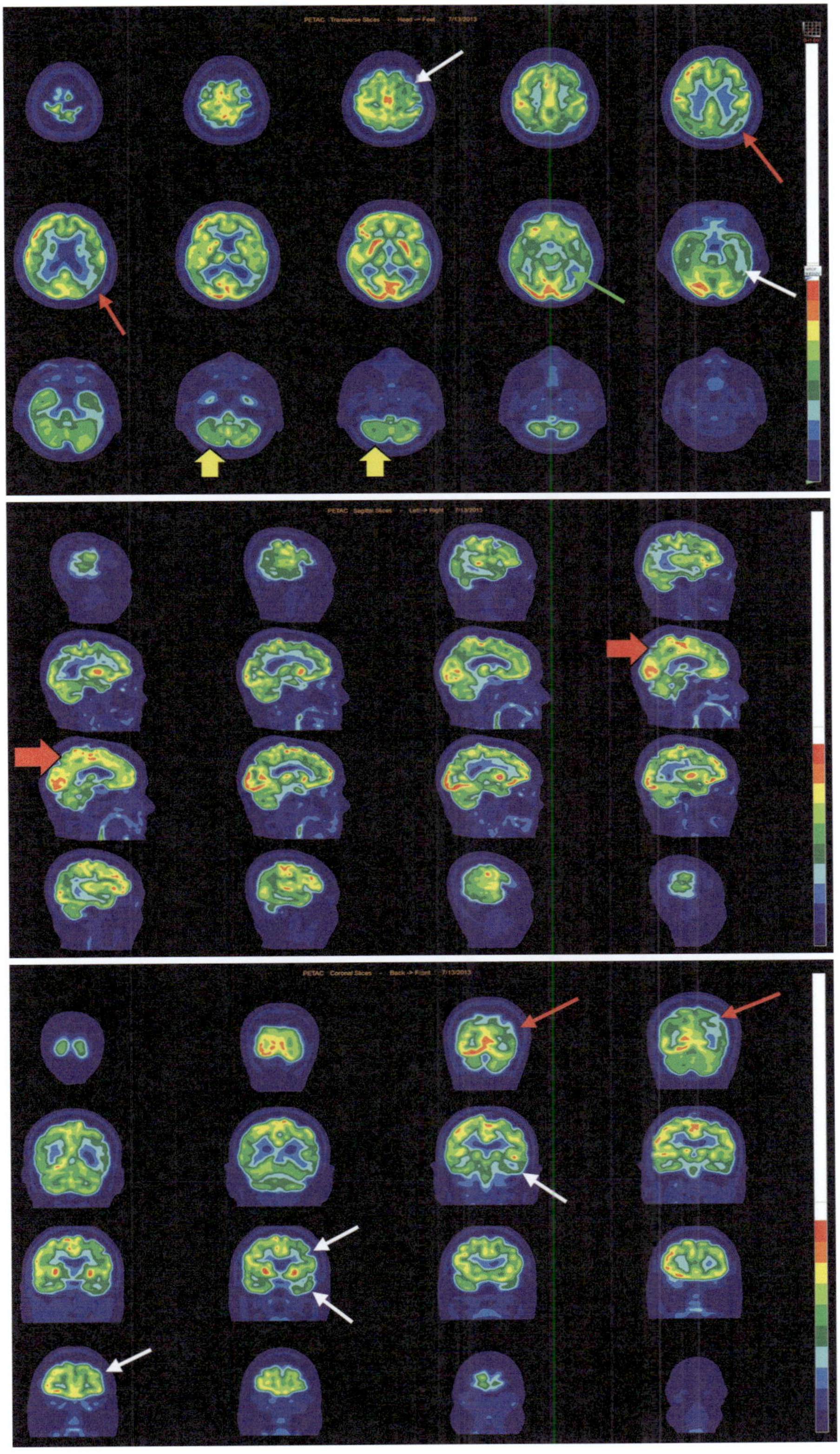

Fig. 1.5 A 69-year-old female with probable late-onset Alzheimer's disease (LOAD)

Case Summary

Progressive short-term memory loss in an elderly patient is concerning for AD. Despite asymmetry, presented in this case are functional neuroimaging characteristics of probable AD, including global and generalized brain atrophy, dominant cortical hypometabolism centered in the parietal lobes including PCG/PCUN, and additional cortical hypometabolism in a spread pattern involving the adjacent temporal, occipital, and frontal lobes. Since the patient's symptoms started after age of 65, this case is consistent with late-onset AD (LOAD), which is the most commonly diagnosed neurodegenerative dementia [12].

Case 1.6 Probable Frontotemporal Dementia (FTD)

Clinical Information

Chief Complaint *Memory loss, behavioral changes, and abnormal MRI findings suspicious for Pick's disease*

The patient is a 65-year-old male presenting with memory loss, behavioral changes for nearly 1 year, and an abnormal brain MRI with findings suspicious for Pick's disease (named after Dr. Arnold Pick, with primary imaging findings of frontal lobe atrophy). Additionally, the patient reports recently developed paranoia for the past 2 months. He denies history of stroke, head injury, or seizures. He is a non-smoker and has no history of alcohol or drug abuse.

Current medications include warfarin 10 mg daily, metformin 1000 mg daily, atorvastatin 20 mg two tablets daily, metoprolol 50 mg daily, losartan 100 mg daily, chlorthalidone 25 mg daily, and insulin glargine 30 units daily by subcutaneous injection.

Past medical history includes obstructive sleep apnea (OSA), treated with continuous positive airway pressure (CPAP), diabetes (on metformin and insulin), hypertension, hyperlipidemia, congestive heart failure, and atrial fibrillation.

There is no family history of dementia.

A recent MR imaging of the brain revealed sulcal and ventricular prominence with frontal lobe predominance as well as nonspecific T_2 hyperintensity with periventricular white matter also with frontal predominance, suspicious for Pick's disease.

Prior laboratory tests showed normal levels of TSH.

The patient's blood glucose level was 146 mg/dL prior to FDG administration for the brain PET study.

FDG PET Findings (Fig. 1.6)

The PET study is technically limited due to the patient's hyperglycemia (146 mg/dL) likely secondary to poorly controlled diabetes despite daily medications including insulin injection and oral metformin. Nevertheless, the images show prominent sulci, lateral ventricles, anterior horns > posterior horns (green arrow), and marked separation of the deep structures (basal ganglia and thalami), all indicating global and generalized brain atrophy.

Moderate to severely decreased FDG activity is identified in the bilateral frontal lobes (red arrows), anterior more prominent than posterior, right slightly more prominent than left. Symmetric, moderate to severely decreased FDG activity is seen in the bilateral temporal lobes (white arrows), anterior more prominent than posterior. Mildly decreased FDG activity is noted in bilateral parietal lobes, whereas FDG activity in the occipital lobes is well preserved.

FDG activity in the bilateral PCG/PCUN is preserved (hatched red arrows), relative to the anterior cingulate gyri (ACG).

FDG activity in the basal ganglia, thalami, and cerebella is symmetric and appears within normal limits.

Discussion

The constellation of anatomic (brain MRI) and metabolic (FDG PET) neuroimaging findings, in conjunction with the patient's clinical presentation, is suggestive of probable frontotemporal dementia (FTD).

Similar to the MRI findings, FDG PET reveals dilated lateral ventricles, anterior horns > posterior horns, in conjunction with prominent sulci and marked separation of basal ganglia and thalami, all indicating global and generalized brain atrophy, which is age-disproportionate for this 65-year-old male patient.

Although the recent MR imaging showed dominant abnormal findings in frontal lobes leading to the impression of Pick's disease, FDG PET shows a similar magnitude of cortical hypometabolism in both frontal and temporal lobes. The more prominent hypometabolism in the anterior and medial frontotemporal lobes is an imaging signature for FTD [3, 8].

The within-lobe metabolic variation is in opposite to the AD spread pattern as discussed in details in Cases 1.4 and 1.5. Additionally, the

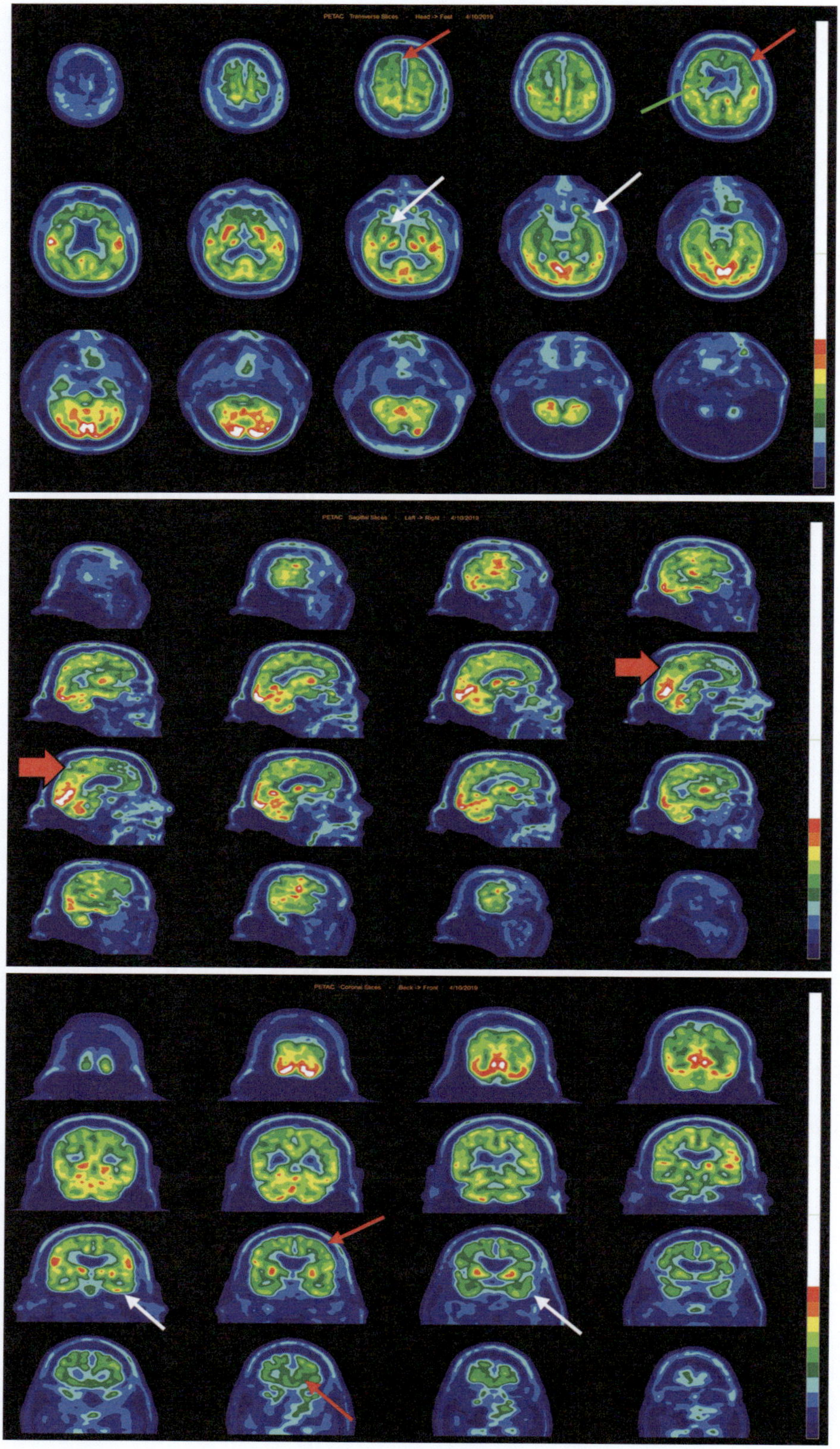

Fig. 1.6 A 65-year-old male with probable frontotemporal dementia (FTD)

relatively preserved metabolism in parietal lobes including PCG/PCUN makes AD less likely.

Case Summary

This case illustrates that functional neuroimaging such as FDG PET could play a complementary rule in the evaluation of demented patients with known abnormal anatomic imaging findings. Although the recent MR imaging showed dominant abnormal findings in frontal lobes leading to the impression of Pick's disease, FDG PET reveals a similar magnitude of cortical hypometabolism in both frontal and temporal lobes, mainly affecting the anterior medial portion of the lobes, which is a neuroimaging signature for FTD. Additionally, FDG PET shows preserved metabolism in the parietal lobes including PCG/PCUN makes AD less unlikely.

Case 1.7 Probable Behavioral Variant FTD (bvFTD)

Clinical Information

Chief Complaint *Memory loss/functional decline and worsening behavioral problems*

The patient is a 61-year-old right-handed male presenting with memory loss, behavioral problems, and speech difficulties for 2–3 years, getting worse and worse per family members. He was brought to the emergency department by police because he was trying to steal lighters in a supermarket. He did not report visual hallucinations or Parkinsonian symptoms. No motor weakness or tremors were noted. There was no prior history of any psychiatric disease.

During his stay in hospital, he exhibited disorganized thoughts, loss of inhibition, loss of speech, and repetitive behaviors, such as repeatedly saying "Did you talk to my son?", and reading same business papers over and over. He refused to take medications. He had minimal interaction with peers, demonstrated increasing isolation and social withdrawal, and had difficulties attending psychiatric therapy group meetings. His judgment was poor because of disinhibition, but his sleep and appetite were good.

The patient used to be a store owner, good with numbers, but has had functional decline and social withdrawal over the last few years. He has a documented history of tobacco, marijuana, and cocaine abuse. He also has a remote history of motor vehicle accidents (ran over by vehicle two times at ages 6 and 12) and a transient ischemic attack (TIA) approximately 30 years ago. He has had hearing loss in left ear for decades.

Current medications include sertraline 50 mg per day, lorazepam 1 mg TID, olanzapine 10 mg per day, haloperidol 5 mg per day, pravastatin 10 mg per day, and aspirin 81 mg per day.

He has no family of history of Alzheimer's disease or behavioral disorders.

Laboratory tests showed that folate, vitamin B_{12}, and TSH were within normal limits.

Brain MRA showed no evidence of vascular stenosis, aneurysm, or occlusion. Brain MRI revealed generalized parenchymal diminution with more prominent atrophy of the temporal lobes. CT of the head/brain showed atrophy of bilateral temporal and frontal lobes and encephalomalacia in the right thalamus.

The patient's blood glucose level was 86 mg/dL prior to FDG administration for the PET study.

FDG PET Findings (Fig. 1.7)

In line with the abnormal CT and MRI findings, FDG PET images show global brain atrophy, as evidenced by marked separation of deep structures (basal ganglia and thalami), sulcal and lateral ventricular prominence (green arrow).

Decreased FDG activity is identified in bilateral frontotemporal lobes, left more prominent than right. Within the frontal lobes (red arrows), decreased FDG activity is more prominent in the anterior and medial portion. Within the temporal regions (white arrows), decreased FDG activity is more prominent in the anterior and medial portion. Mildly decreased FDG activity is noted in the occipital lobes, more prominent in the anterior portion relative to the posterior.

However, FDG activity in the bilateral PCG/PCUN is well preserved (hatched red arrows).

FDG activity is symmetric and preserved in bilateral basal ganglia, whereas bilateral thalamic activity is decreased, right > left, in line with the abnormal CT finding, suggestive of remote right lacunar infarcts.

Discussion

The international consensus criteria for diagnosis of probable behavioral variant FTD (bvFTD) [13] include the following: (1) clinical symptoms meet criteria for possible bvFTD; (2) significant functional decline; (3) neuroimaging (MRI, CT, or PET) results are consistent with FTD. This case meets all of the three criteria for probable bvFTD.

The patient used to be a highly functional businessman and now has exhibited progressive

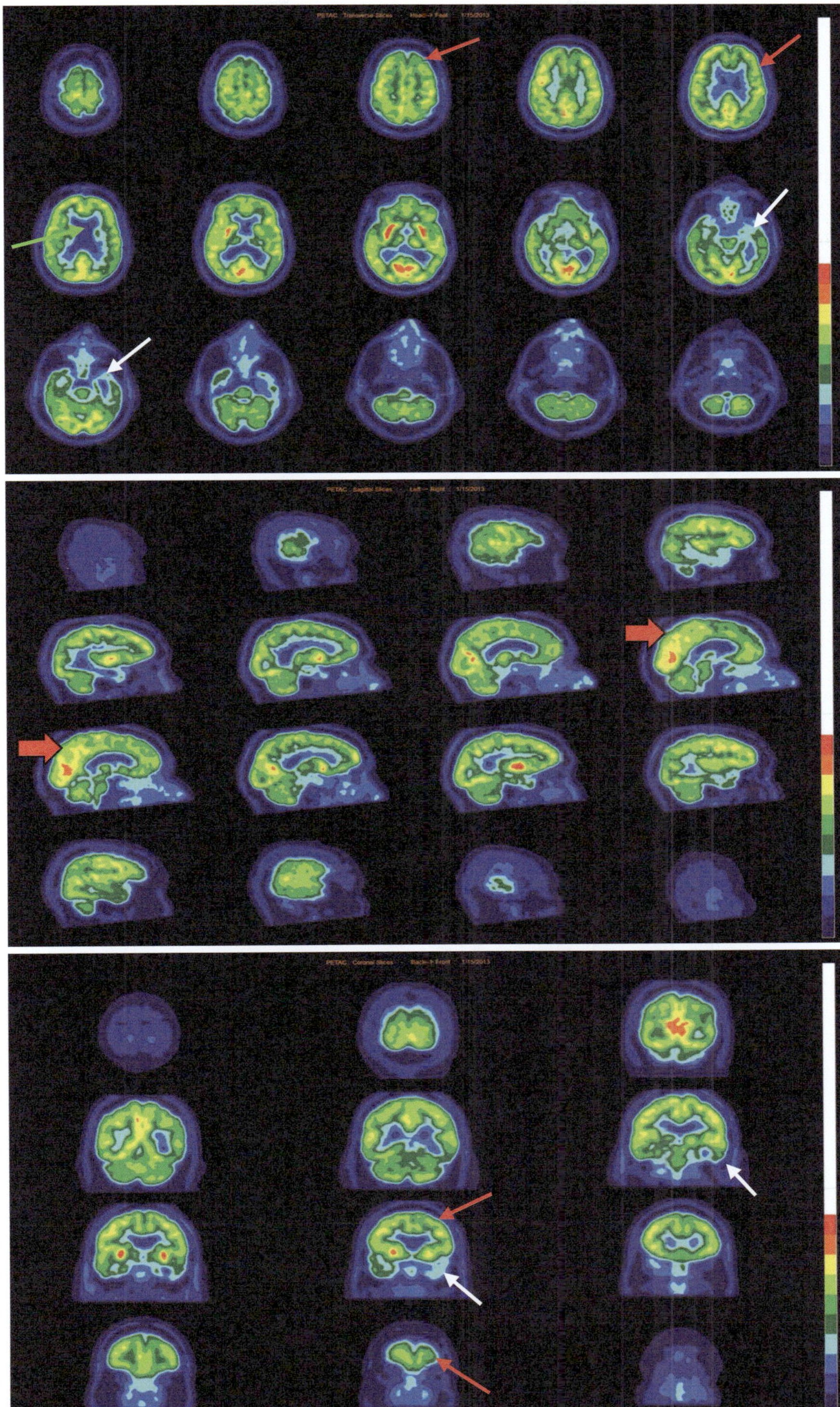

Fig. 1.7 A 61-year-old male with probable behavioral variant FTD (bvFTD)

functional decline over 2–3 years, in addition to socially inappropriate behaviors (*e.g.,* shoplifting, drug abuse), repetitive behaviors verbally and nonverbally, social withdrawal, disorganized thoughts, loss of inhibition, loss of speech, and poor judgment. The FDG PET images show dominant glucose hypometabolism in the bilateral frontotemporal lobes, in a pattern consistent with FTD, despite slight asymmetry.

The well-preserved metabolism in the bilateral PCG/PCUN makes AD less likely.

The bilateral thalamic hypometabolism has unknown etiology, but the right-sided dominant abnormality may relate to ischemic disease, given the history of prior TIA and CT finding of encephalomalacia, raising the possibility of remote right lacunar infarcts.

Case Summary

The triad of complex/profound behavioral problems, worsening functional decline, and PET findings of frontotemporal atrophy/hypometabolism in this case meets the international consensus criteria for diagnosis of probable bvFTD. The preserved metabolic activity in PCG/PCUN makes AD less likely.

Case 1.8 Probable Semantic Variant Primary Progressive Aphasia (svPPA)

Clinical Information

Chief Complaint *Progressive memory loss and severe language difficulty*

The patient is a 58-year-old right-handed female presenting with progressive memory loss and severe language difficulty for 3–4 years. On neurological exam, she scored 25/30 on the MMSE indicating borderline or mild dementia. In contrast, she has severely impaired verbal skills. More specifically, significant impairments were observed with more complex auditory comprehension items. Her written and oral expression were characterized by markedly limited language output that was vague and telegraphic and had frequent errors of repetition. Repetition, however, was intact for single words that were simple and those that were nonsense, with good repetition for simple sentences and increased difficulties as sentences increased in length and complexity. Although her speech is limited in quantity, it is qualitatively of normal volume and fluent, without evidence of halting, effortful speech, or dysarthria. She is currently working full-time as a packer. When asked to describe her job, she said "work is work, packing, and packs things."

The patient had relatively preserved orientation, visuospatial abilities, and nonverbal problem-solving. She does not report hallucinations. However, her niece notices personality changes including social withdrawal, inappropriate affect, and behavioral rigidity.

Current medications include metformin 500 mg per day, atenolol 50 mg per day, atorvastatin 20 mg per day, and lisinopril 10 mg per day.

Past medical history includes hypertension, diabetes, and hyperlipidemia. She reports no appetite or sleep problems. She has no history of drug or alcohol abuse.

She reports no family history of dementia or language issues.

A recent MR imaging of the brain was unremarkable, except for a few nonspecific hyperintense T2 signals in subcortical white matter.

EEG revealed no epileptiform activity of focal cerebral dysfunction.

Recent laboratory tests showed vitamin B_{12}, folate, T3, T4, and TSH in normal ranges.

The patient's blood glucose level was 86 mg/dL prior to FDG administration for the PET study.

FDG PET Findings (Fig. 1.8)

Images show profoundly decreased FDG activity in the bilateral frontal lobes (red arrows) and temporal lobes (white arrows), much more prominent on the left than the right, overall anterior being more affected than the posterior, with preserved FDG activity in the bilateral sensorimotor strips (red triangles). FDG activity in the lateral anterior left parietal lobe is mild to moderately decreased, likely due to disease spread from the frontotemporal regions. FDG activity in the remainder of the cerebral cortices, including the PCG/PCUN (hatched red arrows), is preserved, with enhanced activity in the visual cortices suggesting physiological stimulation.

FDG activity in the left basal ganglion and thalamus (green arrow) is mildly decreased relative to the contralateral.

There is mildly decreased FDG activity in the entire right cerebellum (hatched yellow arrows) when compared to the left, indicating crossed cerebrocerebellar diaschisis.

Discussion

This patient scored 25/30 on the MMSE indicating borderline mild dementia. In contrast to the mild memory issue, she has a profound aphasia, without evidence of halting, effortful speech, or dysarthria, consistent with fluent aphasia. The marked hypometabolism in bilateral frontotemporal lobes, anterior > posterior, left > right, is typical for FTD. Since the patient is right-handed, with anticipated language centers located in the dominant left brain hemisphere, the cortical hypometabolism of the left fronto-

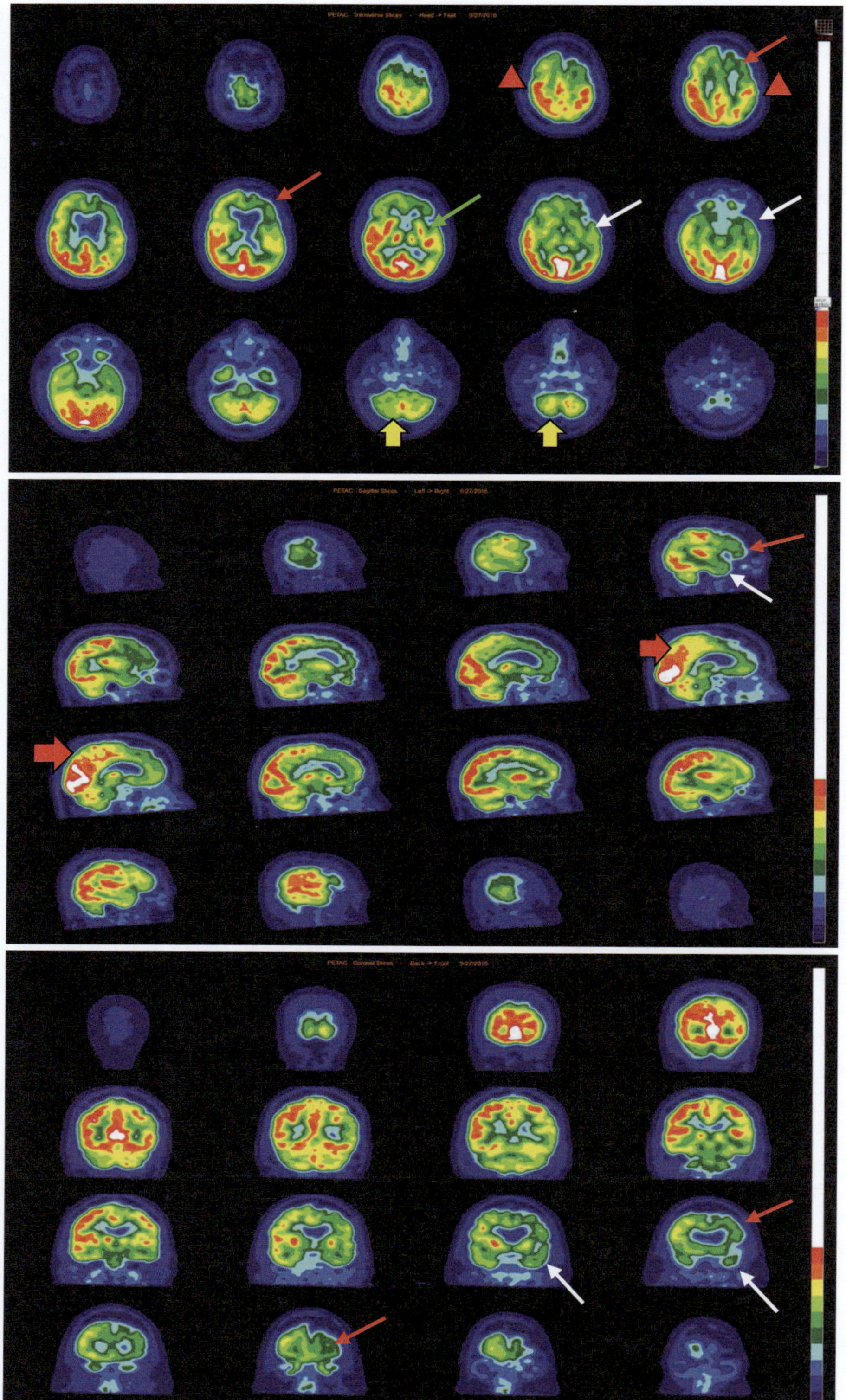

Fig. 1.8 A 58-year-old female with probable semantic variant primary progressive aphasia (svPPA)

temporal lobes may explain her profound language impairment.

This case needs to be differentiated from corticobasal degeneration (CBD), a rare neurodegenerative disease characterized by hypometabolism mainly affecting one side of the frontal lobes, the underlying basal ganglia, and contralateral cerebellum on FDG PET (see Case 1.9 for details). However, in case of CBD, the ipsilateral sensorimotor strip is often affected, but the ipsilateral temporal lobe and contralateral frontal lobe are often spared or less affected. Also, this patient had severe impairment in language, without motor features or higher cortical features that often present in CBD.

The normometabolic activity in PCG/PCUN makes AD less likely.

The mild hypometabolism in the left basal ganglia/thalamus and right cerebellum indicates diaschisis secondary to a presumed neurodegenerative process centered in the left anterior frontotemporal region.

Also, the mild to moderate hypometabolism in the anterior and lateral left parietal lobe is likely due to spread of disease from the left frontotemporal lobes, given the pattern.

The FDG PET findings, in conjunction with the patient's clinical features, meet the criteria for the newly classified semantic variant primary progressive aphasia (svPPA), one of the three variants of PPA. The other two are logopenic variant PPA (lvPPA) and nonfluent/agrammatic variant PPA (navPPA) [5]. Due to substantial inconsistence across institutions, at the present time, svPPA is also referred to as "semantic dementia" or "temporal variant FTD (tvFTD)."

Case Summary

Semantic variant primary progressive aphasia (svPPA) is a subtype of FTD (also referred to as semantic dementia or temporal variant FTD) characterized by profound, progressive fluent aphasia, cognitive impairment, and classic PET findings of dominant cerebral hypometabolism in the left anterotemporal lobe, typically in right-handed patients. Hypometabolic involvement of the adjacent cerebral cortices varies and often follows a spread pattern.

Case 1.9 Probable Corticobasal Degeneration (CBD)

Clinical Information

Chief Complaint *Memory loss and difficulty in speaking for 1 year*

The patient is a 72-year-old female with progressive memory loss and difficulty in speaking for 1 year. She also reports pain and uncomfortable sensation in her legs, especially at night. She is widowed and has no history of smoking or drug/alcohol abuse. She denies history of stroke, head trauma, or seizures.

Mental status exam showed no dysarthria but a nonfluent expressive aphasia, with difficulty in naming and calculating.

Current medications include alprazolam 1 mg per day, amlodipine 5 mg per day, donepezil initially 5 mg per day for 30 days and then increased to 10 mg per day, celecoxib 200 mg per day, atorvastatin 40 mg per day, bupropion 300 mg per day, and aspirin 81 mg per day.

Past medical history includes hypertension, hypercholesterolemia, depression, frontotemporal dementia, drug-induced pancreatitis, psoriasis, and a recent intentional overdose of medication (oxycodone and acetaminophen) due to depression and frustration over her cognitive decline and diagnosis of dementia.

CT of the head/brain showed mildly prominent ventricles and sulci compatible with atrophy. There was hypoattenuation in the periventricular white matter suggestive of chronic small vessel ischemic changes.

A recent MR imaging of the brain revealed nonspecific white matter changes.

Laboratory tests showed TSH and vitamin B_{12} in normal ranges.

The patient's blood glucose level was 109 mg/dL prior to FDG administration for the PET study.

FDG PET Findings (Fig. 1.9)

Images show diffusely decreased FDG activity in the left frontal lobe (red arrows), more profound in the mid and posterior portions including the middle and inferior left sensorimotor strip (red triangles), despite well-preserved activity in the superior portion. In addition, moderately decreased FDG activity is noted in the left basal ganglia (green arrow). Mildly decreased FDG activity is noted in the posterosuperior left temporal lobe (white arrows) and the anterolateral left parietal lobe, suggestive of disease spread from the left frontal lobe.

Mildly decreased FDG activity is noted in the left thalamus and right cerebellum (hatched yellow arrows), relative to the contralateral, suggesting diaschisis.

FDG activity in the bilateral PCG/PCUN (hatched red arrows) is well preserved. FDG activity in the entire right brain hemisphere is essentially preserved (best appreciated on the coronal view in the lower panel), except for the right anterior cingular gyrus that shows mild to moderate hypometabolism.

FDG activity in the left cerebellum is enhanced, with unknown etiology.

Discussion and Follow-Up

The patient's clinical presentation indicates higher cortical features, including general cognitive impairment, depression, and pain/discomfort in her legs. The FDG PET imaging demonstrates dominant cortical hypometabolism in the mid and posterior left frontal lobe including the middle and inferior left sensorimotor strip, in a spread pattern affecting the adjacent anterior left frontal lobe, anterolateral left parietal and posterosuperior left temporal lobe. Moderate hypometabolism is also identified in the underlying left basal ganglia, with evidence of crossed cerebrocerebellar diaschisis in the right cerebellum. The triad of these FDG PET imaging findings is classic for probable CBD [1, 3].

The essentially preserved metabolism in the right frontotemporal lobe, in conjunction with less involvement of the anterior left frontotemporal lobes, makes FTD less likely. The well-preserved metabolism in PCG/PCUN does not support the diagnosis of AD.

Owing to the abnormal FDG PET findings suggesting CBD, the previously prescribed medication of donepezil for the patient has been

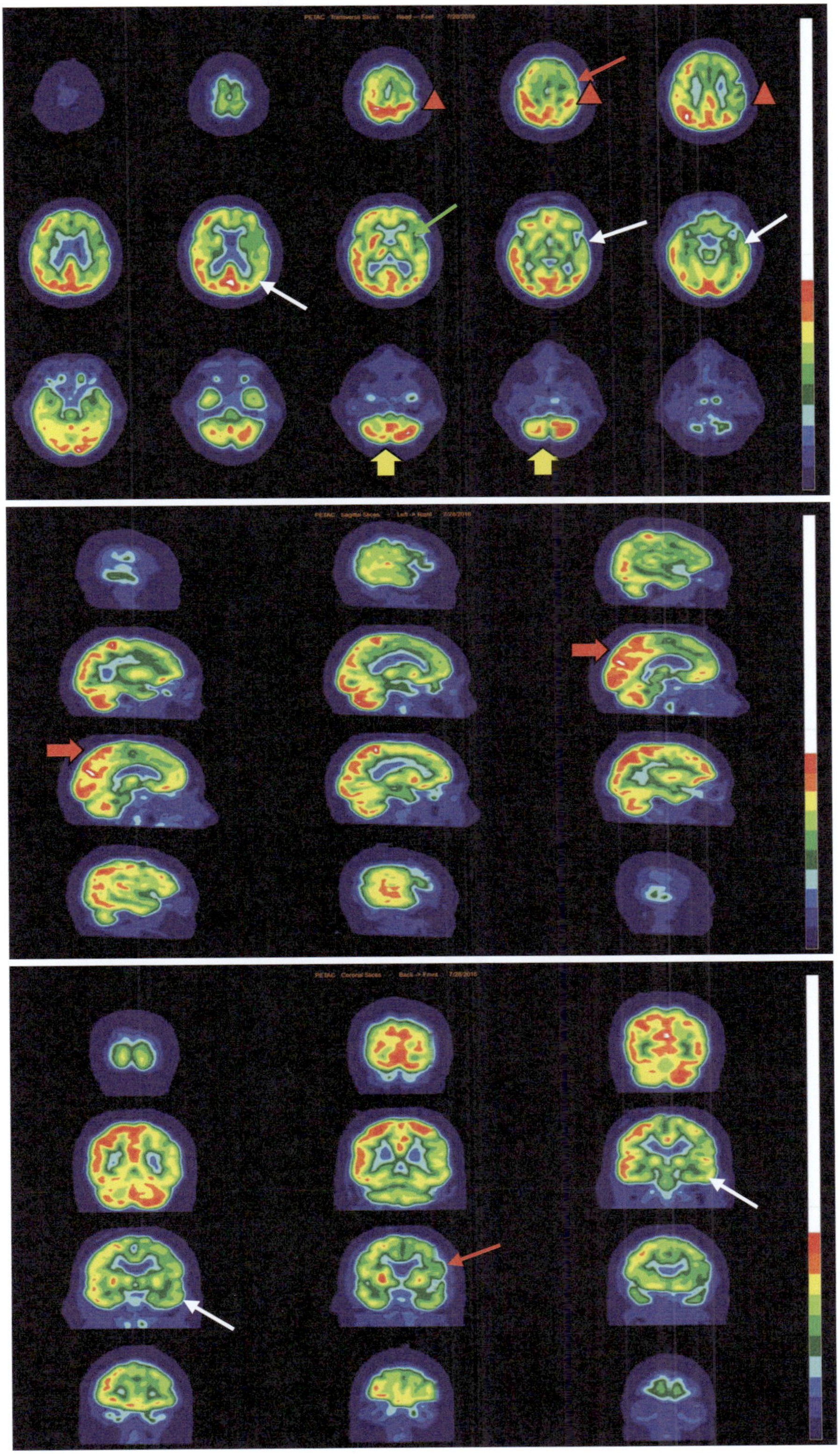

Fig. 1.9 A 72-year-old female with probable corticobasal degeneration (CBD)

stopped. Six months later, the patient was admitted to the emergency department after a fall in the shower, with occipital trauma. CT head showed a superficial extracranial subcutaneous hematoma in the right occipital region. The patient was discharged next day after managing pain with an ice pack. This incident is suggestive of postural instability, a motor feature further supporting the diagnosis of probable CBD.

Case Summary

The triad of hypometabolism involving mid-posterior portion of one of the frontal lobes, the underlying basal ganglia, and the contralateral cerebellum, is typical for probable CBD, which is a rare neurodegenerative disorder with no effective pharmacotherapy and a mean disease duration of approximately 6.6 years [1].

Case 1.10 Probable Dementia with Lewy Bodies (DLB)

Clinical Information

Chief Complaint *Progressive memory loss and worsening hallucinations*

The patient is a 76-year-old right-handed female presenting with short-term memory loss for at least 1 year. Additionally, she complains of hallucinations that were often associated with UTIs (urinary tract infections), but no urgency. She states that her hallucinations were getting worse, now occurring throughout the day and at night. For example, she describes seeing rats in her house even on the ceiling fan. She also sees relatives who died many years ago. She reports that her sleep is good, with no changes in taste or smell. She has no incontinence of bowel or bladder and no pain.

The patient had a high school education plus beauty school training and worked as a beautician. She lost her husband 2 years ago after more than 50 years of marriage.

During the office visit, the patient appears neatly groomed and dressed, without word-finding difficulties or paraphasic errors. Initial neuropsychological evaluation concluded that she had mild depression and mild cognitive impairment secondary to probable microvascular disease/chronic ischemia. Follow-up evaluation revealed that she had progressive dementia with complex visual hallucinations, concerning for "frontotemporal dementia versus diffuse Lewy body dementia."

Current medications include atenolol/chlorthalidone 100/25 mg, half a tablet per day, amlodipine 5 mg per day, lisinopril 10 mg per day, simvastatin 20 mg per day; oxybutynin 5 mg per day, and quetiapine 25 mg per day.

Past medical history includes hypertension and hyperlipidemia, but no history of diabetes or eye disease. She denies liver, kidney, lung, or thyroid disease. She denies any history of psychiatric or psychological intervention. There is no history of drug or alcohol abuse.

There is no family history of Alzheimer's disease.

MR imaging of the brain revealed mild to moderate cerebral atrophy and chronic white matter ischemic changes.

Laboratory tests showed that TSH, vitamin B_{12}, and folate were within normal limits.

The patient's blood glucose level was 90 mg/dL prior to FDG administration for the PET study.

FDG PET Findings (Fig. 1.10)

The images show mild to moderate brain atrophy, as evidenced by well-separated basal ganglia and thalami in addition to prominent cerebral sulci and lateral ventricles (white arrow). Moderately global decreased FDG activity is noted in the cerebral cortices, with relatively preserved metabolic activity in the primary sensorimotor strips (red triangles) and the cerebella. There is further decreased FDG activity corresponding to severe cortical thinning in the bilateral occipital lobes including the primary visual cortices (red arrows), right slightly being more affected than the left. In contrast, FDG activity in the PCG/PCUN is well preserved (middle panel, hatched red arrows). This finding is often referred to as the "cingulate island sign." FDG activity in the bilateral basal ganglia and thalami is within normal limits, despite head-tilting.

Discussion

The PET findings are consistent with generalized brain atrophy and global cerebral hypometabolism, in addition to more profound hypometabolism, along with cortical thinning, in the bilateral occipital lobes including the primary visual cortices. Clinically, patient has chief complaint of progressive memory loss and complex visual hallucinations. Constellation of the abnormal PET findings and clinical presentation is suspicious for dementia with Lewy bodies (DLB) [10].

The relatively preserved FDG activity in PCG/PCUN, in conjunction with decreased FDG activity in the frontal lobes anteriorly and in the occipital lobes posteriorly, is referred to as "cingulate

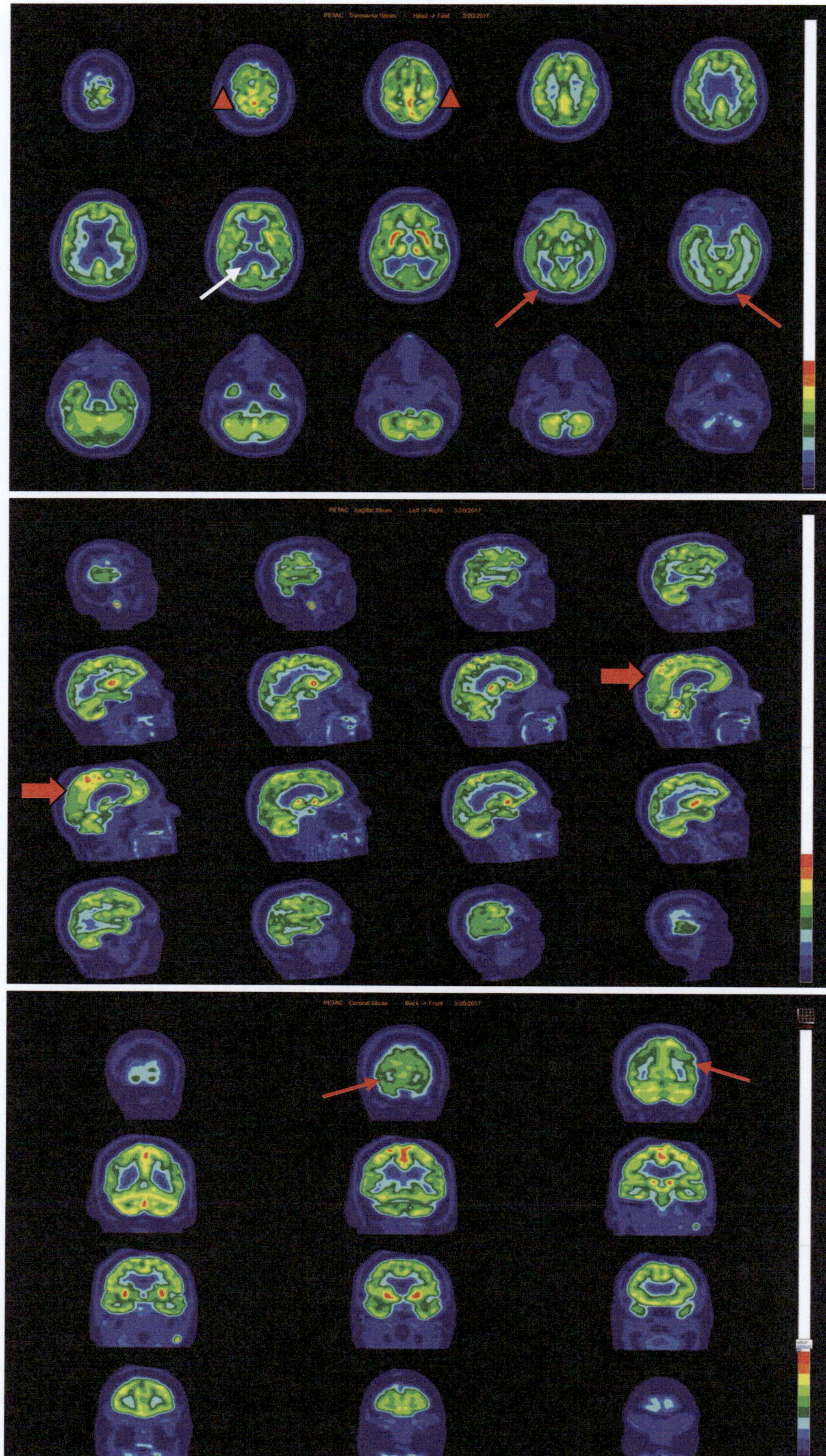

Fig. 1.10 A 76-year-old female with probable dementia with Lewy bodies (DLB)

island sign" [9], which is a highly specific finding to support the diagnosis of probable DLB rather than AD. The differential diagnosis of DLB versus AD is clinically important, as patients with AD could benefit from cholinesterase inhibitor medications, whereas patients with DLB may not. Furthermore, the use of neuroleptics could cause adverse effects in patients with DLB.

DLB has three main clinical features, including cognitive impairment, visual hallucinations, and motor Parkinsonism [10]. The lack of motor Parkinsonism in this patient could be explained by the relatively preserved metabolism in bilateral basal ganglia at the time of the FDG PET study.

Case Summary

Progressive memory loss and worsening visual hallucinations in an elderly patient are two main clinical features suggestive of DLB. This is strongly supported in this case with FDG PET findings of global brain atrophy/hypometabolism, more profoundly hypometabolism in the occipital lobes including the primary visual cortices. In contrast, cortical metabolism in PCG/PCUN is well preserved. This unique imaging finding is often referred to as "cingulate island sign," which is a highly specific imaging biomarker for DLB [9].

Case 1.11 Probable AD with Vascular Pathology

Clinical Information

Chief Complaint *Progressive memory loss, slow walking and talking*

The patient is a 67-year-old female presenting with worsening memory loss for 3–4 years. Her symptoms started a few years ago after a trip to the Middle East, when at that time she felt weakness and fatigue and thought that she had experienced a stroke. Her son, who is with her, states that she has been more confused and slower in walking and speaking than before. She is also having difficulty with recalling information. For example, she cannot remember a person's name, but is able to describe the person. She has weakness of both hands, unable to even hold a spoon to eat. Her son states that she sometimes eats with her fingers because it is easier than eating with a spoon. She often has confusion and does not know where she has placed her clothes or does not remember that she needs to shower with soap. Due to worsening memory loss, she is no longer able to drive and has stopped cooking, although she is still independent in activities of daily living. She denies having delusions or hallucinations, and there is no history of head trauma or seizure. She has been treated with Aricept 5 mg/day initially, which has now increased to 10 mg/day recently. Her son states that the medication is helping minimally.

Neurology exam: MMSE score of 10/30, normal muscle strength and sensation intact bilaterally

Current medications: Aricept 10 mg per day, memantine 10 mg per day, lipitor 20 mg per day, and imodium 2 mg, twice a day

Family history: Alzheimer's disease in her mother and maternal aunt

Social history: No tobacco, alcohol, or drug use

Laboratory tests: normal TSH, folate, and vitamin B_{12}

Imaging:

MRI of the brain 2 years ago: mild diffuse parenchymal volume loss and chronic ischemic changes

Recent CT of the head/brain: remote left lacunar infarctions, otherwise unremarkable

The patient's blood glucose level was 93 mg/dL prior to FDG administration for the PET scan.

FDG PET Findings (Fig. 1.11)

The images show profoundly decreased FDG activity in the bilateral parietal lobes, left > right (red arrows), including the PCG/PCUN (hatched red arrows). In addition, mild to moderate decreased FDG activity is noted in bilateral fronto-tempo-occipital lobes (white arrows) in a spread pattern as the following: within the frontal lobes, left > right, posterior (except for the sensorimotor strips) > anterior, lateral > medial; within the temporal lobes, posterior> anterior, lateral > medial; and within the occipital lobes, superior > posterior, lateral > medial. Decreased FDG activity is also identified in the left basal ganglion and thalamus relative to the contralateral (green arrow), in line with the CT finding of left lacunar infarcts, indicating vascular disease. Minimal decreased FDG activity is noted in the right cerebellum (hatched yellow arrows), indicating crossed cerebrocerebellar diaschisis.

Discussion

The described FDG PET findings have all the metabolic neuroimaging characteristics of probable AD, including the profound hypometabolism in the parietal lobes including PCG/PCUN and involvement of the adjacent temporo-occipito-frontal lobes in a spread pattern. The left dominant hypometabolism could explain patient's slow talking and difficulty with expressive language. However, the asymmetric hypometabolism in the left basal ganglia and thalamus does not follow an AD spread pattern. Instead, the diffuse involvement of the left striatum and thalamus is in line with the recent CT finding of left lacunar infarcts, indicating vascular pathology. The patient's symptom of slow walking is probably a manifestation of vascular parkinsonism.

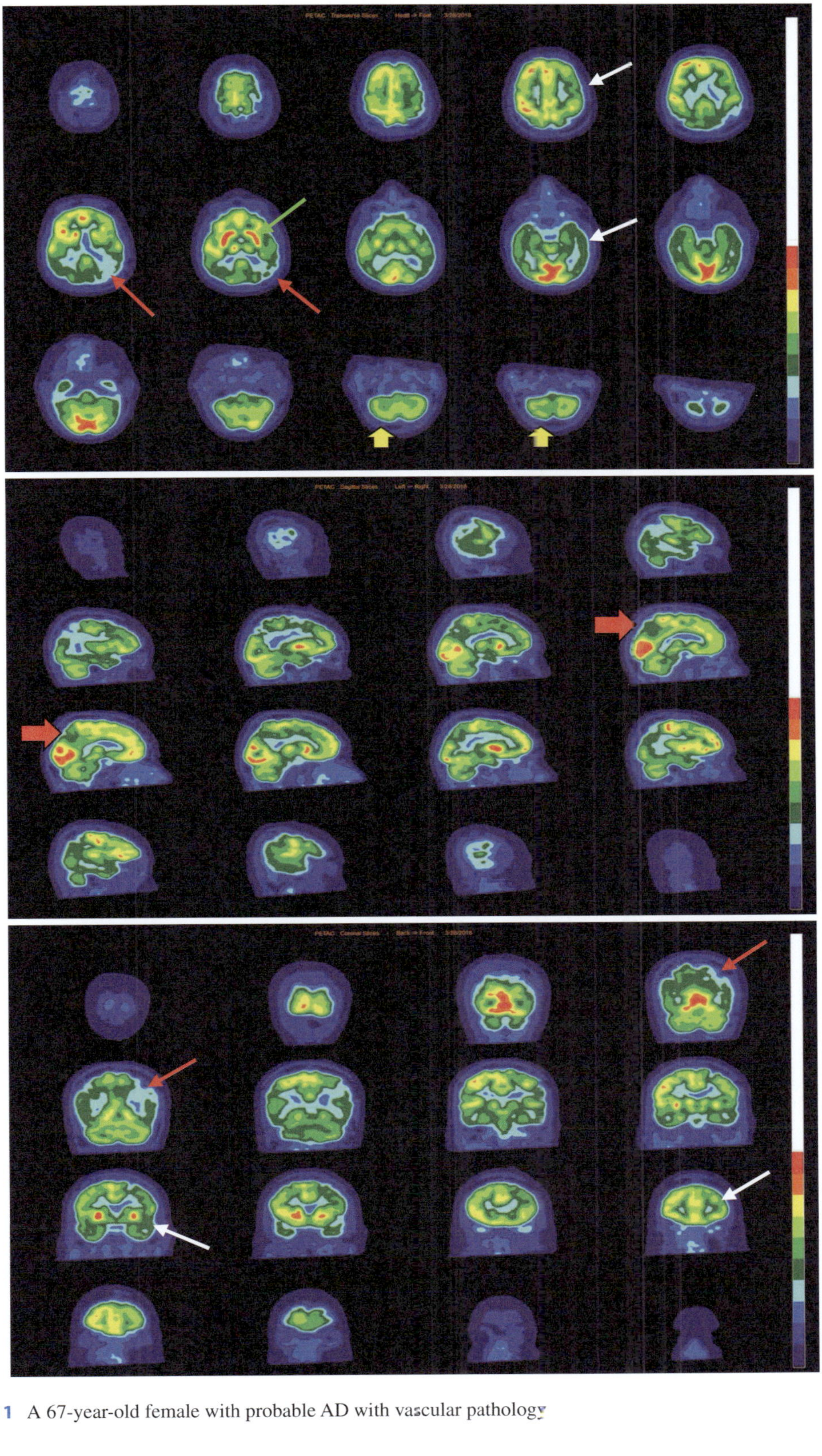

Fig. 1.11 A 67-year-old female with probable AD with vascular pathology

Case Summary

This case again demonstrates FDG PET imaging characteristics of probable AD, including dominant cortical hypometabolism in the parietal lobes including PCG/PCUN, and additional hypometabolic involvement, to a lesser degree, of the adjacent fronto-tempo-occipital lobes in a spread pattern. However, asymmetric hypometabolism, in a non-spread pattern, is identified in the left basal ganglion and thalamus, in line with the recent CT finding of left lacunar infarcts, indicating vascular pathology.

Case 1.12 Dementia Resulting from Traumatic Brain Injury (TBI)

Clinical Information

Chief Complaint *Memory loss and headache post-TBI*

The patient is a 60-year-old female who presents with memory loss and headache since a motor vehicle accident 2 years ago and a fall with head injury and subdural hematoma 12 months ago. She has been experiencing intractable headaches/migraines shortly after the two accidents. Her husband noticed that she repetitively asks the same questions. On her last day of work, she lost her way while driving home on a familiar route, and her husband had to pick her up as a result. At home, she has left the stove on twice, forgets to take out her hairstyling irons, leaves the housework halfway done, and forgets to take her medications. She denies experiencing any hallucinations or seizures, however. There is no history of alcohol or drug abuse. Aricept was prescripted for the treatment of her memory loss, but she could not tolerate it due to worsening insomnia.

Current medications include Relpax (eletriptan) 40 mg twice a day, and Topamax 50 mg twice a day.

Past medical history includes insomnia, anxiety, osteoporosis, and melanoma.

The patient has no family history of dementia.

Brain MRI performed at an outside institution showed subdural fluid collection along the right frontal parietal convexity suggestive of a subdural hematoma, in addition to diffuse thickening and enhancement of the meninges/falx bilaterally. There is no evidence of intracranial mass.

The patient's blood glucose level was 83 mg/dL prior to FDG administration for the PET study.

FDG PET Findings (Fig. 1.12)

Images show no evidence of brain atrophy or cortical scar. However, mild to moderate hypometabolism is identified in the superoanterior portion of the right frontal lobe and the inferolateral portion of the left occipitoparietal lobes (red arrows), likely sequelae of direct and indirect impact brain injuries. Mild hypometabolism is noted in the superomedial parietal lobes and in bilateral temporal lobes, slightly more prominent in the anteromedial portion (white arrows), in a pattern suggestive of normal aging/brain atrophy. Metabolism is well preserved in bilateral PCG/PCUN (hatched red arrows).

Mildly decreased FDG activity is noted in the right cerebellum (also, white arrows), suggesting disachisis. FDG activity in the remainder of the cerebral cortices, basal ganglia, thalami, and left cerebellum is within normal limits.

Discussion

This patient's memory loss and headache were preceded by a motor vehicle accident and a fall with known head injury and subdural hematoma. There is no FDG PET imaging pattern to suggest commonly diagnosed dementias, such as AD, FTD, DLB, or VD. However, there is mild to moderate hypometabolism present in the superoanterior portion of the right frontal lobe concordant with known prior right head injury/subdural hematoma, and in the inferolateral portion of the left occipitoparietal region (opposite to the primary right brain injury), suggestive of sequelae of indirect impact injury. The mild hypometabolism in bilateral superomedial parietal and anteromedial temporal lobes is consistent with normal aging/brain atrophy. The diaschisis in the right cerebellum is mild, without unknown etiology, but may relate to the presumed indirect impact injury in the left brain.

Case Summary

This case illustrates the importance of taking into consideration of history of head injury and anatomic neuroimaging findings in the interpretation of brain FDG PET results. Despite the patient's chief complaint of memory loss for years, there is

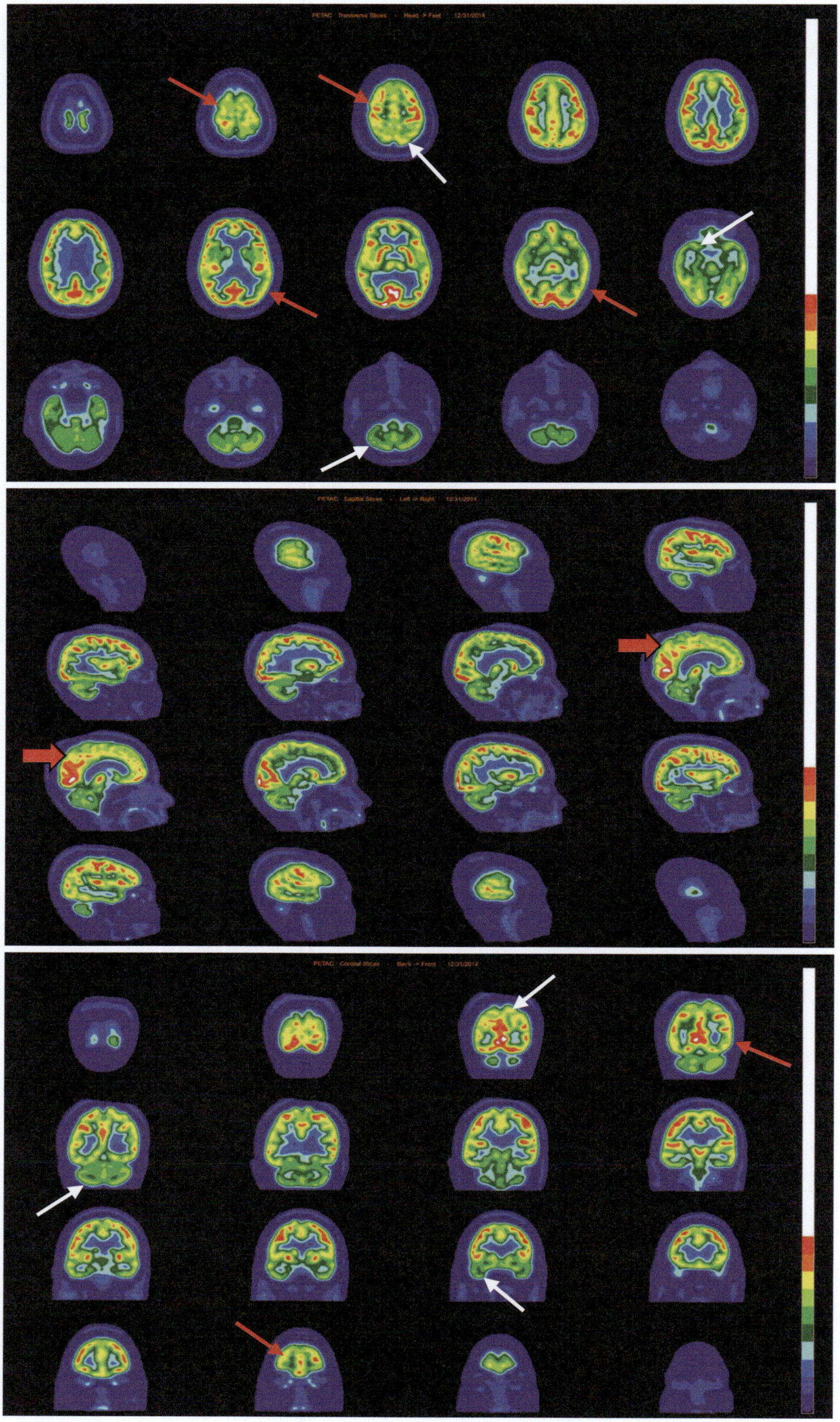

Fig. 1.12 A 60-year-old female with dementia likely secondary to traumatic brain injury (TBI)

no altered metabolic pattern to suggest commonly diagnosed neurodegenerative dementias. However, there is mild to moderate cortical hypometabolism in the superoanterior portion of the right frontal and the inferolateral portion of the left occipitoparietal lobes consistent with the patient's history of known right head injury/subdural hematoma with likely indirect impact injury in the left occipital region. The overall FDG PET findings are suggestive of dementia resulting from TBI.

Case 1.13 Probable Vascular Dementia (VD)

Clinical Information

Chief Complaint *Memory loss and word-finding difficulty for 2 years*

The patient is an 88-year-old ambidextrous female who presents with difficulty with her memory, attention, and word finding over the last 2 years. After the death of her husband recently, she has had increased word-finding difficulty and has become more confused. She also has short-term memory loss and difficulty maintaining new information, to the point that she can no longer pay her bills or drive a car.

The patient denies any focal weakness, double vision, tingling, numbness, dizziness, or tremor. There is no history of head injury or seizure. She scored 8/30 on the Montreal Cognitive Assessment (MOCA) test.

Current medications include aspirin 81 mg daily, lorazepam 25 mg PRN, simvastatin 20 mg daily, levothyroxine 75 mcg daily, metoprolol 50 mg daily, and fexofenadine 180 mg daily.

Past medical history includes arrhythmia, hypertension, hyperlipidemia, hypothyroidism, and chronic kidney disease.

Family history is significant for Alzheimer's disease in her mother diagnosed in her 80s.

Laboratory tests showed normal TSH and vitamin B_{12}.

A recent CT of the head/brain showed diffuse chronic small vessel disease and an age-indeterminate large chronic infarct involving the left basal ganglion.

The patient's blood glucose level was 82 mg/dL prior to FDG administration for the PET study.

FDG PET Findings (Fig. 1.13)

The images show moderate brain atrophy as evidenced by separation of deep structures (basal ganglia and thalami) and prominent sulci and dilated lateral ventricles, left > right. Global cortical hypometabolism is noted, with relatively preserved metabolism in the sensorimotor strips and the primary visual cortices (red triangles). Further decreased FDG activity, along with left frontal cortical thinning and absent FDG activity, is identified in the entire left basal ganglia, suggestive of a large lacunar infarct with involving the adjacent cortex (red arrows). Corresponding to this, there is diffusely decreased FDG activity in the right cerebellum, consistent with crossed cerebrocerebellar diaschisis (hatched yellow arrows). In contrast, FDG activity in bilateral posterior cingular gyri and precuneus (PCG/PCUN) is relatively preserved (hatched red arrows).

Discussion and Follow-Up

Given the patient's history of a left brain infarction and current clinical presentation of severe dementia, FDG metabolic imaging was performed mainly to rule out coexisting neurodegenerative processes. The FDG PET findings confirm a large left lacunar infarction with associated cerebral ischemia in the left middle cerebral artery (MCA) territory. There is also possible involvement of the left anterior cerebral artery (ACA) territory. In addition, the global cortical hypometabolism is concerning for microvascular ischemic disease.

Overall, the PET findings are consistent with vascular dementia [3, 14]. The preserved metabolism in PCG/PCUN makes AD less likely, and the variable hypometabolism in frontotemporal lobes has an overall pattern of brain aging rather than FTD. Given the dominant hypometabolism involving left frontal lobe and left basal ganglion, the differential diagnosis shall include CBD. However, in case of CBD, the metabolism of basal ganglia is less affected relative to the frontal cerebral cortex (see Case 1.9 for details). The severe hypometabolism in the left basal ganglia is consistent with the CT findings of a large left lacunar infarction.

During the follow-up for 1 year, the patient had several hospital admissions due to falls or mental status changes. Neurologic examinations showed worsening dementia with progressive dysphasia.

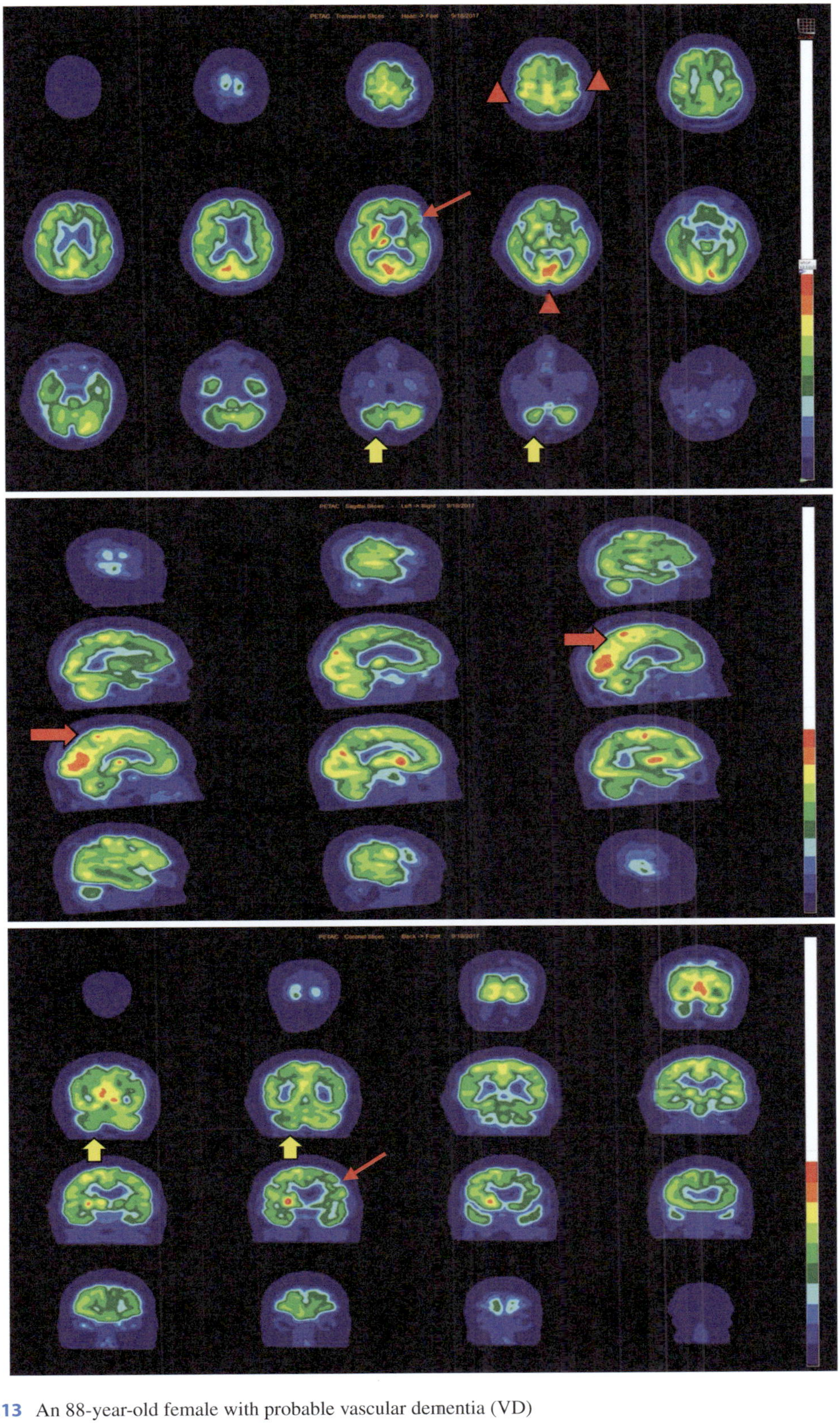

Fig. 1.13 An 88-year-old female with probable vascular dementia (VD)

Case Summary

Clinical diagnosis of VD is often already established based on patients' history, clinical presentation, and anatomic neuroimaging findings. This case reveals metabolic neuroimaging characteristics confirming VD, such as profound hypometabolism in the affected cerebral artery territories, concordant with known brain infarcts in the left brain, as well as crossed cerebrocerebellar diaschisis in the right cerebellum. There are no altered metabolic patterns to suggest AD, FTD, or CBD.

Case 1.14 Possible Mixed Dementia (AD with DLB Pathology)

Clinical Information

Chief Complaint *Progressive memory loss and difficulty with speech*

The patient is a 79-year-old male who presents with memory loss and difficulty with speech for 1 year, which has progressively worsened over the last few months. He reports persistent forgetfulness and often cannot remember what he needs to do. He is unable to add numbers and often fails to balance his checkbook, and for this reason he is no longer able to maintain his finances. He also reports trouble in reading, and difficulty speaking, often unable to articulate what he wants to say. However, he is still able to exercise and lead choir at his church. Neurologic examination showed MMSE score of 16/30. He denies history of stroke, head injury, seizure, or hallucinations.

Current medications include aspirin 81 mg daily, niacin 500 mg twice a day, and omeprazole 40 mg daily.

Past medical history includes hypertension, hypercholesterolemia, CAD (coronary artery disease), spinal stenosis status post lumbar laminectomy, and chronic right foot drop.

Family history is significant for Parkinson's disease and unspecified dementia in his brother.

Prior laboratory tests showed normal TSH, folate, and vitamin B_{12}.

Brain MRI at an outside institution showed age-related brain atrophy and thinning of the corpus callosum with no acute infarct. Brain MRA revealed "no gross cerebral aneurysm."

The patient's blood glucose level was 84 mg/dL prior to FDG administration for the PET study.

FDG PET Findings (Fig. 1.14)

The images show decreased FDG activity, predominantly in the bilateral parietal lobes, right > left (red arrows). In addition, profoundly decreased FDG activity, along with cortical thinning, is noted in the right occipital lobes including the right visual cortex (white arrows). Decreased FDG activity is also noted in the bilateral PCG/PCUN (hatched red arrows), right > left. Mildly to moderately decreased FDG activity is noted in the right superolateral frontal lobe and bilateral temporal lobes (right > left), whereas FDG activity in the bilateral sensorimotor strips, the left frontal cortex, and the left visual cortex is preserved.

FDG activity in bilateral basal ganglia, thalami, and cerebella is within normal limits.

Discussion and Follow-Up

Dominant cortical hypometabolism in the parietal regions of an elderly patient with progressive memory loss and an MMSE score of 16/30 is concerning for AD. Mild to moderate hypometabolism in the frontotemporal lobes has an overall pattern of AD spread. However, additional profound hypometabolism in the bilateral occipital lobes, along with cortical thinning and even involvement of the right visual cortex, does not follow an AD spread pattern, thus raising the possibility of coexisting DLB, despite the lack of typical clinical features such as visual hallucinations.

Given the asymmetric, right-dominant cortical hypometabolism, the differential diagnosis should include ischemic vascular disease/VD. However, prior MRA was unremarkable, and this current FDG PET study does not show any evidence of lacunar or cortical infarcts. Therefore, severe cerebral vascular disease in this patient is less likely. Posterior cortical atrophy (PCA) shall be considered, given the asymmetric and dominant hypometabolic involvement of parietal and occipital lobes, however, there is no anatomic neuroimaging correlate.

During the follow-up, the patient did develop visual hallucinations, with reports seeing his brother who died many years ago. He was treated with Aricept and memantine for several years, without significant improvement. Instead, he had progressive, significant memory decline. In line with his worsening clinical symptoms, a repeat CT of the head/brain showed diffuse brain atrophy, and EEG exam revealed diffuse slowing.

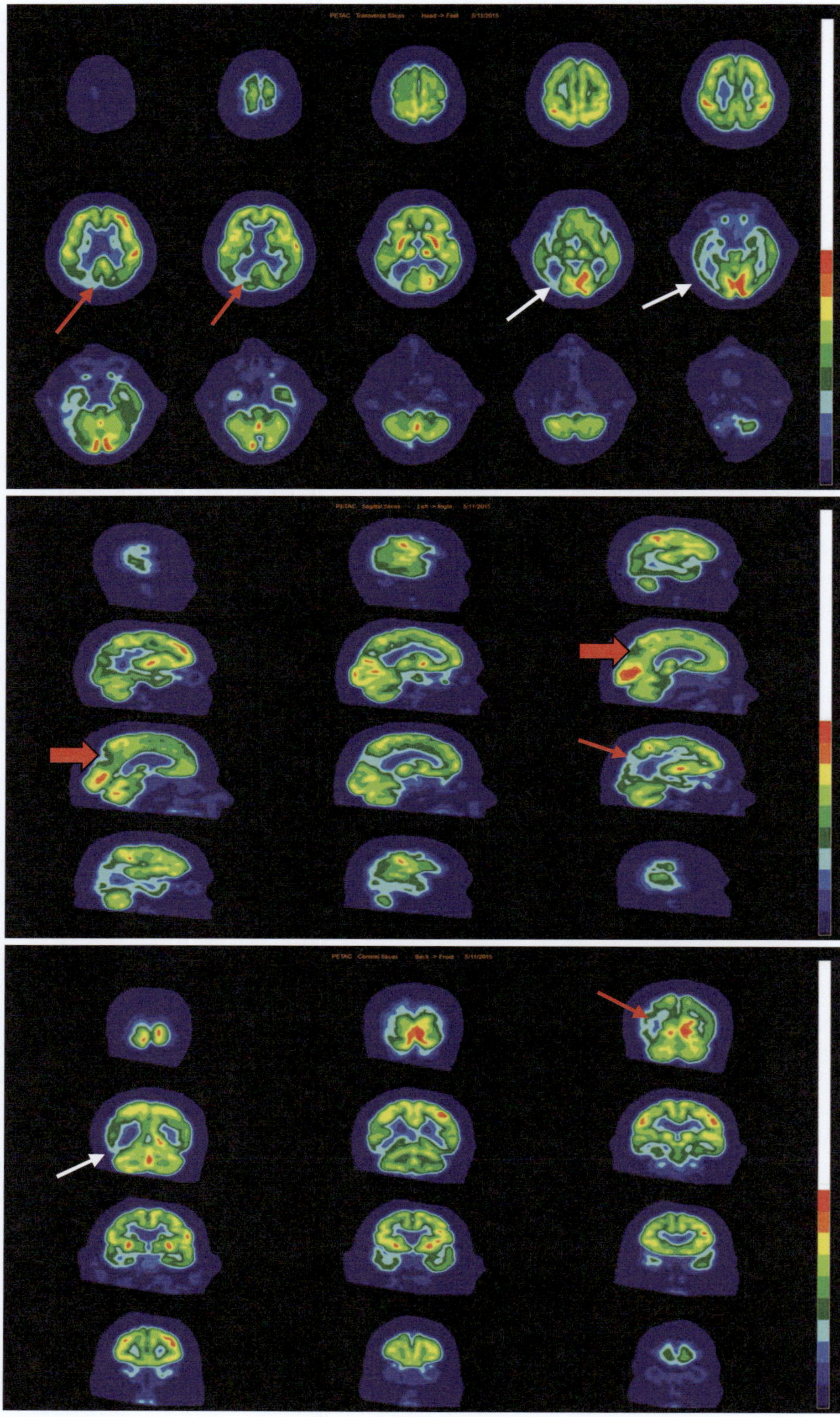

Fig. 1.14 A 79-year-old male with possible AD with DLB pathology

Case Summary

This 79-year-old patient is demented, with MMSE score of 16/30. Although the FDG PET findings of dominant hypometabolism in the parietal lobes and profound hypometabolism/cortical thinning in the occipital lobes are suggestive of mixed dementia including AD and DLB pathology, there was no clinical feature, visual hallucinations at the time of the brain FDG PET study. During the follow-up, however, the development of hallucinations, along with a poor response to pharmacotherapy for AD, worsening memory loss, and diffuse abnormalities on CT and EEG exam, further supports the diagnosis of possible mixed dementia, *e.g.*, AD with DLB pathology.

Case 1.15 Possible Mixed Dementia (FTD with AD Pathology)

Clinical Information

Chief Complaint *Progressive memory loss and word-finding difficulty*

The patient is a 62-year-old right-handed female who was brought in by her husband due to the concern of noticeable cognitive decline for the last 2 years. She initially had difficulty with name recall and later developed additional problems with memory and comprehension. She has become less oriented to time and date with difficulty in completion of simple math problems and performing monetary transactions. She also has notable word-finding difficulties.

Functionally, she used to be an excellent cook but is now unable to follow recipes. She had been very engaged in community volunteer activities, but for the past year, she has been unable to maintain previous leadership roles. She continues to drive, but limits it to local areas during the daytime, though she is adamant that she has no trouble driving.

On neurologic evaluation, she scored 13/30 on the Mini-Mental State Examination (MMSE).

Current medications include aspirin 81 mg daily and vitamin D 1000 units daily.

Past medical history is only notable for osteoporosis and positive ANA (antinuclear antibodies).

There is no family history of dementia.

Laboratory tests show normal TSH, vitamin B_{12}, and vitamin D.

Brain MRI at an outside institution showed "mild atrophy and a few scattered bilateral periventricular white matter changes."

The patient's blood glucose level was 91 mg/dL prior to FDG administration for the PET study.

FDG PET Findings (Fig. 1.15)

The images show prominent sulci and lateral ventricles, posterior horns > anterior horns, suggestive of brain atrophy.

Diffusely decreased FDG activity is identified in bilateral anterior and middle frontal lobes and bilateral temporal lobes (red arrows), left > right, while FDG activity in the posterior portion of the frontal lobes including the primary sensorimotor strips is well preserved. In addition, profoundly decreased FDG activity is seen in the bilateral parietal lobes, left > right, (white arrows). FDG activity in the bilateral PCG/PCUN is also decreased (hatched red arrows), again, left > right.

Mildly decreased FDG activity is noted in the right cerebellum (hatched yellow arrows), consistent with diaschisis.

Discussion and Follow-Up

The FDG PET finding of cortical hypometabolism in the frontotemporal lobes, in conjunction with the patient's progressive memory loss, behavioral changes, functional decline, and expressive aphasia, is suggestive of FTD. Additionally, the profound hypometabolism seen in bilateral parietal lobes including PCG/PCUN, extending into the posterolateral temporal lobes, has an imaging pattern suggestive of AD pathology.

In the ensuing 2-year follow-up, the patient was started on Aricept 10 mg daily and memantine 28 mg daily for the treatment of probable Alzheimer's disease. Despite the pharmacotherapy, her cognitive status declined so profoundly that she lost her ability to perform all ADLs and needed assistance all the time from her husband and an assistant.

Case Summary

The chief complaint of progressive memory loss, functional decline, and difficulty in word finding (expressive aphasia) are classic clinical neurological features suggesting FTD. This is supported by the FDG PET finding of bilateral frontotemporal hypometabolism, left > right. In addition, profound hypometabolism is identified in the bilateral parietal lobes extending into the adjacent posterolateral temporal region, a typical imaging pattern suggesting AD pathology. The diagnosis of mixed dementias is further supported by the patient's poor response to polypharmacotherapy for AD and rapid disease progression during the follow-up.

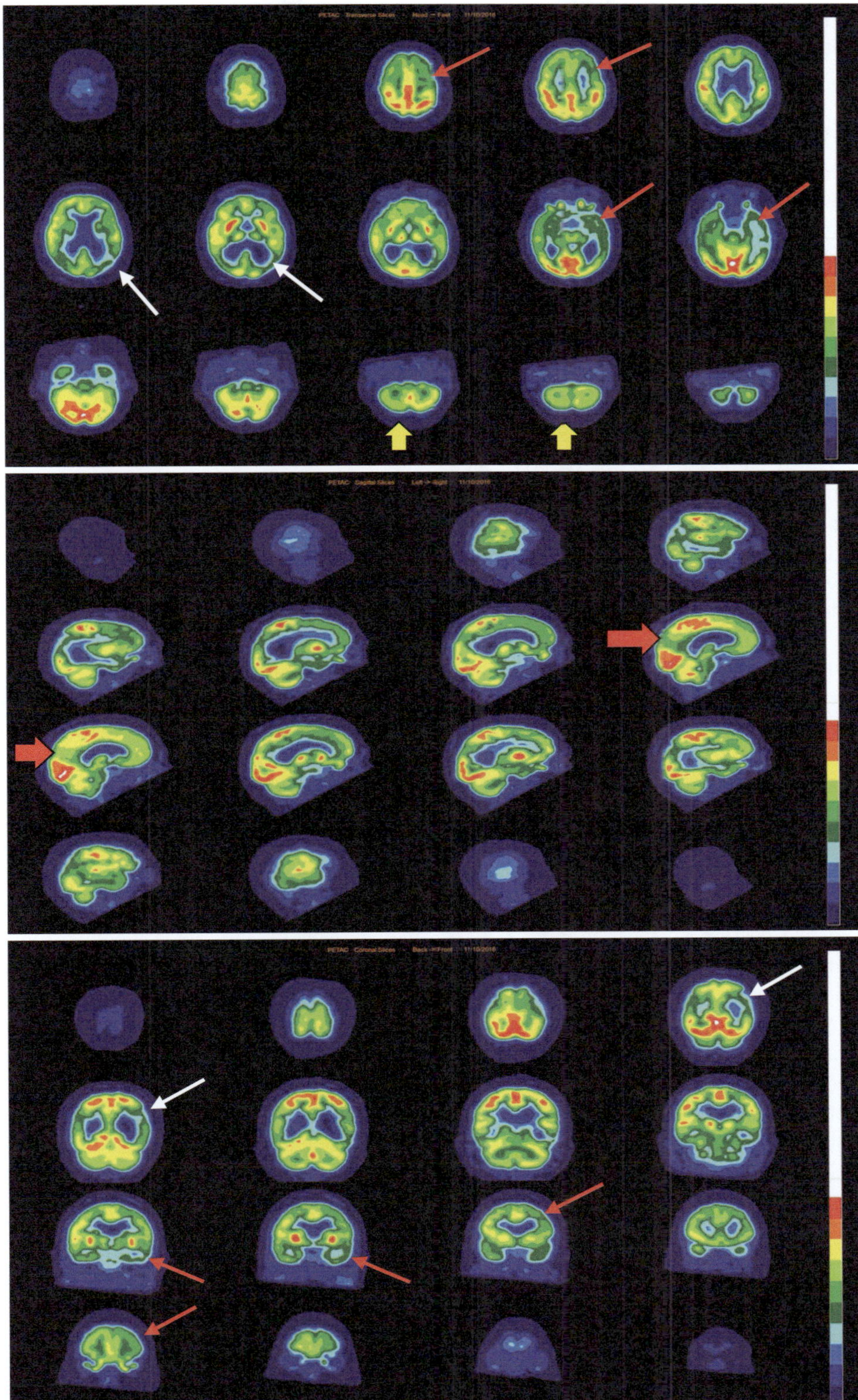

Fig. 1.15 A 62-year-old female with possible FTD with AD pathology

Case 1.16 Dementia Resulting from Major Depressive Disorder (MDD)

Clinical Information

Chief Complaint *Worsening memory loss and chronic fatigue*

The patient is a 71-year-old female presenting with memory difficulty, who was referred for evaluation of "frontotemporal dementia versus pseudodementia due to MDD."

She was diagnosed with major depression in 1995 and first experienced suicidal thoughts in 1999. She also has a comorbid anxiety disorder complicated by panic attacks. She reports generalized fatigue with worsening memory difficulty including short-term memory loss. She frequently forgets what people have told her but denies misplacing objects. She states that she has also recently lost her sense of smell and taste. There were no visual problems or hallucinations.

Neurological evaluation shows apathy on exam with intact language and speech. She scored 29/30 on the MMSE.

Current medications include amlodipine 5 mg per day, aripiprazole 5 mg per day, doxepin 50 mg per day, escitalopram 10 mg per day, lisinopril 40 mg per day, and propranolol 10 mg twice daily.

Past medical history is notable for major depression, anxiety disorder, panic attacks, hypertension, hyperlipidemia, hearing loss, heart murmur, GERD (gastroesophageal reflux disease), bowel disease, constipation, diarrhea, and essential tremor.

Laboratory tests showed normal TSH and folate, but a borderline low level of vitamin B_{12}, which was treated.

CT of the head/brain was unremarkable, except for mild ethmoid sinus disease.

The patient's blood glucose level was 101 mg/dL, prior to FDG administration for the PET study.

FDG PET Findings (Fig. 1.16)

The PET images show sulcal and ventricular prominence, suggestive of mild to moderate generalized brain atrophy. There is moderate to severe global hypometabolism involving all the cerebral cortices including the primary sensorimotor strips and the primary visual cortices (red arrows). However, FDG activity in the PCG/PCUN is relatively preserved (hatched red arrows), which mimics the "cingulate island signal", owing to the diffuse cortical hypometabolism in the surrounding areas.

Mildly decreased FDG activity is noted in the left caudate nucleus (white arrow) with unknown etiology, but concerning for a small lacunar infarct.

FDG activity in the right basal ganglia, bilateral thalami, and cerebella is within normal limits.

Discussion and Follow-Up

The FDG PET finding of generalized brain atrophy is age-disproportionate for this 71-year-old patient. There is also global cerebral hypometabolism without any pattern to suggest commonly diagnosed neurodegenerative dementias. Furthermore, the well-preserved metabolism in bilateral PCG/PCUN makes AD less likely. Although cortical hypometabolism is present in occipital lobes including the visual cortices, this finding is not outstanding when compared to the other cerebral cortices; therefore, DLB is less likely in this patient without any visual problems or hallucinations. The relatively prominent hypometabolism in the anteromedial frontal and anteromedial temporal lobes, in conjunction with the prominent hypometabolism in the superomedial parietal lobes, is likely due to global cortical hypometabolism superimposed on brain atrophy, rather than FTD.

The incidental finding of hypometabolism in the left caudate nucleus is concerning for a small lacunar infarct, though prior CT of the head/brain was unremarkable.

Case Summary

Patients with major depressive disorder (MDD) often present with memory loss in addition to apathy, loss of interest, and generalized fatigue as

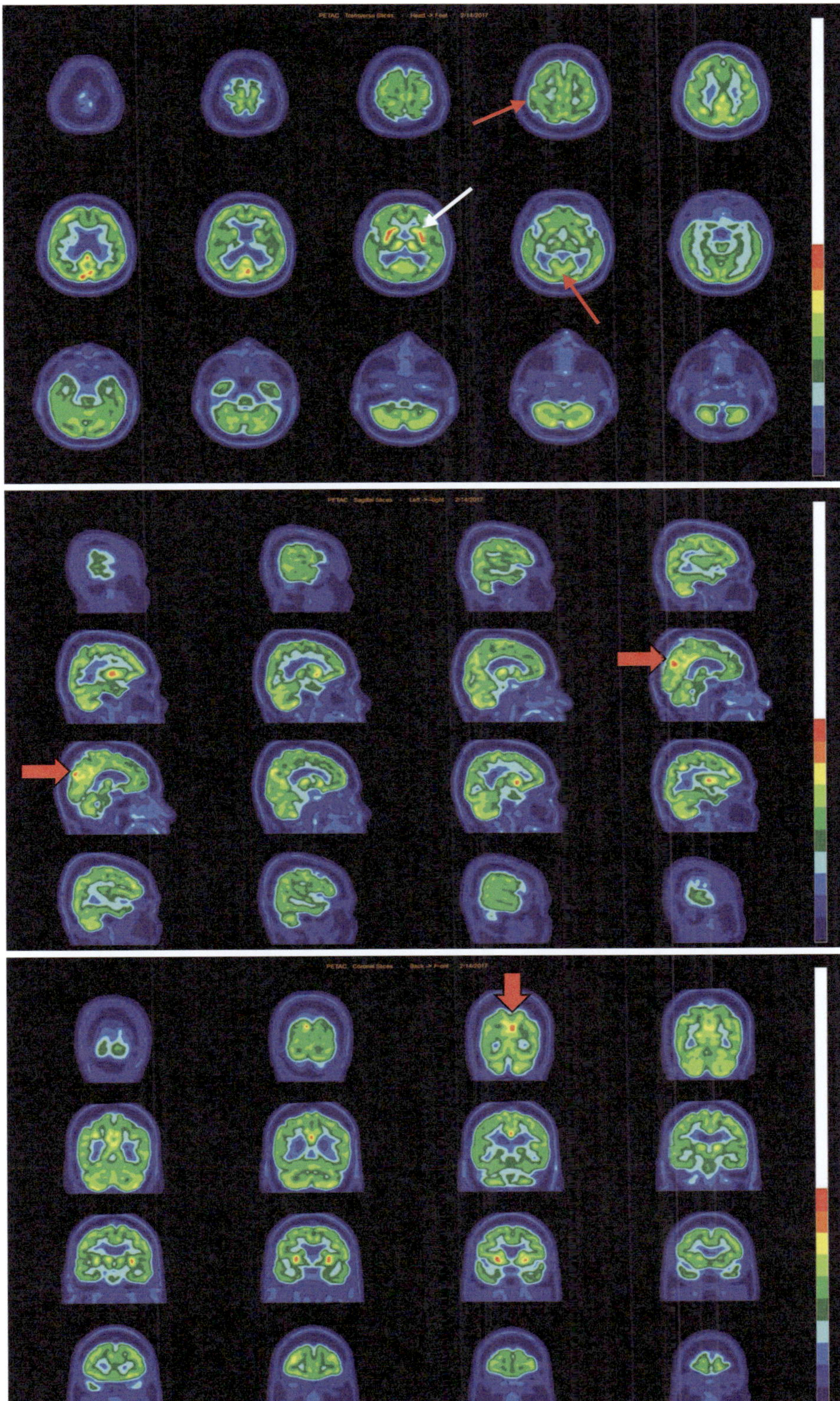

Fig. 1.16 A 71-year-old female with dementia likely secondary to major depression disorder (MDD)

shown in this case. In the absence of anatomic neuroimaging abnormalities, FDG brain PET was requested primarily to rule out coexisting common neurodegenerative dementias. This case shows age-disproportionate and generalized brain atrophy with no discrete PET imaging patterns to suggest AD, FTD, DLB, or VD. Instead, the diffuse and symmetric hypometabolism involving all cerebral cortices including the primary sensorimotor strips and the primary visual cortices is most likely secondary to major depressive disorder (MDD).

Case 1.17 Aphasia Resulting from Brain Arteriovenous Malformation (AVM)

Clinical Information

Chief Complaint *Word-finding difficulty*

The patient is a 54-year-old female who presents to our emergency department after experiencing 2–3 days of sudden-onset word-finding difficulty, nausea, and dizziness. She also reports right arm weakness. She is taking vimpat and lamictal for seizure control. She denies any recent head trauma and has no changes in overall health. She is not on any blood thinners and denies alcohol abuse, tobacco, or illicit drug use.

Current medications include vitamin D 1000 units daily, vimpat 50 mg daily, lamictal 150 mg daily, and vitamin B_{12} 1000 mcg by mouth daily.

Past medical history includes seizure disorder and known left brain AVM/aneurysm treated with multiple Gamma Knife procedures and embolization.

She has no family history of dementia or aphasia.

CT of the head/brain in the emergency department showed a known large AVM centered in the left parietal lobe with extensive surrounding vasogenic edema causing an approximately 8 mm rightward midline shift. Possibility of ischemia in the left frontal lobe/acute stroke cannot be excluded.

Brain MRI revealed a large complex hemorrhagic lesion with areas of remote and subacute blood products associated with cystic changes in the left parieto-occipital lobe and in the splenium of the corpus callosum.

EEG exam was consistent with left hemisphere slowing and some sharp wave forms, but no ictal events.

The patient's blood glucose level was 105 mg/dL prior to FDG administration for the PET study.

FDG PET Findings (Fig. 1.17)

The PET images show a large area of absent or nearly absent FDG activity occupying the entire left parieto-occipital lobes (red arrows), with involvement of the posterior left frontal lobe, and the posterior superior portion of the left temporal lobe, corresponding to the known complex vascular lesion with posttreatment changes on the anatomic neuroimaging studies (CT and MRI). In addition, mild to moderately decreased FDG activity indicating vasogenic edema is noted in the remainder of the left frontotemporal lobes, including the inferior frontal lobe (white arrows), which is often referred to as the Broca's area. In contrast, FDG activity in the right hemisphere cerebral cortices is enhanced, likely representing functional compensation. Decreased FDG activity is noted in the left thalamus (green arrow) and the right cerebellum (hatched yellow arrows) consistent with diaschisis. FDG activity in the bilateral basal ganglia, the right thalamus, and the left cerebellum is within normal limits.

Discussion and Follow-Up

This patient's sudden-onset expressive aphasia was preceded by known left brain AVM/aneurysm status post multiple rounds of treatment with Gamma knife and embolization. The FDG PET findings of profound hypometabolism centered at the known AVM site in the left parieto-occipital lobes are consistent with posttreatment changes. In addition, mild to moderate hypometabolism, likely secondary to vasogenic edema, is identified in the surrounding left hemispheric cortices including the Broca's area, which may explain the patient's chief complaint of word-finding difficulty (expressive aphasia). The patient's other symptoms, such as nausea and right arm weakness, likely due to increased intracranial pressure.

There is no metabolic imaging pattern to suggest a neurodegenerative process. Instead, enhanced metabolism is noted in the entire right brain hemisphere, suggestive of functional compensation.

During her hospital stay, all the symptoms including aphasia gradually improved following treatment with decadron. She was discharged 5 days later with a final clinical diagnosis of expressive aphasia secondary to AVM-associated left brain vasogenic edema.

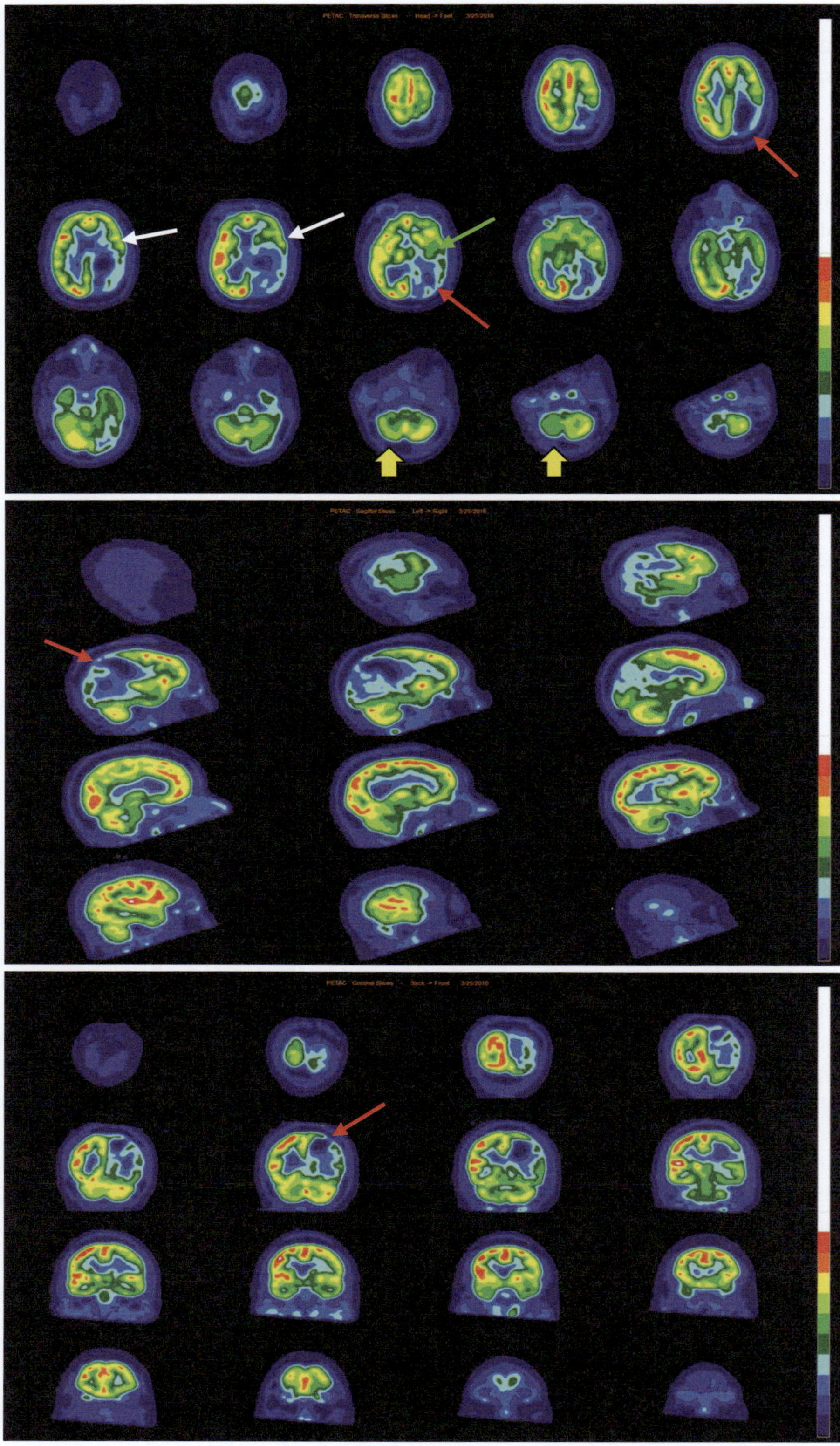

Fig. 1.17 A 54-year-old female with aphasia likely secondary to arteriovenous malformation (AVM)

Case Summary

This case emphasizes the importance of clinical history and anatomic neuroimaging findings in the interpretation of brain FDG PET images. The profound hypometabolism centered in the left parieto-occipital lobes well corresponds to the patient's known AVM/aneurysm site with extensive posttreatment changes. Additionally, mild to moderate hypometabolism, likely due to vasogenic edema, is identified in the surrounding areas including the inferior left frontal lobe, often referred to as the Broca's area, thus explaining the patient's chief complaint of expressive aphasia, which resolved after effective treatment with decadron.

Case 1.18 Dementia and Aphasia Resulting from Primary CNS Lymphoma (PCNSL)

Clinical Information

Chief Complaint *Sudden-onset confusion, memory loss, and aphasia*

This is a 67-year-old female in generally good health who presents with confusion, memory loss, and aphasia that started 2 days ago. MR imaging of the brain showed "two nodular foci of enhancement in the right frontal lobe and multifocal ill-defined areas of enhancement in the left temporal lobe associated with moderate vasogenic edema and localized mass effect." Multiple stereotactic biopsies of the right frontal lobe "lesions" at 3, 6, 9, 10, ad 12 o'clock showed "fragments of white matter with mild reactive changes," per pathology report from an outside institution. There is no history of head injury, seizure, or stroke.

Current medications include zantac 150 mg daily, losartan 100 mg daily, indapamide 1.25 mg daily, levetiracetam 250 mg twice a day, antivert 12.5 mg daily, and aspirin 81 mg daily.

Past medical history includes hypertension, diabetes, hyperlipidemia, dizziness, and anxiety disorder.

There is no family history of dementia.

A recent laboratory test showed normal TSH.

The patient's blood glucose level was 132 mg/dL prior to FDG administration for the PET study.

FDG PET Findings (Fig. 1.18)

The images show two highly FDG-avid left brain masses, one located in the posterosuperior left temporal lobe (white arrows) and the other at the junction of the left frontotemporoparietal region (red arrows), in addition to mild to moderate diffusely decreased FDG activity in the remainder of the left brain hemisphere, suspicious for left brain malignant tumors with mass effect or vasogenic edema or both. The maximal SUVs (standardized uptake values) of the two masses were 25.3 and 25.6, respectively, in comparison with maximal SUV of 10–12 in the contralateral normal-appearing brain parenchyma. Inconsistent with the recent MRI findings, there was no focal abnormality in the right frontal lobe (red triangles). FDG activity in bilateral PCG/PCUN (hatched red arrows) and the anterior cingulate gyri is well preserved. Diffusely decreased FDG activity is noted in the right cerebellum (hatched yellow arrows), consistent with crossed cerebrocerebellar diaschisis.

Discussion and Follow-Up

This patient presents with sudden-onset memory loss accompanied by confusion and aphasia. Although the initial MR imaging showed multiple lesions involving the right and left brain hemispheres, multiple biopsies of the right frontal lobe "lesions" were negative/inclusive at an outside institution. The FDG PET metabolic imaging findings, however, are highly suggestive of two malignant tumor masses, both in the left brain, with mass effect or vasogenic edema leading to likely Broca's (expressive) aphasia. Furthermore, there is no focal metabolic abnormality in the right frontal lobe, further supporting the negative pathology, per report. In this particular case, FDG PET was a superior imaging modality to clarify the presence of tumor masses when compared to MRI.

Four days after the abnormal FDG PET scan, the patient underwent a left brain biopsy which was positive for diffuse large B-cell lymphoma (DLBCL) with 100% c-MYC positivity. Cytogenetics were negative for double-hit lymphoma. Tumor cells were CD20, B6, and MUM1 positive, per pathology. MR imaging of the cervical, thoracic, and lumbar spine was negative for lymphomatous involvement. Similarly, FDG PET CT showed no lymphomatous involvement in the periphery.

The patient was treated with 12 cycles of chemotherapy followed by autologous stem cell transplantation. She has been in complete remission over the past 2 years.

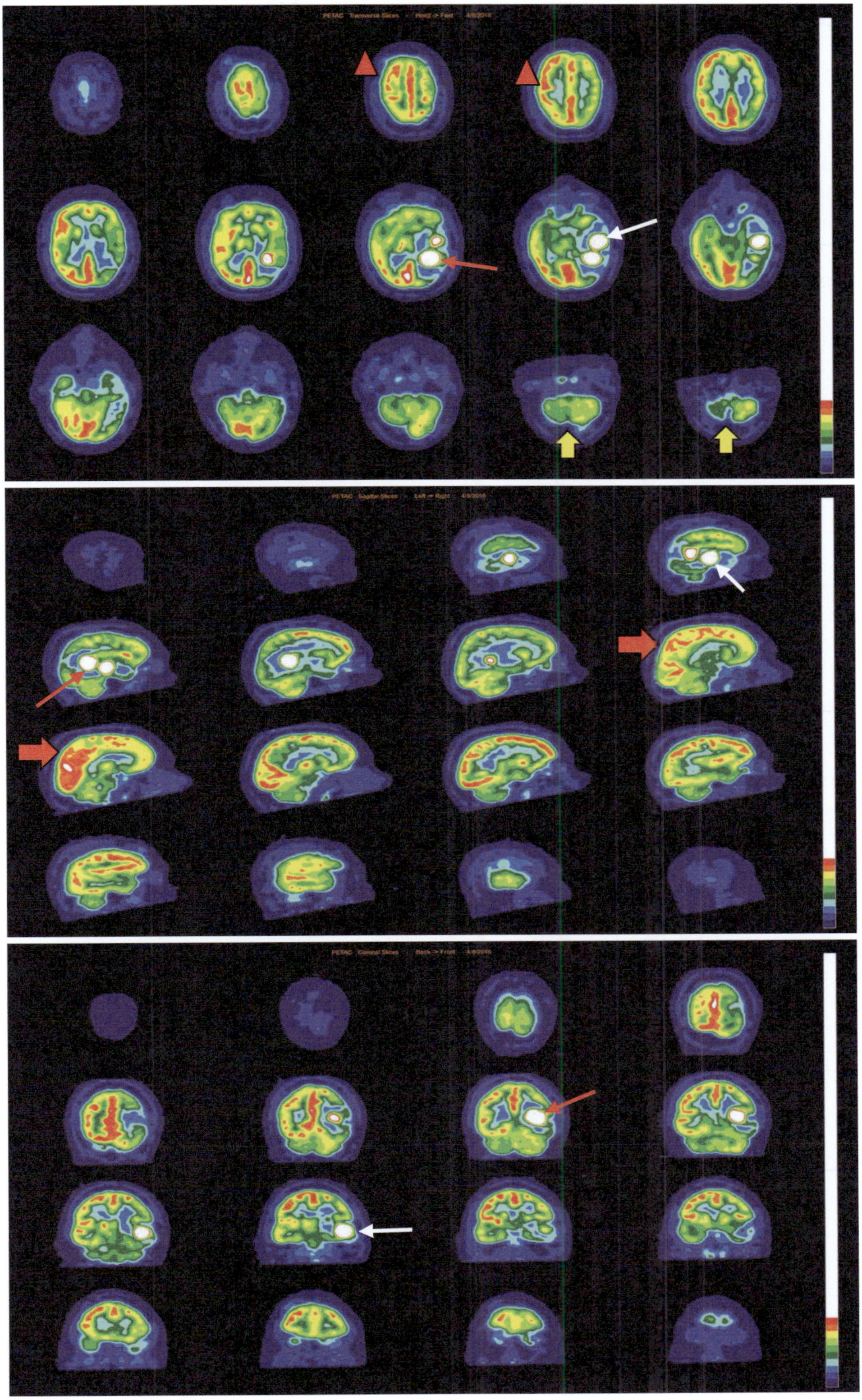

Fig. 1.18 A 67-year-old female with dementia and aphasia due to primary CNS lymphoma (PCNSL)

Case Summary

Dementia resulting from malignant brain tumors is a rare neurological condition. The combination of memory loss and expressive aphasia in this patient suggests involvement of the dominant hemisphere, often the left brain hemisphere in right-handed patients. The two discrete left brain masses with intense FDG avidity on PET imaging are highly suggestive of malignant tumors, which were later biopsy-proven to be primary CNS lymphoma (PCNSL). In addition, the FDG PET imaging effectively ruled out any additional lesions or involvement in other portions of the brain, which is important for clinical management of this patient who had prior MRI findings suspicious for contralateral brain (right frontal lobe) "lesions" with negative/inconclusive biopsies.

Case 1.19 Dementia of Unknown Type

Clinical Information

Chief Complaint *Progressive memory loss for 8 years and mood issues/depression for decades*

The patient is a 56-year-old right-handed female who presents with progressive memory loss for 8 years according to her son, despite her denial of any progression. She forgets where she is at times and what she is speaking about. Sometimes, she misplaces things and often loses objects around the house. She cannot recall things that she said 1 hour ago and often mixes up names, calling her son by his brother's name or a cousin's name instead. In addition, she has an extensive history of depression and mood disorders. She admits that her depression is not well controlled, and so she has recently started taking a new medication, Wellbutrin. She states that she has had intermittent lightheadedness, which can occur while sitting down or standing up, and is often associated with blurred vision for a couple of seconds. She denies loss of consciousness or seizure-like activity. She also admits to having lower extremity neuropathy and an unsteady gait, for which she uses a cane for walking. She denies vertigo or hallucinations. On neurologic exam, her MMSE score was 28/30.

She used to work as a cardiovascular nurse and now is on disability leave. She is divorced with two children. She had an extensive smoking history but quit 2 years ago. She also had a history of alcohol abuse/dependence and quit 7 years ago.

Current medications include Wellbutrin 75 mg daily, dexlansoprazole 60 mg daily, benztropine 0.5 mg twice a day, tamsulosin 0.4 mg daily, gabapentin 300 mg every 8 hours, lisinopril 5 mg daily, sennosides 8.6 mg two caps a day, insulin aspart total of 11 units per day, divalproex 500 mg two tabs a day, omeprazole 40 mg twice a day, and aspirin 81 mg daily.

She has a complex past medical history including schizoaffective disorder, obsessive-compulsive disorder, depression, hyperlipidemia, insulin-dependent diabetes mellitus type 2, COPD (chronic obstructive pulmonary disease), CKD (chronic kidney disease), GERD (gastroesophageal reflux disease), arthritis, and spondylolisthesis. She also reports a remote history of a closed head injury but denies history of seizure or stroke.

Family history is significant for dementia in her mother at age 70 and obsessive-compulsive disorder in her grandmother.

MR imaging of the brain a year ago showed small vessel ischemic demyelination and otherwise unremarkable. EEG exam was normal.

Laboratory tests show normal vitamin B_{12} and TSH.

The patient's blood glucose level was 113 mg/dL prior to FDG administration for the PET study.

FDG PET Findings (Fig. 1.19)

The images show sulcal and ventricular prominence indicating mild brain atrophy. There is global cerebral hypometabolism including the primary visual cortices with relatively preserved activity at the primary sensorimotor strips (red triangles). Metabolism in PCG is also mildly decreased but relatively preserved (hatched red arrows) when compared to the anterior cingulate gyri (ACG). However, FDG activity in bilateral PCUN is moderately decreased (hatched red arrows).

FDG activity in bilateral basal ganglia and thalami is within normal limits despite head-tilting.

In contrast, FDG activity in the cerebella is diffusely increased, especially in the region of the cerebellar vermis (red arrows).

There is an incidental finding of focally increased FDG activity at the anterior floor of the mouth (white arrows), with unknown etiology and uncertain clinical significance.

Discussion and Follow-Up

The FDG PET study was requested to evaluate "possible early-onset Alzheimer's disease (EOAD)"; however, imaging interpretation is confounded by the complex history of psychiatric disorders and by the fact that the patient is

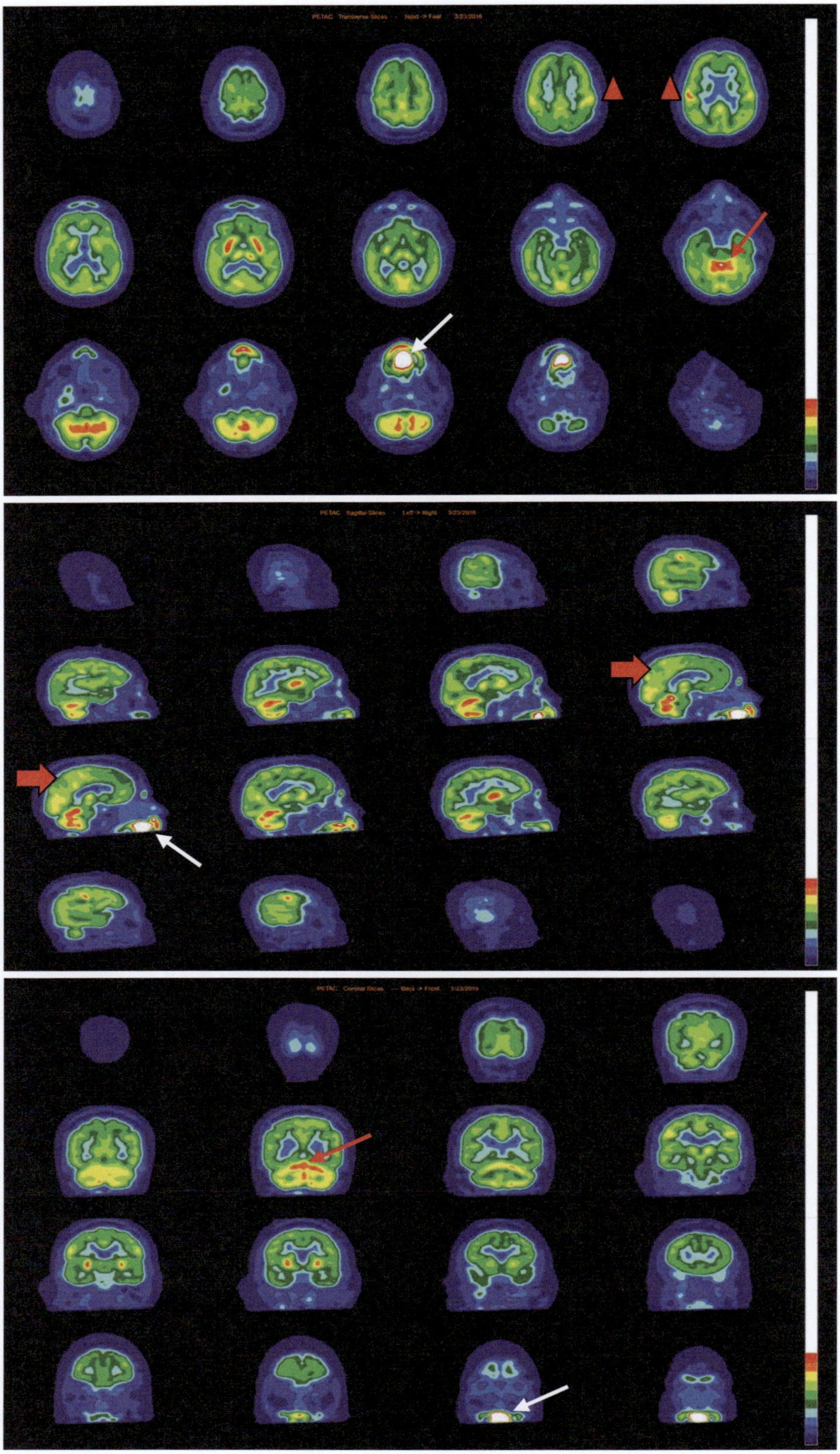

Fig. 1.19 A 56-year-old female with dementia of unknown type

currently on multiple psychiatric medications. Although the global cerebral hypometabolism is likely due to or related to depression, this cannot explain the PET finding of brain atrophy that is age-disproportionate for this 56-year-old patient. The relatively preserved metabolism in PCG makes AD less likely, although there is moderately decreased metabolism in the bilateral PCUN. The absence of hallucination or behavior/language issues, in line with the lack of regional metabolic abnormality in the frontotemporal and occipital regions, makes DLB or FTD less likely. The diffuse cerebellar hypermetabolism has an unknown etiology, though a speculated autoreactive immune process versus sequelae of schizoaffective disorder is considered. Another consideration of the cerebellar hypermetabolism especially in the vermis region is alcoholic encephalopathy.

During the ensuing 3-year follow-up, she had multiple admissions to our hospital due to suicidal/homicidal ideation, confusion, falls, syncope, or altered mental status/encephalopathy. The patient had two follow-up CTs of the head/brain, both showing no acute processes. However, her memory impairment and decline were getting worse. She continued to misplace objects around the house and developed very poor short-term memory. Her son reported that she could not recall things that were said or discussed with her even 1 hour earlier. Cholinesterase inhibitor medication was not prescribed because in the setting of unspecified dementia, it was best to avoid drug-drug interactions with the patient's antipsychotic medications and to avoid the potential for dysrhythmia.

Case Summary

Brain atrophy and global cortical hypometabolism in this 56-year-old patient are abnormal and age-disproportionate. There are no typical altered metabolic patterns to suggest any commonly diagnosed neurodegenerative dementias, such AD, FTD, DLB, or VD. Therefore, this patient's dementia is of an unknown type, which was supported by the follow-up data.

Case 1.20 Negative Amyloid Brain PET Scan

Clinical Information

Chief Complaint *Memory loss for 1 year*

The patient is a 76-year-old male who presents with memory loss for 1 year, concerning for AD. He denies history of stroke, seizure, or head injury.

Past medical history is notable for anemia, allergic rhinitis, osteoporosis, obesity, and colon cancer.

The patient has no family history of dementia.

Recent CT the head/brain showed age-related brain volume loss, otherwise unremarkable.

Laboratory tests showed normal TSH, free T3, folate, and vitamin B_{12}.

The patient's blood glucose level was 68 mg/dL prior to F-18 Vizamyl administration for the brain PET scan.

F-18 Vizamyl PET/CT Imaging Findings (Fig. 1.20)

The beta-amyloid PET images show highest tracer intensity in the pons (white arrow), followed by bilateral thalami (red arrow). Both findings are normal. Nonspecific mild to moderate tracer uptake is noted in the white matter and cerebella, with no significant uptake in the gray matter. Of note, there are some asymmetric tracer uptake in the bilateral frontal lobes, most likely due to brain atrophy as shown on the concurrent CT.

Discussion and Follow-Up

Since F-18 Vizamyl is normally distributed to the pons with highest intensity, therefore, on the 10-step color display, beta-amyloid PET images need to be normalized using the pons as a reference color of red. After normalization, the images indicate a negative amyloid PET scan, as evidenced by a clear gray/white matter contrast and no significant tracer distribution to the gray matter. Review of concurrent or available CT or MR imaging is very helpful in the clarification of brain atrophy-associated blurring between the gray and white matter.

During the follow-up for 1 year, there were no major memory issues in this patient.

Case Summary

A negative amyloid brain PET scan is characterized by nonspecific mild to moderate tracer distribution only in the white matter, no significant tracer activity in the gray matter. As a result, there is a clear gray/white matter contrast. Negative beta-amyloid scans make the diagnosis of Alzheimer's disease – the most common type of neurodegenerative dementia unlikely at the time of the PET imaging; however, non-AD dementing disease cannot be excluded [4].

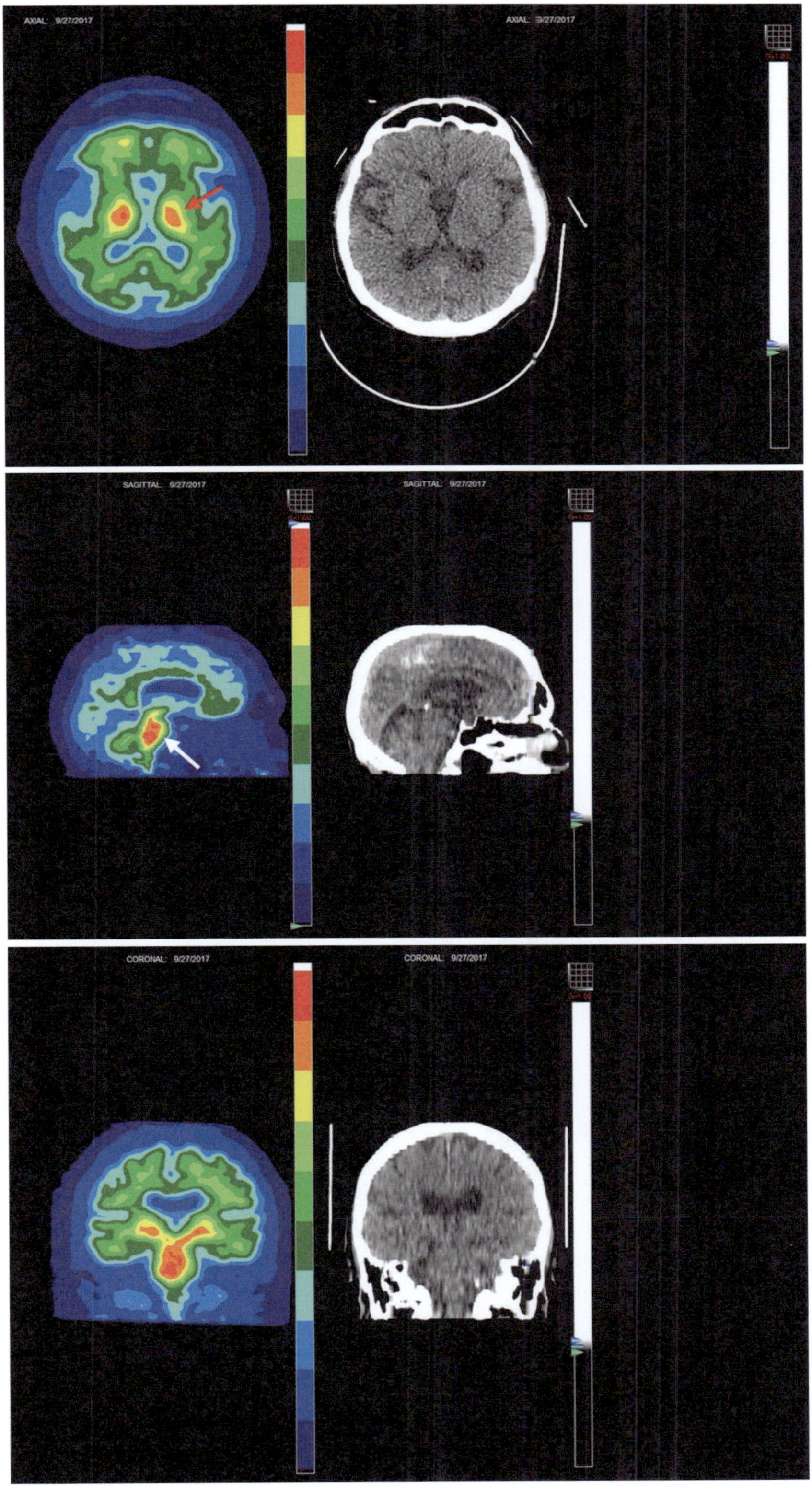

Fig. 1.20 A 76-year-old male with memory loss and negative amyloid brain PET

Case 1.21 Positive Amyloid Brain PET Scan

Clinical Information

Chief Complaint *Progressive memory decline for years*

The patient is a 71-year-old male who presents with progressive memory decline. Over the past few years, he has been often forgetting to take medications and misplacing his keys and cell phone.

He is a gas station owner and still functionally able to run his business and to take care of the finances. He is still able to drive, but within the last year, he has been in two accidents, which were caused by the patient's distraction. On neurological exam, he achieved MMSE score of 22/30.

He denies history of stroke, head trauma, or seizure.

Past medical history includes hypercholesterolemia, hearing loss, GERD (gastroesophageal reflux disease), and arthritis.

Family history is significant for Alzheimer's disease in his brother.

Two recent brain perfusion SPECT scans with and without premedication of Diamox (a cerebral vascular dilating agent) showed left temporal and parietal ischemic disease.

Recent MR imaging of the brain showed chronic ischemic changes in the white matter and incident findings suggestive of prior subarachnoid hemorrhage.

F-18 Vizamyl PET Imaging Findings (Fig. 1.21)

The PET images show moderate- to high-intensity tracer uptake in multiple cerebral cortical gray matter regions, including the bilateral frontal lobes, bilateral temporal lobes, and bilateral occipital lobes (hatched red arrows), with relative sparing of the primary visual cortices. Among the involved cortices, the frontal lobes have highest tracer intensities.

Nonspecific, high-intensity tracer uptake is noted in the pons (white arrow) and the thalami (red arrow), which is in a normal distribution pattern.

Discussion and Follow-Up

This is a positive beta-amyloid brain PET scan characterized by significant tracer distribution to multiple areas of the cortical gray matter with blurring of the gray/white matter contrast.

A positive amyloid PET scan is not by itself indicative of AD, although it raises concerns for an amyloid-associated neurodegenerative process, such as AD, FTD, or DLB. Moreover, a positive beta-amyloid PET scan could occur in some elderly individuals with no memory impairment [4, 11].

During the ensuing 20-month follow-up, the patient received memantine 5 mg every morning and 10 mg every evening. Despite the treatment, his family members report that the patient's short-term memory loss has worsened, and he often takes days off of work and stays alone at home. He is still able to drive but only for short distances from home.

Case Summary

A positive amyloid brain PET scan is characterized by moderate- or high-intensity tracer uptake in the gray matter, nonspecific uptake in the white matter, and a blurring gray/white matter contrast. A positive scan raises concerns for amyloid-associated neurodegenerative dementias, although it is not diagnostic of AD, and it could occur in some elderly individuals with no memory impairment.

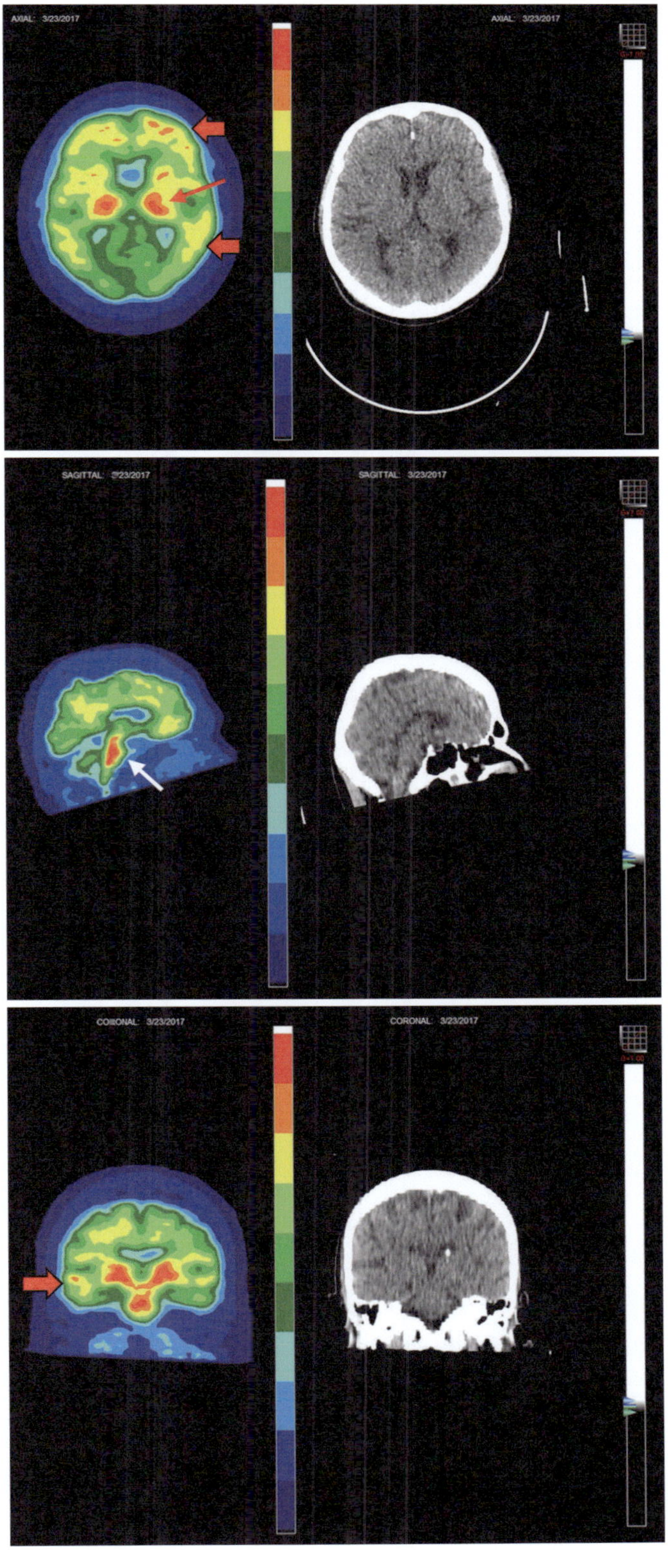

Fig. 1.21 A 71-year-old male with decline in memory and positive amyloid brain PET

References

1. Armstrong MJ, Litvan I, Lang AE, et al. Criteria for the diagnosis of corticobasal degeneration. Neurology. 2013;80:496–503.
2. Bertz V, Mosconi L, Pupi A. Brain: Normal variations and benign findings in FDG PET/CT imaging. PET Clin. 2014;9(2):129–40.
3. Brown RK, Bohnen NI, Wong KK, et al. Brain PET in suspected dementia: pattern's of altered FDG metabolism. Radiographics. 2014;34:684–701.
4. Filippi L, Chiaravalloti A, Bagni O, et al. ^{18}F-labeled radiopharmaceuticals for the molecular neuroimaging of amyloid plaques in alzheimer's disease. Am J Nucl Med Mol Imaging. 2018;8(4):268–81.
5. Gorno-Tempini ML, Hillis AE, Weintraub S, et al. Classification of primary progressive aphasia and its variants. Neurology. 2011;76:1006–14.
6. Herholz K. Guidance for reading FDG PET scans in dementia patients. Q J Nucl Med Mol Imaging. 2014;58:332–43.
7. Ishii K. PET approaches for diagnosis of dementia. Am J Neuroradiol. 2014;35(11):2030–8.
8. Kato T, Inui Y, Nakamura A, et al. Brain fluorodeoxyglucose (FDG) PET in dementia. Ageing Res Rev. 2016;30:73–84.
9. Lim SM, Katsifis A, Villemagne VL, et al. The 18F-FDG cingulate island sign and comparison to 123I-beta CIT SPECT for diagnosis of dementia with Lewy bodies. J Nucl Med. 2009;50(10):1638–45.
10. Mak E, Su L, Williams GB, O'Brien JT. Neuroimaging characteristics of dementia with lewy bodies. Alzheimers Res Ther. 2014;6(2):18–27.
11. Marcus C, Mena E, Subramaniam RM. Brain PET in the diagnosis of alzheimer's disease. Clin Nucl Med. 2014;39:e413–26.
12. Peterson R, Graff-Radford J. Alzheimer disease and other dementias. In: Daroff RB, Jankovic J, Maxxiotta JC, Pomeroy SL, editors. Bradley's neurology in clinical practice. 6th ed. Philadelphia: Elsevier Saunders; 2012. p. 1380–421.
13. Rascovak K, Hodges JR, Knopman D, et al. Sensitivity of revised diagnosis criteria for the behavioral variant of frontotemporal dementia. Brain. 2011;134(9):2456–77.
14. Shivamurthy VKN, Tahari AK, Marcus C, et al. Brain FDG PET and the diagnosis of dementia. Am J Radiol. 2015;204:W76–85.
15. Silverman DHS, Mosconi L, Ercoli L, et al. PET scans obtained for evaluation of cognitive dysfunction. Semin Nucl Med. 2008;38(4):251–61.
16. Silverman DHS. Brain F-18 FDG PET in the diagnosis of neurodegenerative dementias: comparison with perfusion SPECT and with clinical evaluation lacking nuclear imaging. J Nucl Med. 2004;45:594–607.
17. Zhu X-C, Tan L, Wang H-F, et al. Rate of early onset of alzheimer's disease: a systematic review and meta-analysis. Ann Transl Med. 2015;3(3):38–43.

2 Single Photon Emission Computed Tomography (SPECT) in Dementias

Case 2.1 Probable Normal Aging

Clinical Information

Chief Complaint *Memory difficulty for 7 years with recent decline*

The patient is an 81-year-old female presenting with memory difficulty that started 7 years ago with recent worsening. She states that she cannot express herself as she used to and finds herself being more forgetful. However, she is still able to live independently and continues to drive and pay bills by herself. She denies history of head trauma, seizure, or stroke.

Neuropsychological evaluation showed intact attention, processing speed, memory, and reasoning functions. But there was evidence of mild decline in unassisted recall of single words and names. She scored 29/30 on the MMSE.

Past medical history includes hypertension, arrhythmia, syncope, headache, and osteoporosis. There is no family history of dementia or AD. Brain MRI and MRA were unremarkable. CT of the head/brain showed mild and diffuse brain atrophy.

Laboratory tests showed TSH, folate, and vitamin B_{12} in normal ranges.

SPECT Imaging Findings (Fig. 2.1)

The images show mild sulcal prominence but no evidence of dilated lateral ventricles, suggestive of minimal to mild brain atrophy. The space between the deep structures (basal ganglia/thalami) is within normal limits. Despite heterogeneity likely due to motion artifact during imaging acquisition, tracer activities in the bilateral frontal and occipital lobes, the basal ganglia, and cerebella are essentially symmetric. The highest tracer activity is noted in the basal ganglia, the primary visual cortices, and the cerebella, whereas tracer activity in the temporal lobes is lowest.

There is mildly decreased tracer activity indicating hypoperfusion in the bilateral superomedial parietal lobes (red arrows) and in the anteromedial temporal lobes (white arrows). However, tracer activity in the bilateral PCG/PCUN (posterior cingulate gyri/precuneus) is well preserved (hatched red arrows).

Tracer activity in the right thalamus is asymmetrically increased (green arrow) relative to the left, with unknown etiology and uncertain clinical significance.

D. Wu, *Clinical Nuclear Medicine Neuroimaging*, https://doi.org/10.1007/978-3-030-40893-0_2

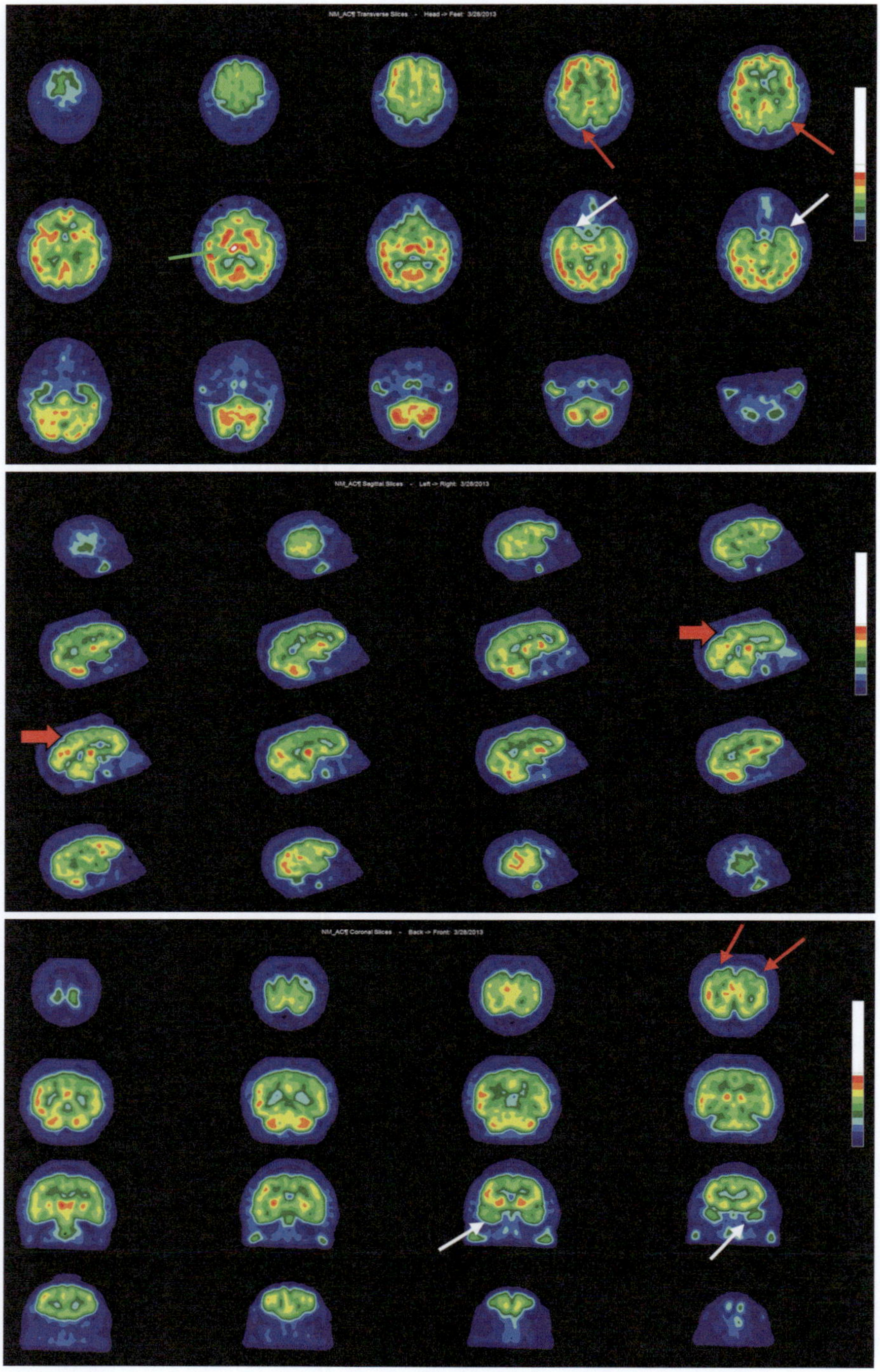

Fig. 2.1 An 81-year-old female with probable age-appropriate brain aging

Discussion and Follow-Up

Although the patient has complained memory difficulty for many years, she achieved a MMSE score of 29/30, indicating that she is actually not demented. Indeed, she is living independently and continues to drive and pay bills by herself. Therefore, the pretest likelihood of a severe neurodegenerative disease is low.

Like the imaging review process in PET studies as detailed in Chap. 1, I recommend to display brain perfusion SPECT images in a 10-step color spectrum. Since the basal ganglia normally have highest tracer activity in adult brains, the color of the basal ganglia regions needs to be adjusted to red. The transaxial imaging slides (the upper panel) are displayed from superior to inferior or from the head to feet. The sagittal slides (the middle panel) are from left to right, while the coronal slides (the lower panel) are from posterior to anterior or back to front. The PCG/PCUNs are actually the deep medial (vertical) parietal lobes, only separated by the posterior interhemispheric fissure, and best appreciated on the sagittal view. They are the two adjacent slides in the center of symmetrically displayed sagittal images.

Unlike FDG PET imaging that normally shows lowest tracer activity in the cerebella, brain perfusion SPECT imaging often shows normal highest tracer activity in the cerebella [3, 10]. The mechanism of this scintigraphic finding is poorly understood, but it is likely multifactorial. Like FDG PET imaging, tracer activity in the temporal lobes on SPECT imaging generally has a normal regional variation as the following: posterior, superior, and lateral > anterior, inferior, and medial (mesial).

The brain perfusion SPECT images shall be reoriented in the same way as the brain FDG PET images (see Case 1.1 in Chap. 1 for details).

After color normalization and image reorientation, the SPECT images of this particular case show an essentially normal pattern of perfusion tracer distribution. More specifically, the highest tracer activity is noted in the bilateral basal ganglia and cerebella, whereas the lowest activity is seen in the temporal lobes. The increased tracer activity in the right thalamus has an unknown etiology and is of uncertain clinical significance. There is no evidence of cortical or lacunar infarcts, making VD less likely. Mild cortical hypoperfusion is noted in the superomedial parietal lobes and the anteromedial temporal lobes. These cortical regions are the common sites of brain atrophy. In line with the CT findings, the minimal to mild brain atrophy is likely age-appropriate for this 81-year-old patient. The well-preserved perfusion in the bilateral PCG/PCUN makes AD less likely. The normoperfusion in the frontal and occipital lobes does not support the diagnosis of FTD or DLB.

During the follow-up for 4 years, the patient's mild cognitive impairment/difficulty has been persistent but stable, without pharmacotherapy.

Case Summary

Brain perfusion imaging evaluation of dementias is often a challenge, because of normal aging and age-appropriate brain atrophy that are easily overestimated. This case demonstrates an essentially normal pattern of brain perfusion, with highest tracer activity in the basal ganglia and cerebella and lowest activity in the temporal lobes, especially in the mesial temporal regions. Only mild hypoperfusion is identified in the bilateral superomedial parietal lobes and antero-inferior temporal lobes, which are common sites for brain atrophy, likely age-appropriate in this 81-year-old patient. The overall SPECT imaging findings are consistent with probable normal aging, which was further supported by clinical follow-up data.

Case 2.2 Possible MCI

Clinical Information

Chief Complaint *Worsening memory loss for 3 years*

The patient is a 68-year-old male presenting with worsening memory loss and incomprehension for 3 years. His wife states that he started experiencing mild cognitive impairment after a stroke in 1997 and at that time he was also diagnosed with residual mild vascular dementia, which was stable for nearly 20 years. Over the last 3 years, however, he has had difficulty remembering what people have told him, and he asks the same questions repeatedly. For example, he would ask multiple times if his taxes were done, even getting into his car to drive to where he files his tax return, despite having completed it several days ago. In addition to memory loss, he was found to have intermittent confusion. He is still driving and occasionally cooks at home. He remains fully independent in his ADL (activities of daily life). Neurological exam revealed normal attention, registration, and concentration. Language exam was normal for naming, repetition, expression, and reception. Cognitive testing showed MMSE score of 28/30.

Current medications include aspirin 81 mg daily, atorvastatin 10 mg every night, carvedilol 10 mg twice daily, fluoxetine 40 mg daily, lisinopril 40 mg daily, and pantoprazole 40 mg daily.

Past medical history is notable for stroke in 2006, anxiety, depression, essential hypertension, hyperlipidemia, GERD (gastroesophageal reflux disease), OSA (obstructive sleep apnea), a remote motor vehicle accident with closed head injury in 1997, prostate hypertrophy, and pulmonary artery aneurysm.

There is no family history of dementias.

A recent MR imaging of the brain revealed age-appropriate brain volume with normal ventricular morphology, but moderate senescent findings in periventricular and deep white matter, compatible with chronic small vessel ischemia.

Laboratory tests showed TSH, folate, and vitamin B_{12} in normal ranges.

The patient underwent a baseline brain perfusion SPECT study and then a Diamox challenge study with 15 days apart.

SPECT Findings

The images on the baseline study (Fig. 2.2a) show essentially symmetric brain hemispheres. There is no evidence of brain atrophy. Mildly decreased tracer activity is noted in bilateral superomedial frontoparietal, superolateral occipital, and anteromedial temporal lobes (red arrows). The decreased tracer activity in the bilateral superolateral occipital lobes is slightly more prominent on the left. Asymmetrically decreased tracer activity is identified in the right caudal nucleus (the upper panel of Fig. 2.2a, white arrow), whereas tracer activity in the bilateral thalami is relatively increased (green arrow). Tracer activity in the bilateral PCG/PCUN is well preserved (hatched red arrows).

Tracer activity in the remainder of the cerebral cortices and bilateral cerebella is within normal limits.

On the challenge study with Diamox (Fig. 2.2b), there is globally increased perfusion as expected. The prior mildly decreased tracer activity in the superomedial parietal lobes and the superolateral occipital lobes has resolved, whereas the minimally decreased tracer activity in the superomedial frontal and the anteromedial temporal lobes is persistent (red arrows). The prior perfusion defect in the right caudate nucleus has resolved as well (the upper panel of Fig. 2.2b, white arrow). Again, tracer activity in the bilateral PCG/PCUN is well preserved (hatched red arrows), and the hyperperfusion to the bilateral thalami is persistent (green arrow).

Discussions

Although this 68-year-old patient complains of worsening memory loss for 3 years, his MMSE score is 28/30, indicating that he is not demented. Indeed, he is fully independent in his ADL and

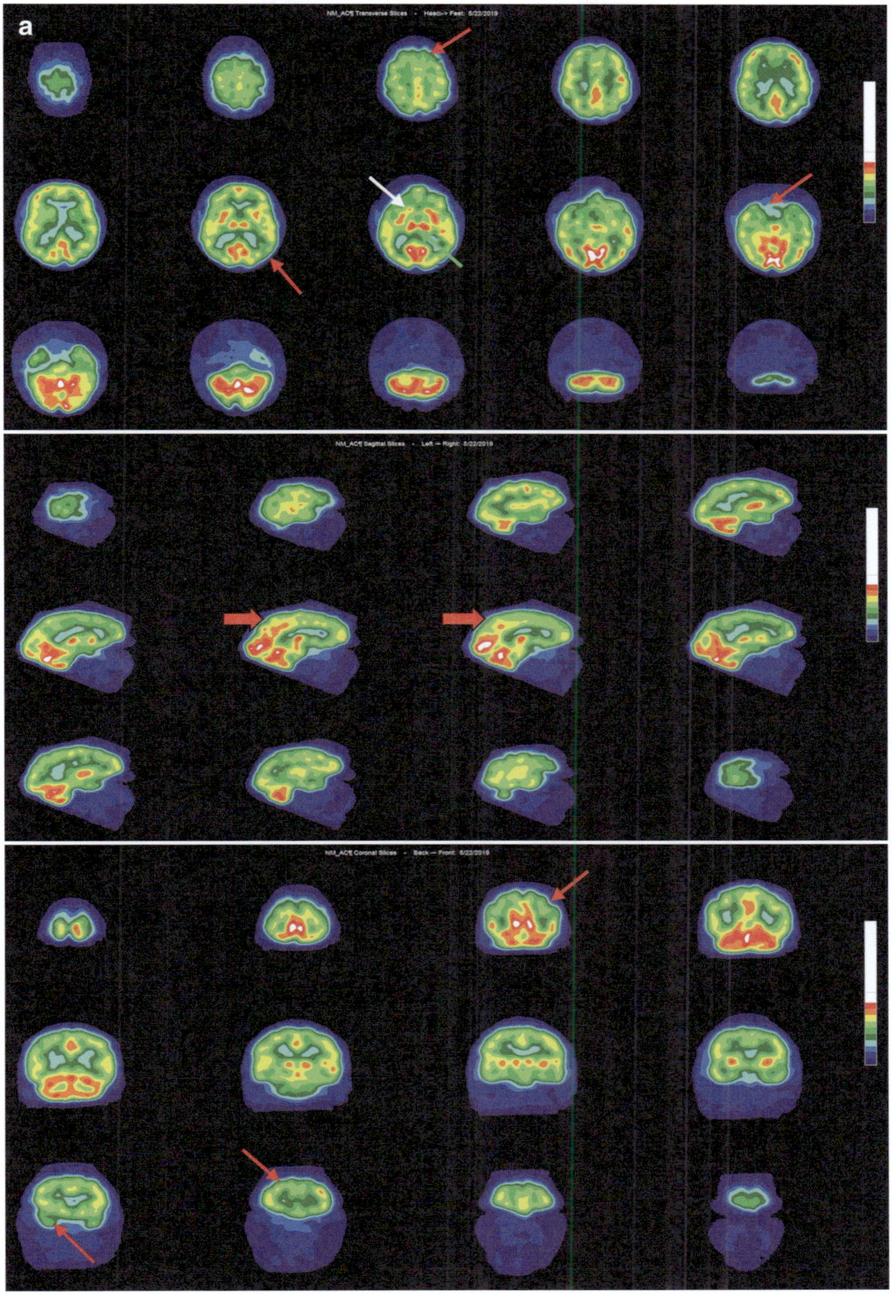

Fig. 2.2 (**a**) An 68-year-old male with possible MCI – a baseline brain perfusion SPECT. (**b**) An 68-year-old male with possible MCI – a challenge study with Diamox

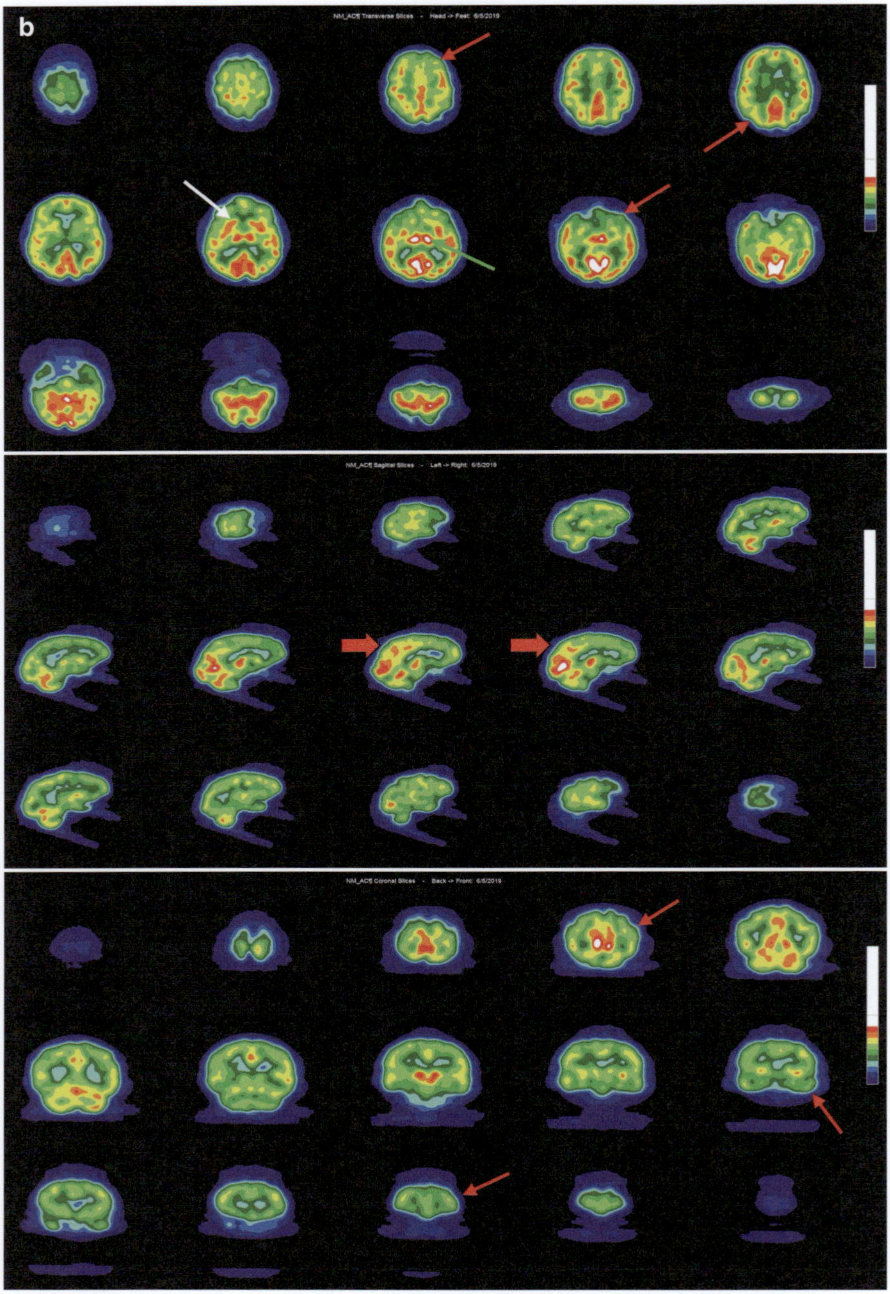

Fig. 2.2 (continued)

had an essentially unremarkable neurological exam. However, he has a complex past medical history including prior stroke and a remote closed head injury. Brain SPECT perfusion studies at baseline and with Diamox challenge were recently requested for evaluation of "mixed dementia" by his geriatrician.

The abnormal finding of right caudate nucleus hypoperfusion on the baseline study, later resolved on the challenge study with Diamox, is in line with his history of prior stroke and indicates an old lacunar infarct with a good vascular reserve. However, this small and solitary lesion, in the context of his clinical presentation, is not severe enough for consideration of VD.

The mild hypoperfusion in the frontoparieto-temporal lobes has an atypical pattern for AD or FTD. Instead, the improved perfusion on the Diamox challenge study is suggestive of a vascular nature. Furthermore, the preserved perfusion in bilateral PCG/PCUN makes AD less likely.

The mild hypoperfusion in the bilateral superolateral occipital lobes, left > right, is concerning for early-stage DLB. However, the good response to Diamox challenge and lack of clinical features (no visual hallucinations and/or Parkinsonism) make DLB less likely.

The persistent mild hypoperfusion in the superomedial frontal and the anteromedial temporal lobes raises concerns of direct or indirect TBI (traumatic brain injury), given the remote history of closed head injury. However, the pattern is atypical, and the findings are too subtle to consider dementia secondary to TBI.

Case Summary

Despite the patient's complex medical history and chief complaint of worsening memory loss for 3 years, the brain perfusion SPECT studies show no evidence of brain atrophy. There are multiple areas of mild cortical hypoperfusion, with improvement in some of them after Diamox challenge, but there are no imaging features suggesting FTD, DLB, or VD. The normal perfusion of the bilateral PCG/PCUN also makes AD less likely. There is no typical pattern to suggest TBI either, although the patient had a remote history of closed head injury. The right caudate nucleus hypoperfusion on the baseline study, resolved on the Diamox challenge study, is suggestive of prior lacunar infarct with a good vascular reserve. The overall imaging findings, in conjunction with the clinical presentation, are consistent with possible MCI, likely secondary to ischemic vascular disease.

Case 2.3 Possible Late-Onset Alzheimer's Disease (LOAD)

Clinical Information

Chief Complaint *Progressive memory loss and functional decline for 2 years*

The patient is a 72-year-old female who denies any memory problems, but her two daughters, who accompany her, have noticed that she has had progressive memory loss/forgetfulness. As a matter of fact, the patient's cognitive status has declined to the point that she needs a reevaluation for her driving license. Also, her daily functions have declined gradually over the past 2 years. Neuropsychological evaluation revealed a broad pattern of cognitive decline, with MMSE score of 25/30.

Current medications include melatonin 3 mcg daily, tramadol 50 mg daily, venlafaxine 150 mg daily, Depakote 125 mg twice a day, and a multivitamin tablet daily.

Past medical history includes depression, anxiety disorder, panic attack, paranoia, hypertension, and hyperlipidemia.

The patient reports that several family members have had dementia or Alzheimer's disease.

CT of the head/brain was unremarkable. Brain MRI showed mild generalized brain atrophy with mild chronic ischemic white matter changes, without mass or mass effects nor acute infarct.

Laboratory tests showed folate, vitamin B_{12}, TSH, and free T4 in normal ranges.

SPECT Imaging Findings (Fig. 2.3)

The images demonstrate a dominant area of cortical hypoperfusion in the bilateral parietal lobes, right > left (red arrows). Further, perfusion to the bilateral PCG/PCUN is also mild to moderately decreased, again right > left (hatched red arrows). In the remainder of the right brain hemisphere, mild to moderate cortical hypoperfusion is noted, in a spread pattern, involving the adjacent right superolateral frontal and occipital lobes and the right posterolateral temporal lobe (white arrows). Within the right frontal lobe, perfusion to the primary sensorimotor strip (red triangles) is relatively preserved or less affected.

Radioactive tracer activity in the bilateral basal ganglia, thalami, and the primary visual cortices is symmetric and within normal limits, suggestive of normoperfusion. Tracer activity in the left frontotemporal and occipital lobes is also preserved, except for minimal to mildly decreased tracer activity in the left medial anterior frontal and left inferomedial temporal lobes, likely due to brain atrophy.

Discussion and Follow-Up

Clinically, the patient presents with progressive memory loss and functional decline for 2 years. Neuropsychological evaluation revealed a broad pattern of cognitive decline.

On the brain perfusion SPECT images, despite the presence of asymmetry, the dominant hypoperfusion is identified in the parietal lobes, right > left, with involvement of the adjacent right frontal, temporal, and occipital lobes in a spread pattern. Further, perfusion of the bilateral PCG/PCUN is also mild to moderately decreased, right > left. The constellation of the clinical presentation, abnormal neuropsychological evaluation results, strong family history, and the typical SPECT brain perfusion findings, is suggestive of probable AD [1, 2, 5].

Given the involvement of the frontotemporal lobes, FTD needs to be considered. As mentioned earlier, the hypoperfusion within the right frontal lobe is more prominent in the superior and lateral aspects relative to the medial and inferior. Within the right temporal lobe, the hypoperfusion is more prominent in the posterior and lateral than the medial and anterior. The imaging pattern is suggestive of disesae spread from the right parietal lobe, rather than FTD. The minimal hypoperfusion to the anteromedial left frontal and anteromedial left temporal lobes is likely due to brain aging/atrophy.

The right-sided dominant hypoperfusion raises concerns for cerebral vascular disease.

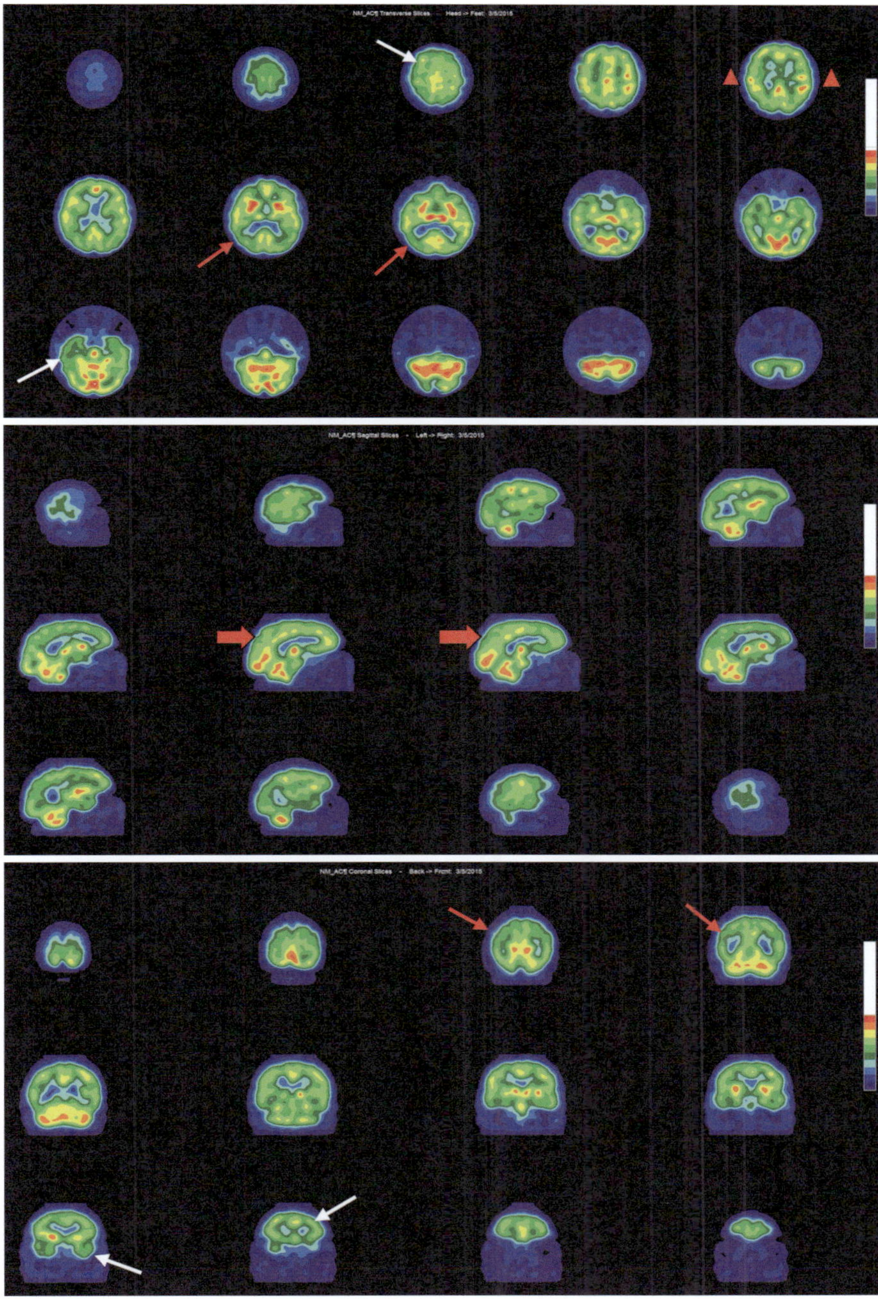

Fig. 2.3 A 72-year-old female with possible late-onset Alzheimer's disease (LOAD)

However, the involvement of the left parietal lobe, and the preserved perfusion to the right basal ganglion and thalamus is supportive of AD rather than VD [4, 7].

In the follow-up over the past 2.5 years, the patient was treated with Aricept, initially 5 mg daily, titrated up to 10 mg daily. She tolerates the medication well, with overall stable memory, and increased social activities, per family members.

Case Summary

This 72-year-old female patient presents with progressive memory loss and functional decline for 2 years. She had abnormal neuropsychological evaluation and a positive family history for dementia and AD. Brain perfusion SPECT study shows imaging characteristics of probable AD, including dominant cortical hypoperfusion in the parietal lobes including the PCG/PCUNs, with involvement of the adjacent frontotemporal and occipital lobes in a spread pattern. The imaging diagnosis of probable AD is further supported by the clinical follow-up data, *e.g.,* a favorable response to pharmacotherapy with a central acetylcholinesterase inhibitor (Aricept). Since the patient started to have symptoms in her early 70s, later than the cutoff age of 65, this case is consistent with probable late-onset AD (LOAD) – the most commonly diagnosed neurodegenerative dementia [1, 2, 5].

Case 2.4 Probable Early-Onset Alzheimer's Disease (EOAD)

Clinical Information

Chief Complaint *Progressive memory loss for 8 years*

The patient is a 58-year-old female presenting with worsening memory loss that started 8 years ago. She denies history of stroke or seizure. She reports no focal weakness, numbness, or tingling. There is no visual loss, diplopia, or hallucinations. She reports a very difficult relationship with her husband. She feels that her poor spouse relationship/stress is causing or contributing to some of her memory dysfunction. She has never smoked and denies history of drug abuse or alcohol dependence.

Current medications include citalopram 20 mg daily and hydroxyzine 25 mg daily.

Past medical history includes anxiety disorder, chronic kidney disease, and gastroesophageal reflux disease (GERD).

She has no family history of dementia.

Brain MRI of 2 years ago was read as unremarkable.

Laboratory tests showed TSH, vitamin B_{12}, and folate in normal ranges.

SPECT Imaging Findings (Fig. 2.4)

The images show prominent sulci and mildly dilated posterior horns of the lateral ventricles (green arrow), suggestive of brain atrophy. Dominant hypoperfusion is identified in the bilateral parietal lobes (red arrows), including the PCG/PCUNs (hatched red arrows), right > left. Moderate hypoperfusion is also present in the frontotemporal and occipital lobes (white arrows). Within the frontal lobes, the posterior and lateral portion is more affected than the anterior and medial portion, with preserved perfusion to the primary sensorimotor strips (red triangles), best appreciated on the transaxial view (the upper panel). Hypoperfusion is also seen in the temporal lobes; the posterior and lateral portion is more affected than the anterior and medial portion. Similarly, in the occipital lobes, hypoperfusion is more prominent in the superior/posterior and lateral than the anterior and medial, with well-preserved perfusion to the primary visual cortices. The imaging pattern is suggestive of disease spread from the parietal regions. Despite slight head-tilting, normoperfusion is seen in the bilateral basal ganglia, thalami, and cerebella.

Discussion

The chief complaint of progressive memory loss in a 58-year-old female patient is extraordinary. Neurological evaluation yielded a low index of suspicion for underlying neurodegenerative disorders, mainly due to the patient's age, history of anxiety disorder, her difficult spousal relationship, and unremarkable MRI brain. Laboratory tests showed no reversible causes of dementia.

The brain perfusion SPECT images, however, are markedly abnormal and show age-disproportionate brain atrophy with global and regional cerebral hypoperfusion, which are highly suggestive of a neurodegenerative process. The most severe cortical hypoperfusion is identified in the bilateral parietal lobes including the PCG/PCUNs. Additional involvement of the adjacent frontotemporal and occipital lobes is in a spread pattern. All the imaging findings are typical for probable AD [1–3, 5]. The significant involvement of the bilateral frontal lobes indicates advanced disease [4, 7].

Approximately 1 month after the brain perfusion SPECT study, the patient underwent a follow-up brain MRI, which was initially read unremarkable again. Due to the scintigraphic abnormalities of the SPECT imaging, the MRI was reviewed and found to have "significant generalized volume loss since the prior (MRI) study of 2.5 years ago," per an amended report. Due to the functional and anatomic neuroimaging findings, the patient was treated with memantine for 1.5 years, and her memory issue has been stable, per family members.

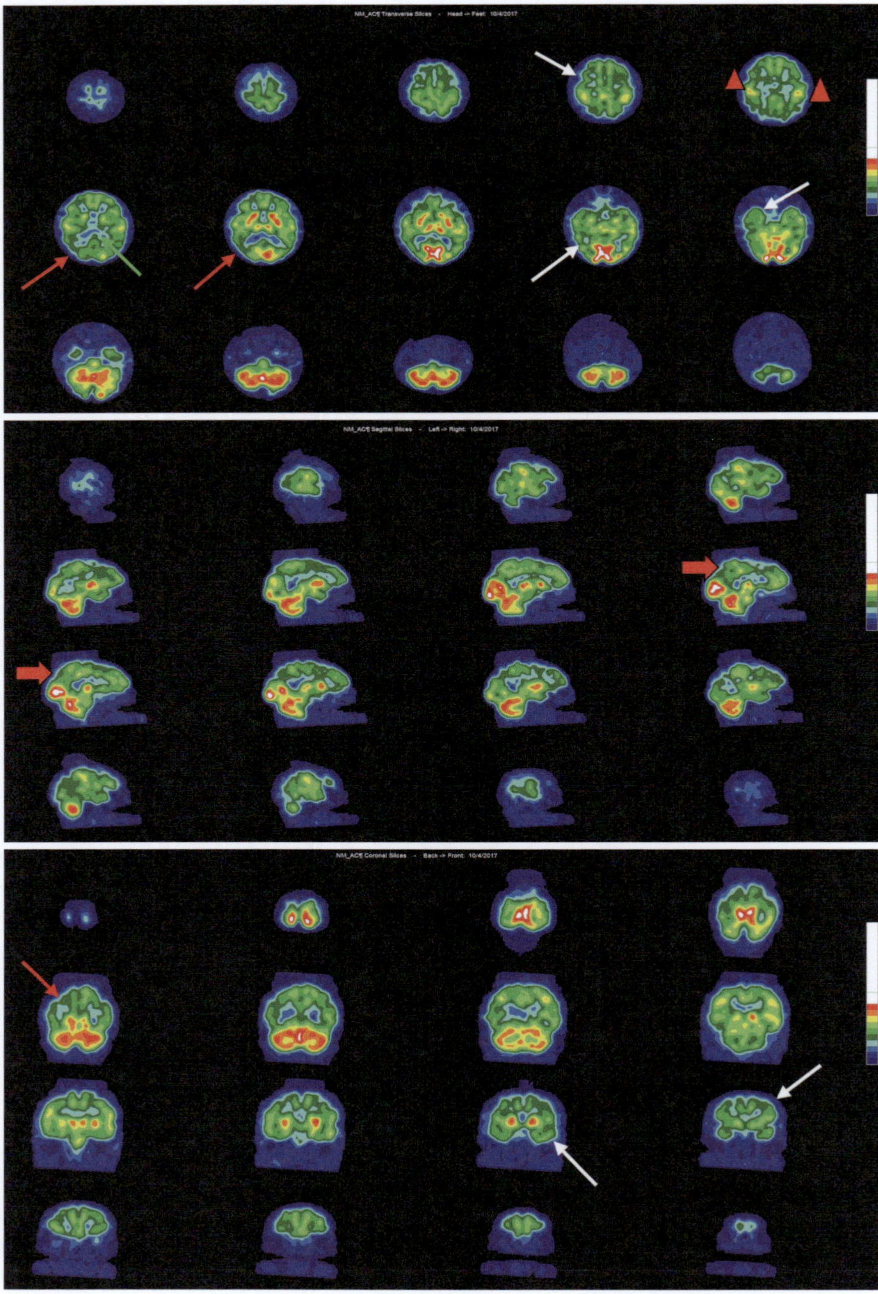

Fig. 2.4 A 58-year-old female with probable early-onset Alzheimer's disease (EOAD)

Case Summary

Although this 58-year-old patient has had progressive memory loss for more than 8 years, her prior brain MRI was normal. In contrast, the brain perfusion SPECT imaging is markedly abnormal and reveals age-disproportionate brain atrophy and global and dominant regional cerebral hypoperfusion, most prominent in the parietal lobes, with involvement of the adjacent temporal-occipital-frontal regions in a spread pattern. The constellation of the clinical presentation and SPECT imaging findings is highly suggestive of probable AD. The substantial bilateral frontal lobe involvement indicates advanced disease. Since the patient's symptoms started prior to the cutoff age of 65, this case is consistent with early-onset AD (EOAD). The diagnosis of advanced neurodegenerative AD in this patient was supported by a follow-up brain MRI which showed "significant generalized volume loss since the prior (MRI) study of 2.5 years ago" and a favorable response to pharmacotherapy.

Case 2.5 Probable Frontotemporal Dementia (FTD)

Clinical Information

Chief Complaint *Memory loss for 7 years*

The patient is a 78-year-old male presenting with memory loss for at least 7 years, for which he has gave up driving. He does not remember his home addresses in Michigan or Florida, although he remembers the names of his children and grandchildren as well as their occupations. Preceding to his memory loss, he had a fall 7 years ago with subsequent loss of consciousness and brain hemorrhage. Over the last half a year, he had two falls with a right shoulder fracture. Due to shuffling gaits, he uses a cane as an assistive device to ambulate, although he often forgets to use his cane at home. He has no history of seizure. Neurologic examination revealed no evidence of aphasia, but his MMSE score was 20/30.

Current medications include memantine 10 mg daily, Xarelto 20 mg daily, and Zocor 20 mg daily.

Past medical history includes transient ischemic attacks (TIAs), depression, prior fall with head injury 7 years ago, and two recent falls over the last half year with shoulder fracture, hypertension, dyslipidemia, and atrial fibrillation.

There is no family history of dementias or AD.

Laboratory tests show normal TSH, folate, and vitamin B_{12}.

The patient underwent a baseline brain SPECT perfusion and then a challenge study with Diamox one week later.

SPECT Imaging Findings

The baseline images (Fig. 2.5a) show mild to moderate decreased tracer activity in all of the cerebral cortices, including the sensorimotor stripes and the primary visual cortices. In addition, more profound hypoperfusion is identified in the bilateral anteroinferior frontal/orbitofrontal lobes (red arrows) and the anteromedial temporal lobes (white arrows), best appreciated on the coronal view (Fig. 2.5a, the lower panel). When compared to the right basal ganglia, perfusion to the left basal ganglia is minimally decreased (green arrow). Tracer activity in the bilateral thalami and cerebella is essentially symmetric and likely within normal limits. Relative to the anterior cingulate gyri, perfusion to the bilateral PCG/PCUNs is preserved (hatched red arrows).

The challenge study with Diamox (Fig. 2.5b) showed global increased/improved perfusion as expected. However, the cortical hypoperfusion in bilateral frontotemporal lobes remains (red and white arrows) in the same pattern, *e.g.,* left being more affected than the right, anterior/inferior being more affected than the posterior and superior in the frontal lobes, and anterior/medial being more affected than the posterior and lateral in the temporal lobes. Also, the minimal hypoperfusion to the left basal ganglia is persistent, whereas tracer activity in the right basal ganglia, bilateral thalami, and cerebella is globally increased, especially the left thalamus. In contrast to the persistent hypoperfusion in the anterior cingulate gyri, the perfusion to bilateral PCG/PCUNs is significantly improved and well preserved (hatched red arrows).

Discussion and Follow-Up

The two sets of SPECT imaging at baseline and with Diamox challenge show persistent, dominant cortical hypoperfusion to the frontotemporal lobes. The findings are neuroimaging characteristics of FTD [5], despite lack of clinical features associated with FTD such as behavioral/personality changes and/or language issues at the time of the SPECT imaging studies.

The baseline imaging study shows mild to moderate global cortical hypoperfusion, which is improved on the challenge study with Diamox, indicating preserved cerebrovascular reserve (CVR). This is likely secondary to depression, given the involvement of bilateral sensorimotor strips and primary visual cortices, although a generalized ischemic vascular process needs to be considered.

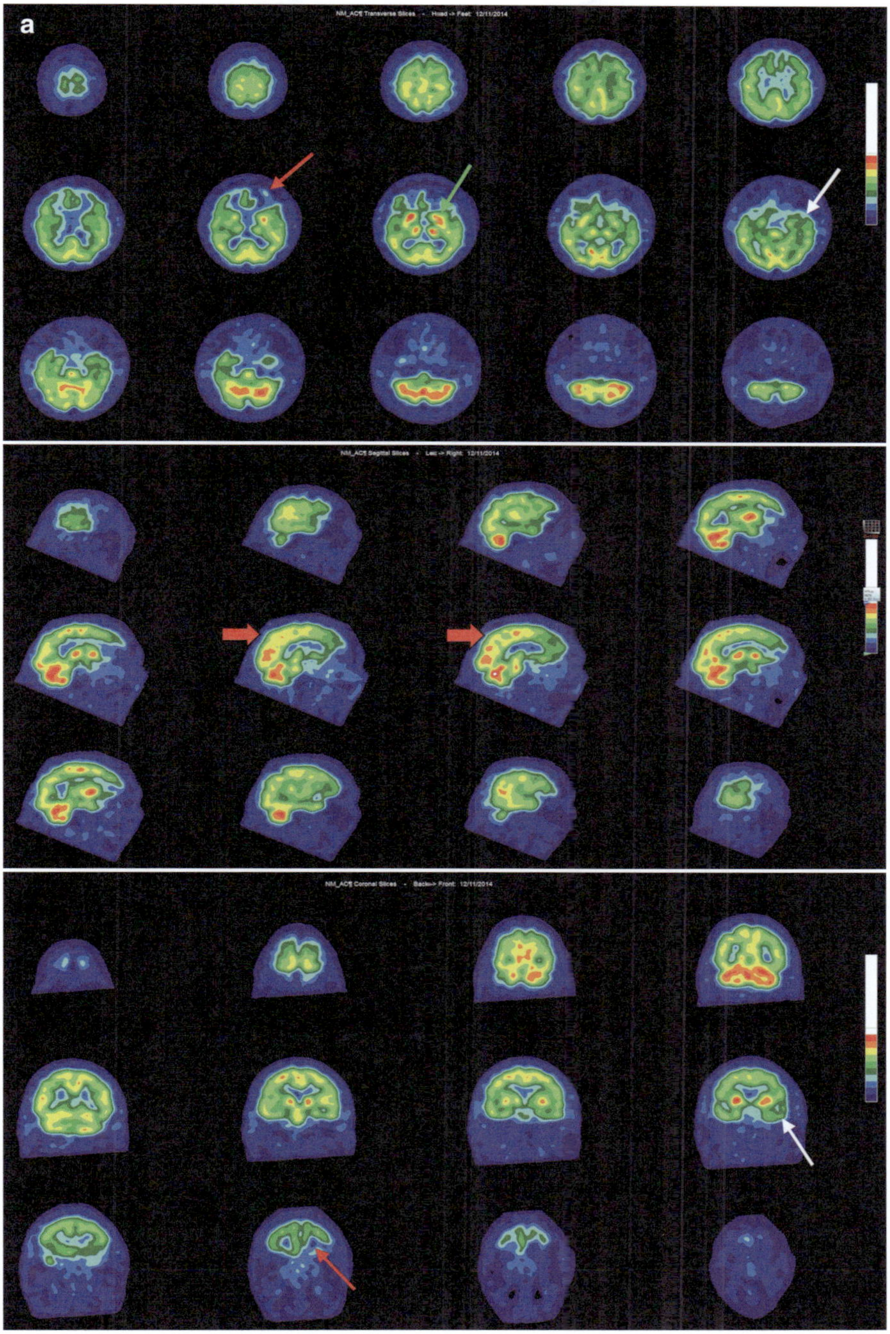

Fig. 2.5 (**a**) A 78-year-old male with probable FTD – a baseline study. (**b**) A 78-year-old male with probable FTD – a challenge study with Diamox

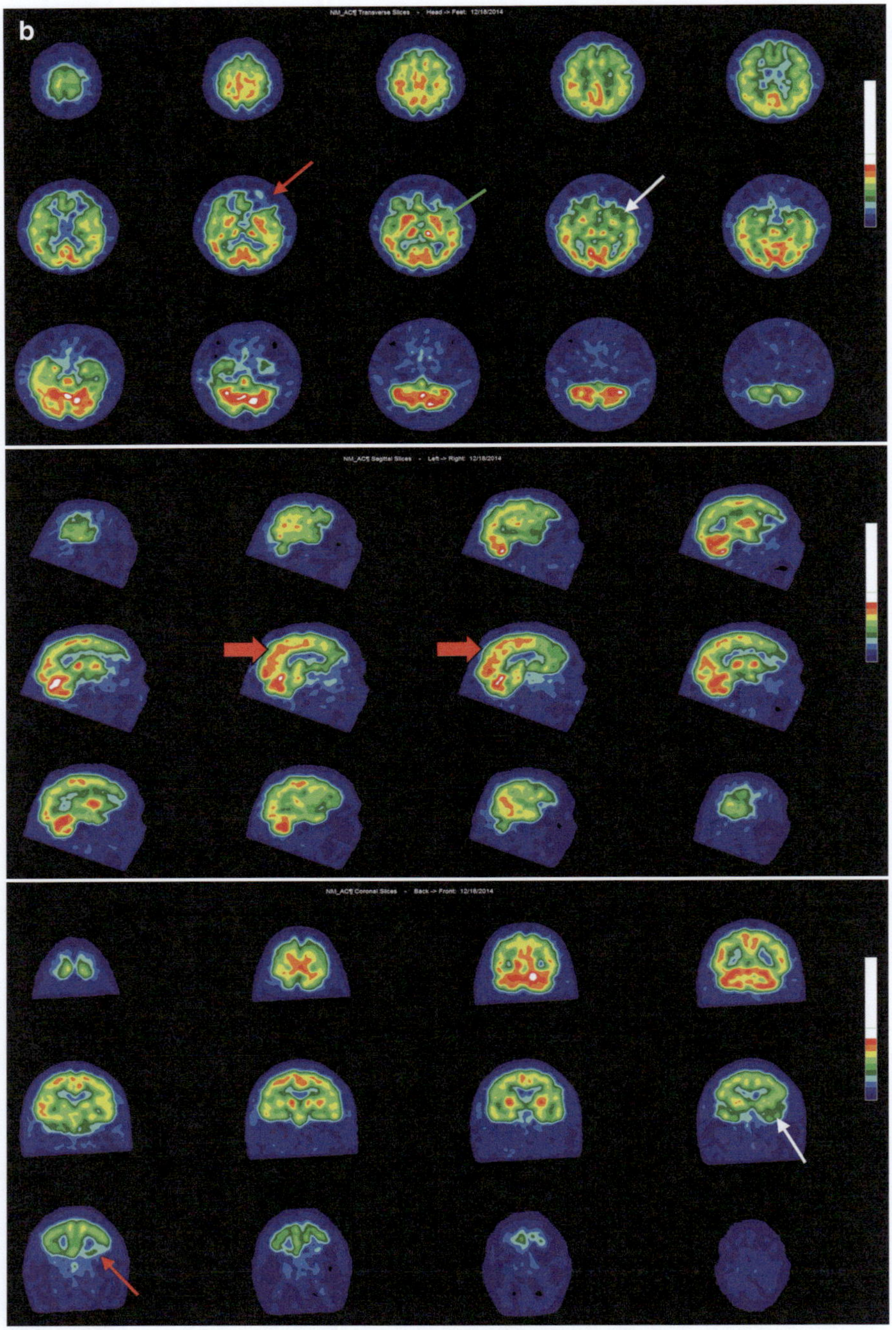

Fig. 2.5 (continued)

The prior fall/brain injury preceding to the onset of memory loss in this patient raises concerns for dementia secondary to traumatic brain injury (TBI). Since the patient lives in two states (Michigan and Florida), his prior anatomic neuroimaging studies were unavailable for review. Despite the limitation, the multi-lobe involvement of hypoperfusion is in favor of a neurodegenerative dementia rather than brain injury.

The relatively preserved perfusion to the bilateral PCG/PCUNs makes AD less likely. The minimal hypoperfusion to the left basal ganglia likely due to neurodegenerative involvement may explain symptoms of shuffling gaits and recent falls. However, there is no evidence of cortical or lacunar infarcts to suggest VD.

After the abnormal SPECT imaging studies, the patient was treated with memantine, 10 mg daily. But the medication was stopped 1 year later, due to lack of benefits. Further follow-up showed that the patient developed increasing behavioral issues/changes. For example, he would urinate in inappropriate locations and would become aggressive in the morning with improvement throughout the rest of the day. He scored MMSE score of 15/30 approximately 4 years after the SPECT imaging studies; at that time his MMSE score was 20/30, indicative of progression of dementia.

Case Summary

Despite confounding factors such as prior head injury and lack of typical clinical features at the time of the brain perfusion studies, the SPECT imaging findings on both baseline and Diamox-challenging studies are suspicious for underlying FTD in this patient, as evidenced by dominant and persistent cortical hypoperfusion to bilateral frontotemporal lobes. The imaging impression of probable FTD was supported by clinical follow-up data, such as a poor response to pharmacotherapy, worsening dementia over times, and newly developed behavioral issues/changes, which are common clinical features of FTD.

Case 2.6 Probable Behavioral Variant Frontotemporal Dementia (bvFTD)

Clinical Information

Chief Complaint *Behavior issues and short-term memory loss*

The patient is a 75-year-old female with an extensive history of depression and anxiety presenting with behavior issues and memory loss. She is accompanied by her son, who reports that her long-term memory appears intact, but she is forgetful about daily events. Recently, she has forgotten to turn the stove off several times after cooking. Three years ago, she went to a gas station and completely forgot how to pump gas which caused her to give up driving. Notably, her son also reports that she was started on donepezil some time ago to help with her memory loss, but there is no improvement in her memory.

In addition to memory problems, she has been an avid gambler for many years and even lost her house due to gambling 2 years ago. Her son also reports that she is a pathologic liar.

She denies head injury and there is no history of stroke or seizure. She is a former smoker but denies history of drug abuse or alcohol dependence.

Neurologic evaluation revealed that she has coarse tremors, and she scored 24/30 on the MMSE.

Past medical history is notable for depression, anxiety disorder, hypertension, and hypothyroidism.

Current medications include citalopram 20 mg daily, aspirin 81 mg daily, donepezil 10 mg daily, levothyroxine 25 mcg daily, olanzapine 5 mg daily, pantoprazole 40 mg daily, tolterodine 2 mg daily, vitamin B_{12} 500 mcg daily, and propranolol 40 mg daily.

Family history is negative for dementia or AD.

MR imaging of the brain was read unremarkable.

Laboratory tests showed TSH, folate, and vitamin B_{12} in normal ranges.

SPECT Imaging Findings

The baseline SPECT images (Fig. 2.6a) show brain atrophy, as evidenced by separation of the deep structures (basal ganglia and thalami), prominent sulci and lateral ventricles (green arrow). Moderate hypoperfusion is identified in the bilateral frontal lobes (red arrows), and mild hypoperfusion is seen in the anterior and inferior temporal lobes (white arrows). Perfusion to the bilateral occipital lobes and parietal lobes including the PCG/PCUNs (hatched red arrows) is preserved. Symmetric normoperfusion is seen in bilateral basal ganglia, thalami, and cerebella.

The challenge study with Diamox (Fig. 2.6b) shows persistent cortical hypoperfusion to the bilateral frontal lobes (red arrows) and inferior/anterior temporal lobes (white arrows), despite global improved perfusion as expected. Perfusion to the bilateral basal ganglia and thalami, the remainder of cortices including the PCG/PCUNs (hatched red arrows), and the cerebella is unchanged when compared to the baseline study. Again, the lateral ventricles are prominent (green arrow) indicating brain atrophy.

Discussion and Follow-Up

Clinically, the patient's behavioral issues are more prominent than her memory loss/impairment as evidenced by pathologic lying and gambling addiction even after the loss of her house. In contrast, she scored 24/30 on the MMSE, indicating only borderline or mild dementia. Although her brain MRI was reported unremarkable, brain perfusion SPECT imaging studies without and with Diamox challenge show age-disproportionate brain atrophy and persistent hypoperfusion to the bilateral frontotemporal lobes, with frontal lobes being more affected than the temporal lobes. These functional neuroimaging findings are concordant with the clinical presentations, suggestive of behavioral variant FTD (bvFTD) [9].

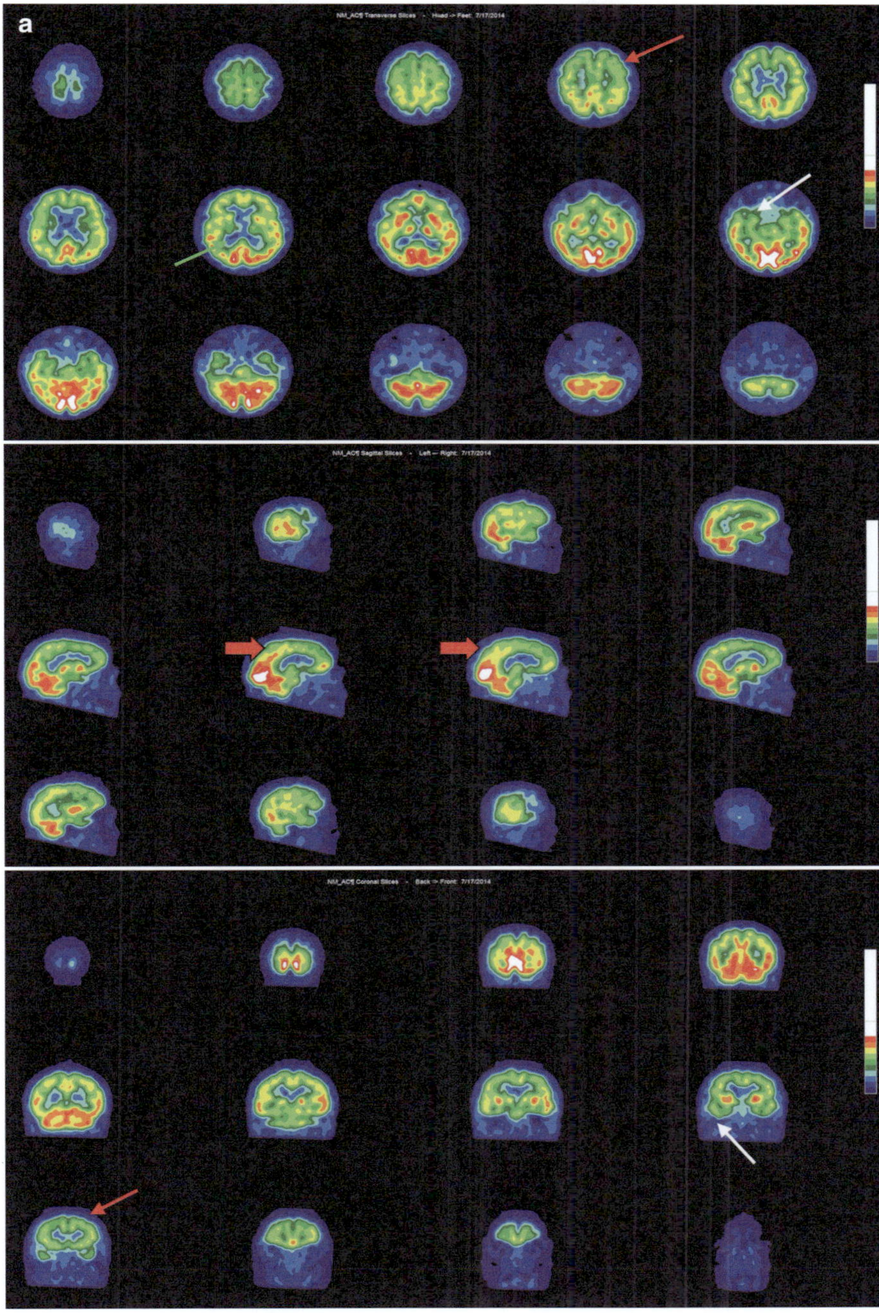

Fig. 2.6 (**a**) A 75-year-old female with probable bvFTD – a baseline study. (**b**) A 75-year-old female with probable bvFTD – a challenge study with Diamox

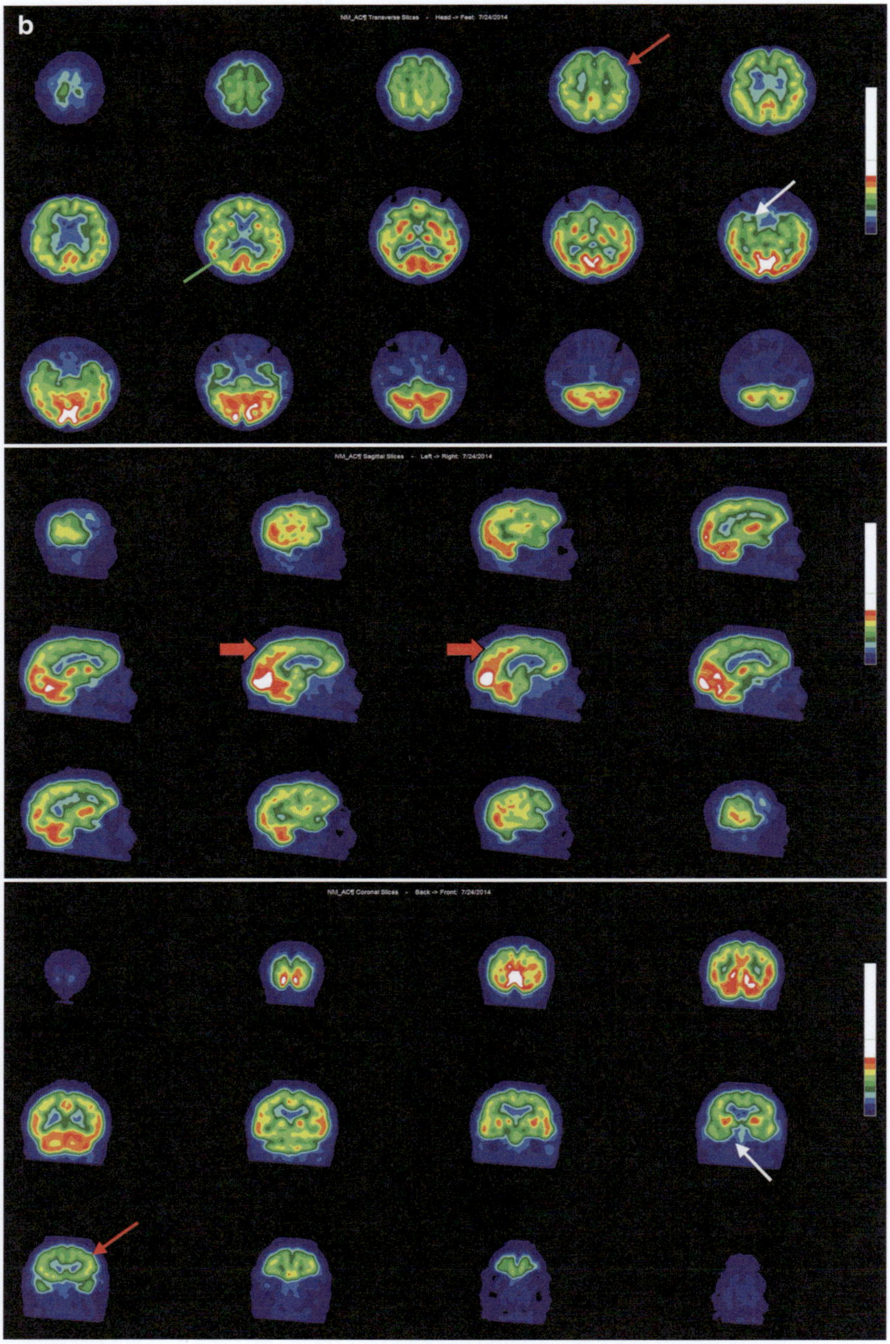

Fig. 2.6 (continued)

The patient's current medications include donepezil, a central acetylcholinesterase inhibitor for cognition enhancement, which is commonly used for the treatment of patients with AD. Apparently, this medication did not improve patient's memory according to her son. This negative treatment response is in line with the preserved perfusion to bilateral parietal lobes including the PCG/PCUN that makes AD less likely.

In addition to her memory loss and mood complaints, the patient's behavioral problems made her family feel overwhelmed. A few months after the abnormal brain perfusion SPECT studies, she was admitted to an assistant living facility.

Case Summary

This is an elderly female patient with marked behavioral issues and mild memory loss. Despite the reported unremarkable MRI, brain perfusion SPECT studies without and with Diamox challenge show age-disproportionate brain atrophy and persistent cortical hypoperfusion to bilateral frontotemporal lobes. In contrast, normoperfusion is seen in the parieto-occipital regions including the PCG/PCUNs. The constellation of the SPECT imaging findings and the patient's clinical presentation is suggestive of bvFTD, a subtype of FTD which is also referred to as frontal variant FTD (fvFTD) [9].

Case 2.7 Probable Dementia with Lewy Bodies (DLB)

Clinical Information

Chief Complaint *Progressive memory loss and hallucinations*

The patient is an 81-year-old male physician presenting with intermittent visual hallucinations and memory loss for 2 years. He has recently had increasing difficulty with his finances. He describes instances where he is not able to calculate tips after eating at restaurants with friends. He reports an instance in which he was having a meal with his wife, who deceased many years ago.

The patient is a psychiatrist. His colleagues have noticed his functional decline and told him that they would report him to the state authority if he did not get an evaluation. He denies any falls, gait changes, or weakness/tremor. Neurologic examination showed MMSE score of 23/30.

Current medications include amlodipine 5 mg daily, aspirin 81 mg daily, escitalopram 10 mg daily, losartan 100 mg daily, pravastatin 40 mg daily, and vitamin D 1000 units daily.

Past medical history is notable for seizures, TIA (transient ischemic attack), depression, anxiety, panic attacks, hypertension, hyperlipidemia, and prostate cancer.

There is no family history of dementia.

Brain MRI showed moderate volume loss of brain parenchyma. Brain MRA was unremarkable. CT of the head/brain was reported normal.

Laboratory tests show TSH, free T_4, folate, and vitamin B_{12} in normal ranges.

SPECT Imaging Findings

The baseline study images (Fig. 2.7a) show separation of the deep structures (basal ganglia and thalami), prominent sulci and lateral ventricles (green arrow), and posterior horns > anterior horns, all indicating brain atrophy. There is global, mild to moderate cortical hypoperfusion including the primary sensorimotor strips. Additionally, predominant cortical hypoperfusion is identified in the bilateral occipital lobes including the primary visual cortices (red arrows). In contrast, perfusion to the bilateral PCG/PCUNs is preserved (hatched red arrows) relative to the anterior cingulate gyri. Finally, there is a small, subtle defect between the right caudate nucleus and putamen (white arrow), and the right thalamic perfusion is also slightly decreased relative to the left.

The perfusion images with Diamox challenge (Fig. 2.7b) show unchanged global and regional cortical hypoperfusion, still predominant in the bilateral occipital lobes (red arrows), whereas perfusion to the bilateral PCG/PCUNs is again preserved (hatched red arrows). Brain atrophy is noted, as evidenced by separation of basal ganglia/thalami as well as prominent sulci and lateral ventricles (green arrow). The known small defect in the right basal ganglion and the minimally decreased perfusion to the right thalamus have improved (whilte arrow), suggestive of a preserved vascular reserve in the region.

Discussion and Follow-Up

This 81-year-old male patient presents with progressive memory loss, visual hallucination, and MMSE score of 23/30. These clinical features are concerning for DLB.

Consistent with the MRI finding of brain parenchymal volume loss, brain SPECT perfusion studies without and with Diamox consistently showed brain atrophy and mild to moderate global cortical atrophy, again raising concerns of underlying neurodegenerative diseases. Additionally, predominant cortical hypoperfusion is identified in the bilateral occipital lobes including the primary visual cortices. The constellation of these neuroimaging findings and clinical presentation is suggestive of dementia with Lewy bodies (DLB) [11].

Although cerebral hypoperfusion extends into the adjacent parietal regions, perfusion to the cingulate gyri/precuneus is well preserved. This finding, in conjunction with hypoperfusion in the cuneus regions posteriorly and the anterior cingulate gyri, is referred to as "cingulate island sign" (CIS), which is a highly specific imaging biomarker for DLB rather than AD [8, 11].

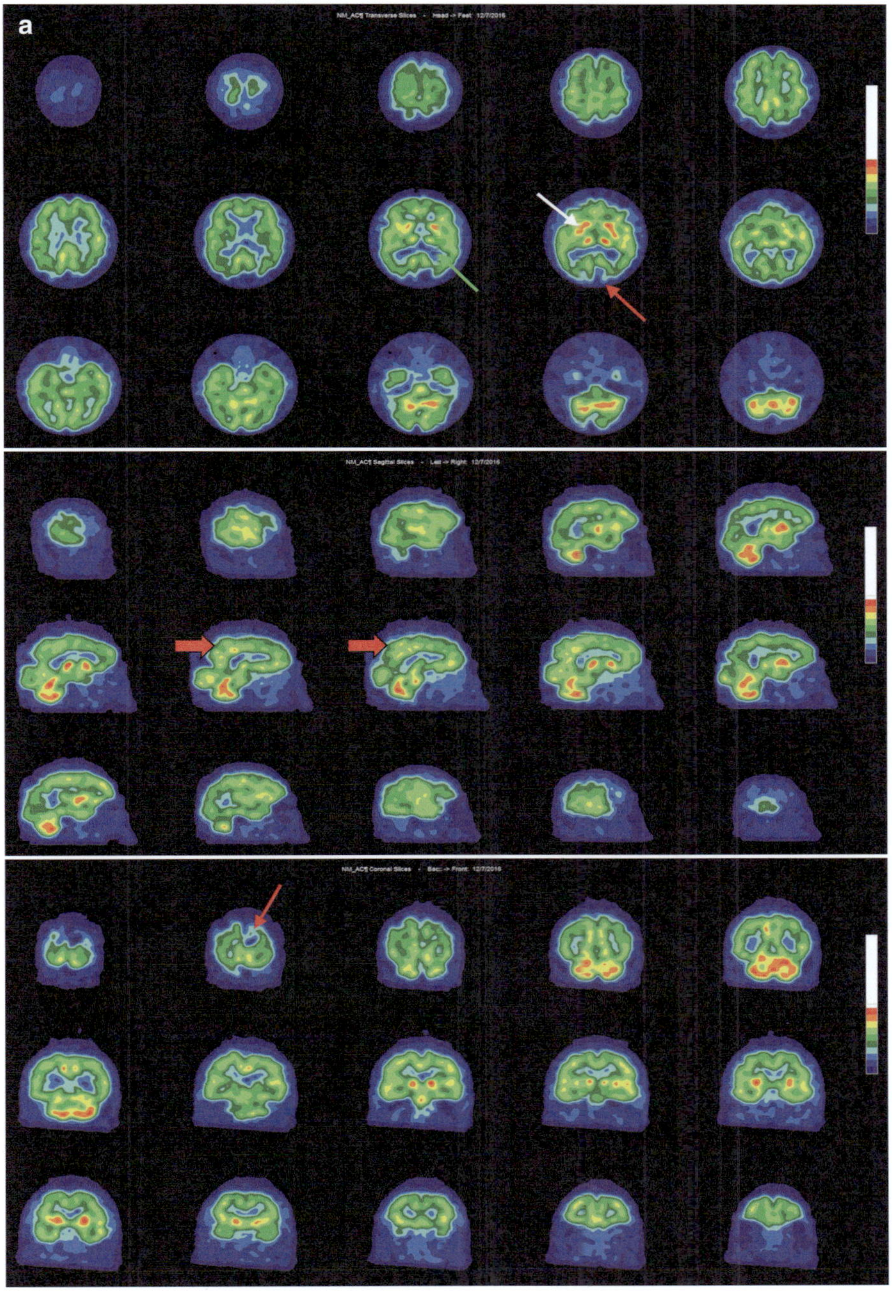

Fig. 2.7 (**a**) An 81-year-old male with probable DLB – a baseline study. (**b**) An 81-year-old male with probable DLB – a challenge study with Diamox

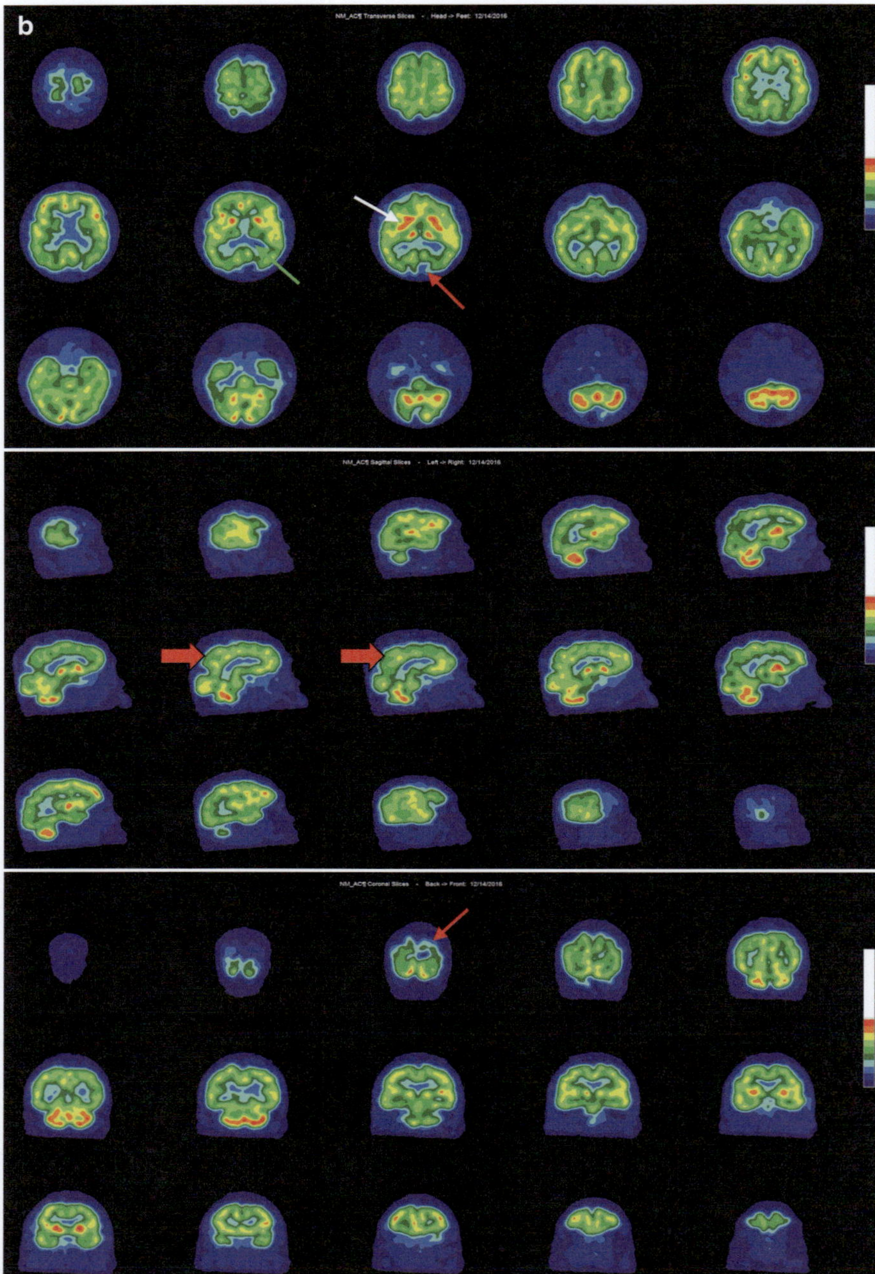

Fig. 2.7 (continued)

The small perfusion defect in the right basal ganglia is suggestive of a prior lacunar infarct. The finding is improved on the challenge study with acetazolamide, indicating a good vascular reserve in the region.

Case Summary

The progressive memory loss, complex visual hallucinations, and functional decline in this 81-year-old patient with MMSE score of 23/30 are clinical features concerning for DLB. Consistently, the SPECT imaging findings of predominant cortical hypoperfusion in the occipital lobes including the primary visual cortices, and the relatively preserved perfusion in the PCG/PCUNs, also called "cingulate island sign" (CIS), are neuroimaging characteristic of DLB rather than AD [8].

Case 2.8 Probable Primary Progressive Aphasia (PPA) with AD Pathology

Clinical Information

Chief complaint *Progressive difficulties in word-finding for years*

The patient is a 67-year-old right-handed female presenting with intermittent speech disturbances and progressive difficulties in word-finding/self-expression for 2–3 years. She states that she has had to "fight to get her words out." In addition, she has noted changes in her handwriting. She has had no difficulty chewing or swallowing, however.

The patient reports no diplopia, visual changes, hallucinations, vertigo, headaches, weakness, sensory symptoms, or problems with balance. She reports she was in a motor vehicle accident 2 years ago but denies head injury or whiplash. She has no history of stroke, TIA, seizure, or serious head injury. The patient has a college education and is self-employed as a painter, but she has not been able to work for half a year.

Current medications include acetaminophen-codeine 300–15 mg every 4 hours, alprazolam 0.5 mg PRN, sertraline 100 mg daily, and simvastatin 10 mg daily.

Past medical history is notable for social anxiety disorder, hyperlipidemia, and GERD (gastroesophageal reflux disease).

Family history is positive for language problems in her mother.

On neuropsychological exam, she was found out to have broad cognitive impairment in both language and nonlanguage functions, with MMSE score of 18/30.

Brain MRI showed mild to moderate volume loss with no acute infarct. EEG examination showed no seizure activities.

Laboratory tests showed TSH, free T3, and free T4 in normal ranges.

The patient underwent a baseline brain SPECT perfusion and a Diamox challenge study, with approximately 3 months apart.

SPECT Imaging Findings

The baseline SPECT images (Fig. 2.8a) show asymmetric, predominant hypoperfusion of the entire left temporal lobe (red arrows). In addition, profound hypoperfusion is present in the bilateral parietal lobes (white arrows), left being more affected than the right. Hypoperfusion is also noted in the bilateral PCG/PCUNs (hatched red arrows), relative to that of the anterior cingulate gyri. Mild to moderate hypoperfusion is also seen in the adjacent superior posterior left frontal lobe and superior lateral left occipital lobe. Mild hypoperfusion is noted in the left basal ganglion (green arrow) when compared to the right.

Although the challenge study with Diamox shows expected global increased perfusion (Fig. 2.8b), the predominant hypoperfusion to the entire left temporal lobe remains (red arrows). The profound hypoperfusion to the bilateral parietal lobes (white arrows), including the PCG/PCUNs (hatched red arrows), is also persistent. Mild to moderate hypoperfusion remains in the adjacent left frontal and occipital lobes. In contrast, perfusion to the left basal ganglion is improved (green arrow) when compared to the baseline study.

Discussion and Follow-Up

The clinical presentation of progressive difficulties in word-finding for 2–3 years in this 67-year-old patient is a classic clinical feature of primary progressive aphasia (PPA), also referred to as semantic variant PPA (svPPA) [6]. The clinical diagnosis is confirmed by the brain perfusion SPECT studies without and with acetazolamide challenge, which show persistent, predominant hypoperfusion to the entire left temporal lobe, a dominant language region in this right-handed patient.

As mentioned earlier, neuropsychological exam of the patient revealed broad cognitive impairment in both language and nonlanguage functions, with MMSE score of 18/30. This indi-

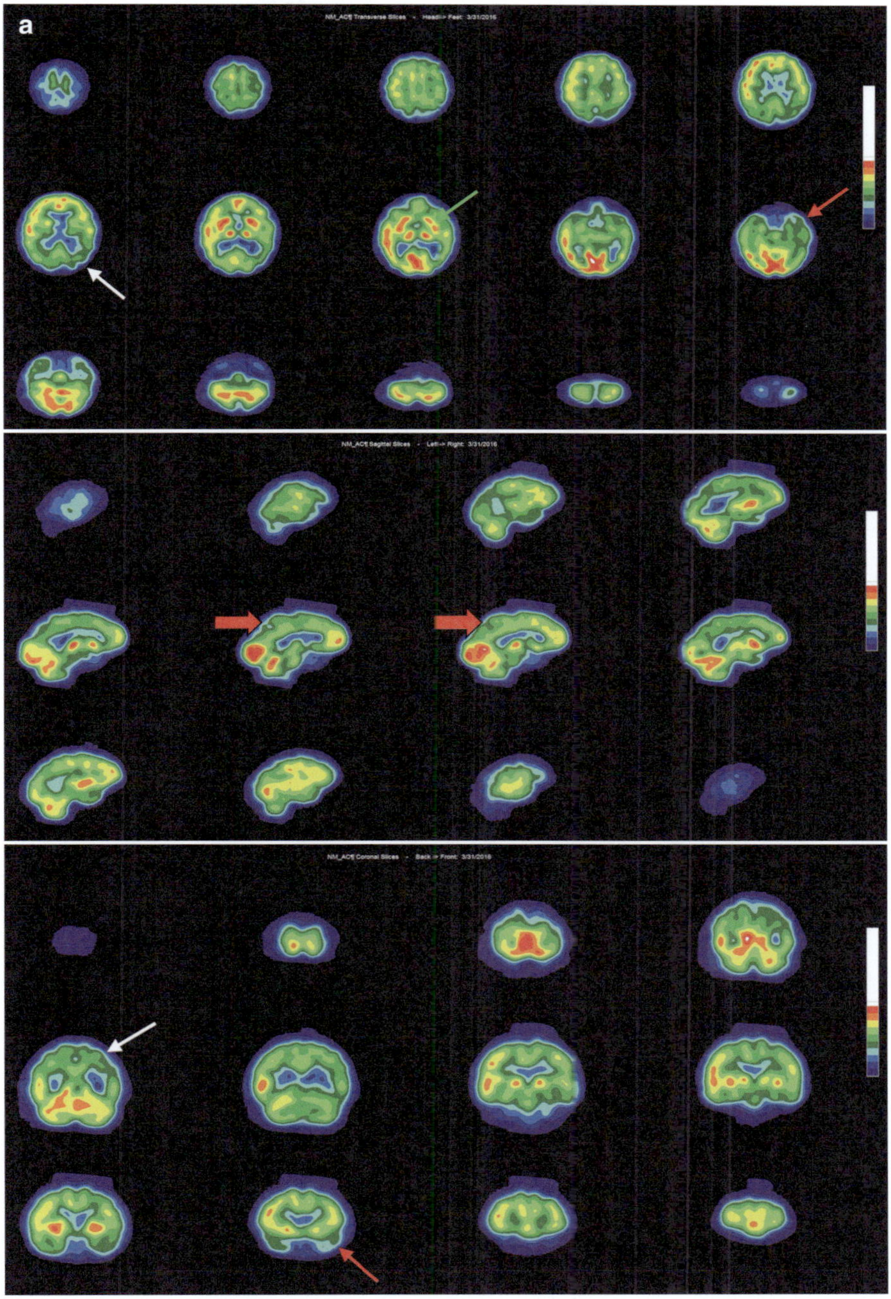

Fig. 2.8 (**a**) A 67-year-old female with probable PPA and AD pathology – a baseline study. (**b**) A 67-year-old female with probable PPA and AD pathology – a challenge study with Diamox

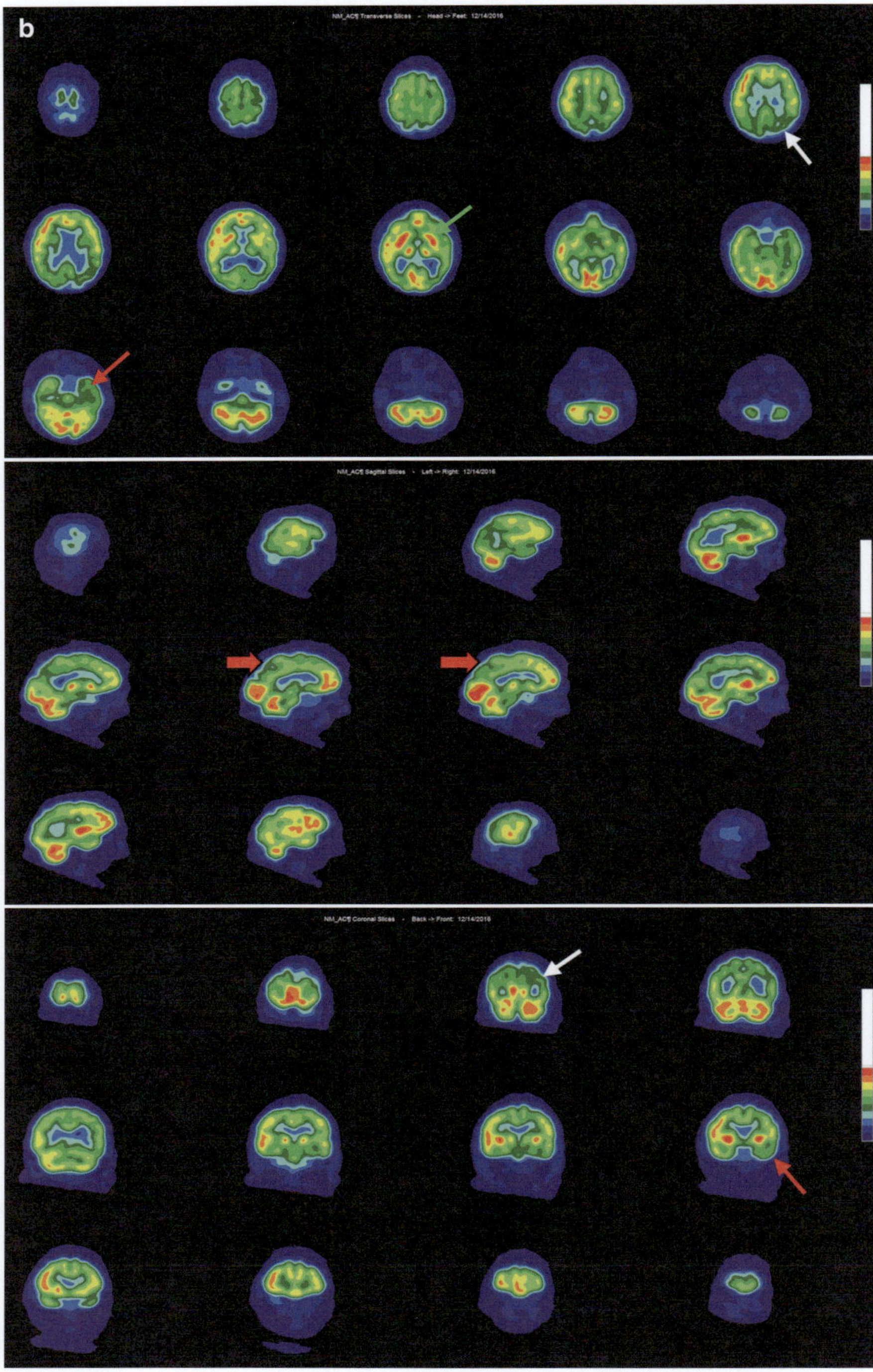

Fig. 2.8 (continued)

cates the patient's cognitive impairment extends beyond the language domain.

On the brain SPECT studies, additional profound hypoperfusion was identified in the bilateral parietal lobes including the PCG/PCUNs, with the left side being more affected than the right. Mild to moderate hypoperfusion is also noted in the adjacent left superior posterior frontal lobe, and left superior and lateral occipital lobe, suggestive of a spread pattern from the left parietal region. These imaging features, in conjunction with the abnormal MRI finding of volume loss and the broad cognitive impairment in nonlanguage functions on neurological exam, are suggestive of AD pathology.

The mild hypoperfusion to the left basal ganglion is likely due to disease spread from a neurodegenerative process from the left temporal region (*e.g.*, PPA), though ischemic vascular disease cannot be excluded, given the improved perfusion on the challenge study with Diamox.

After the abnormal SPECT brain perfusion studies, the patient was started on Aricept 10 mg daily, with transient improvement in speech/expression for approximately 1 year. After that, however, her language difficulties became deteriorated. A follow-up neurologic examination 1 year later showed a deteriorating MMSE score of 16/30. Also, she had worsening aphasia and more difficulties in word-finding and expressing, indicating disease progression.

Case Summary

The clinical presentation of progressive difficulties in word-finding and self-expressing for years in this patient is concerning for primary progressive aphasia (PPA) [6]. Brain perfusion SPECT studies without and with Diamox challenge show persistent, predominant cortical hypoperfusion to the left temporal lobe in this right-handed patient, in support of the clinical diagnosis of PPA. Additional SPECT findings have imaging features suggesting AD pathology, including hypoperfusion to the bilateral parietal lobes and PCG/PCUNs, as well as the involvement of the adjacent frontal and occipital lobes in a spread pattern. The imaging diagnosis of PPA with coexisting AD pathology is in line with the neuropsychological exam findings of broad cognitive impairment in both language and nonlanguage functions. This was further supported by a favorable, though transient, response to donepezil, a central acetylcholinesterase inhibitor for the treatment of patients with AD.

Case 2.9 Possible Vascular Dementia (VD) with bvFTD Pathology

Clinical Information

Chief Complaint *Memory loss and aggressive behaviors*

The patient is an 81-year-old female who presents to the office with her daughter. Her daughter, who is always with her for office visits, reports that her mother has had memory loss for years that has been worsening recently. Her daughter reports that the patient is no longer capable of driving. However, the patient adamantly denies this and says she still can drive.

The daughter says that her mother has had episodes of paranoia and gets agitated easily. She has been verbally and physically aggressive to her husband and her children. She has also had a diminished appetite and weight loss. There is no history of head injury or seizure.

Past medical history is notable for anxiety disorder and hypothyroidism for which she is on thyroid replacement therapy. She is a former smoker but has no history of alcohol or drug use.

During the office encounter, the patient notably repeated herself several times in a short period of time. Neurologic examination revealed MMSE score of 19/30.

CT of the head/brain showed mild prominence of the lateral ventricles, basal cisterns, and cortical sulci consistent with age-appropriate atrophy and deep white matter and periventricular hypodensities likely from chronic ischemic demyelination. No large territorial infarct was seen on the CT scan.

Laboratory tests show TSH, free T3, and free T4 in normal ranges.

SPECT Imaging Findings (Fig. 2.9)

The images show prominent lateral ventricles and sulci indicating brain atrophy. There is diffusely decreased tracer activity and possible a small infarct in the left basal ganglia (purple arrows), suggestive of multiple, small lacunar infarcts. Additionally, multiple small cortical defects are identified involving at least the bilateral parietal, the right occipital, the right medial frontal, and left forefrontal lobes (white arrows) suggestive of cortical punctate infarcts. There is mildly decreased perfusion to the left thalamus relative to the contralateral. Despite the cortical punctate infarcts, there is overall preserved perfusion to the bilateral parieto-occipital lobes including the PCG/PCUNs (hatched red arrows). In contrast, moderate to severe hypoperfusion is identified in the bilateral forefrontal lobes, left being more prominent than the right (red arrows). Minimally decreased perfusion to the left temporal lobe is also noted when compared to the right.

Discussion and Follow-Up

Despite the lack of evidence of a large territory infarct, per report, the CT of head/brain showed findings highly suggestive of severe ischemic vascular disease. Consistently, brain perfusion SPECT study revealed several small lacunar infarcts and multiple, bilateral punctate cortical infarcts, suggestive of small vessel ischemic disease. Mild hypoperfusion is noted in the left deep structures (basal ganglia and thalamus) and the left temporal lobe when compared to the contralateral, suggestive of left hemispheric ischemic disease.

In addition to the abnormalities suggesting infarcts and ischemia, the SPECT study also revealed profound hypoperfusion to bilateral frontal lobes. In conjunction with the patient's behavioral issues, this is suggestive of behavioral variant FTD (bvFTD) pathology [6].

During the ensuring 10-month follow-up, the patient developed gait and mobility problems indicating Parkinsonism. Additionally, her memory loss worsened, and her functionality further declined.

Case Summary

Brain SPECT perfusion imaging interpretation is challenging in this patient due to scant clinical information and limited anatomic neuroimaging

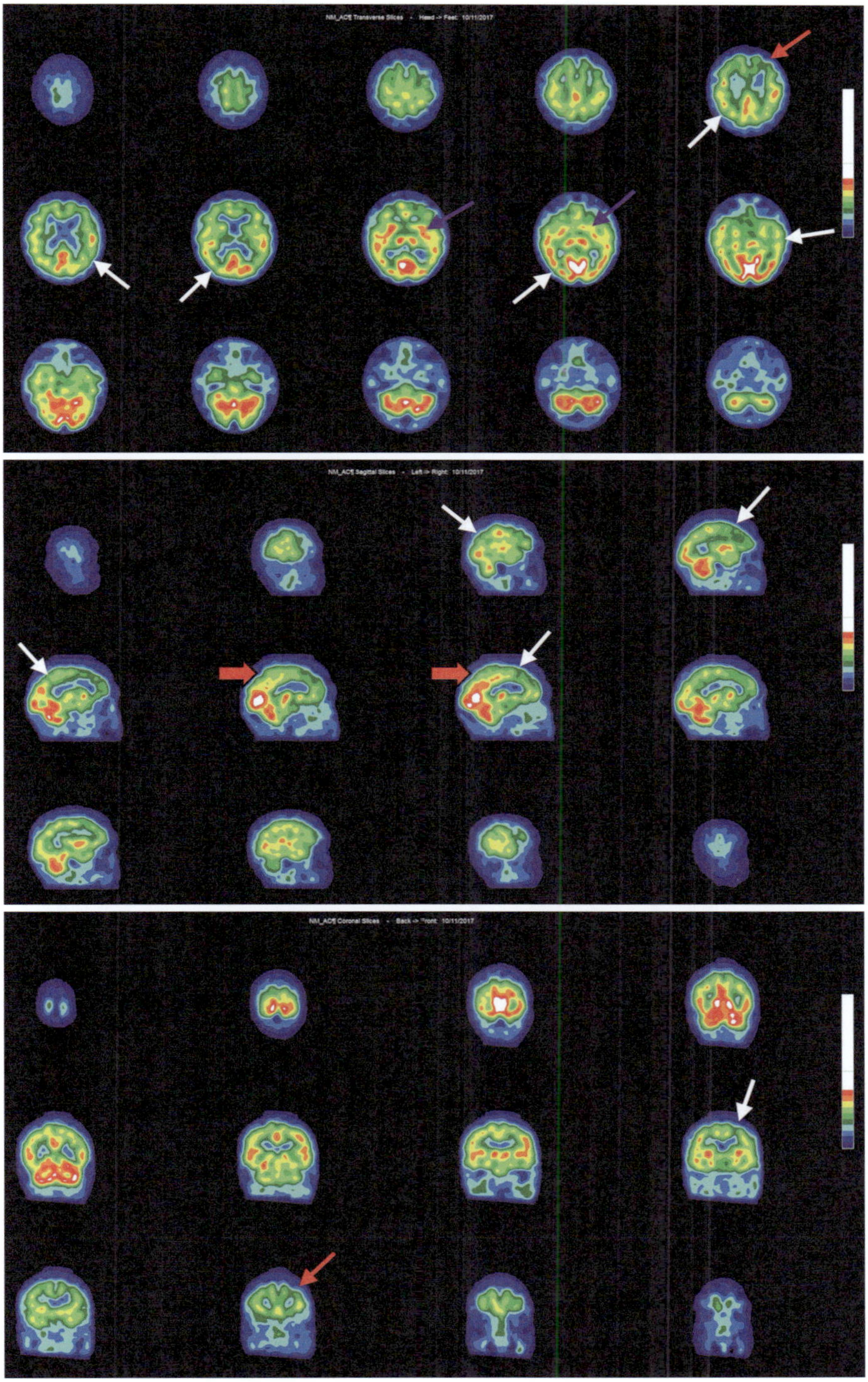

Fig. 2.9 An 81-year-old female with possible VD with bvFTD pathology

studies. Consistent with abnormal but vague CT brain findings, brain perfusion SPECT images show several small lacunar infarcts, multiple cortical punctate infarcts, and asymmetric hypoperfusion to the left temporal lobe and deep structure, suggestive of VD. Additionally, the constellation of the outstanding behavioral issues in clinical presentation and profound hypoperfusion to the bilateral forefrontal lobes is suggestive of bvFTD pathology. The imaging diagnosis of probable mixed dementia (VD with bvFTD pathology) was further supported by limited clinical follow-up data.

Case 2.10 Probable Posterior Cortical Atrophy (PCA)

Clinical Information

Chief Complaint *Progressive memory loss and frequent falls*

The patient is an 84-year-old right-handed female presenting with worsening memory loss for several years. In addition, she has had significant mobility issues with gait shuffling and frequent falls with broken teeth and head injuries. Her daughter, who is with her, reports that her mother's memory problem and mobility issues started around the same time, with periods of confusion often worsening in the evening. Her daughter also reports that her mother sometimes has hallucinations, mostly auditory. For example, a few months ago, the patient complained of hearing "crackling" noises, but her family members did not. The patient used to have significant behavioral issues and has been on risperidone for treatment for years without benefits.

Current medications include clonazepam 0.5 mg twice a day, citalopram 20 mg daily, risperidone 0.25 mg daily, and multivitamins.

Past medical history is notable for hypertension, depression, anxiety, and dizzy spells.

There is no family history of dementia.

Neurological exam showed MMSE score of 10/30.

Recent laboratory tests showed TSH, folate, and vitamin B_{12} in normal ranges.

SPECT Imaging Findings

The baseline study images (Fig. 2.10a) show severe cortical hypoperfusion to the entire right occipitoparietal lobe (red arrows), though the right visual cortex is less affected. Mild to moderate hypoperfusion is seen in the right frontotemporal cortices (white arrows), in a spread pattern. Note that the right sensorimotor strip is also affected. In contrast, perfusion to the left hemispheric cortices is overall preserved, with the exception of mild hypoperfusion to the left parietal lobe. Perfusion to the bilateral PCG/PCUNs (hatched red arrows) is higher than the anterior cingulate gyri, but lower than the cuneus regions. Therefore, there is no cingulate island sign (CIS). Perfusion to the bilateral thalami and cerebella is essentially symmetric and is within normal limits; however, mild hypoperfusion is noted in the right basal ganglia (green arrow) compared to the left.

The challenge study with Diamox (Fig. 2.10b) shows globally increased perfusion as expected, with more prominent perfusion in the primary visual cortices and the cerebella, especially bilateral thalami. However, the predominant hypoperfusion remains in the right occipitoparietal lobes (red arrows). Also, the mild to moderate hypoperfusion to the right frontal and temporal lobes is persistent (white arrows), still in the same spread pattern. In contrast, perfusion to the left parietal lobe is improved when compared to the baseline study. Again, perfusion to the bilateral PCG/PCUNs (hatched red arrows) is higher than the anterior cingulate gyri, but lower than the cuneus regions.

Discussion and Follow-Up

This 84-year-old right-handed female presents with progressive memory loss and mobility issues. The scintigraphic finding of asymmetric cortical hypoperfusion to the entire right hemisphere with predominance in the occipital and parietal region, in conjunction with the clinical features (vision and coordination issues), is suggestive of posterior cortical atrophy (PCA) [12]. PCA is a rare neurodegenerative condition often associated with AD and is considered as a variant of AD. In addition, the improved perfusion to the left parietal lobe and persistently decreased perfusion to the right basal ganglia and thalamus on the challenge study with Diamox are suggestive of vascular pathology, with variable vascular reserves. The involvement of the right basal ganglion may explain the patient's mobility symptoms, suggesting Parkinsonism.

Given the clinical presentation of memory loss and the imaging feature of dominant occipital hypoperfusion, DLB needs to be considered. However, DLB is characterized by global and

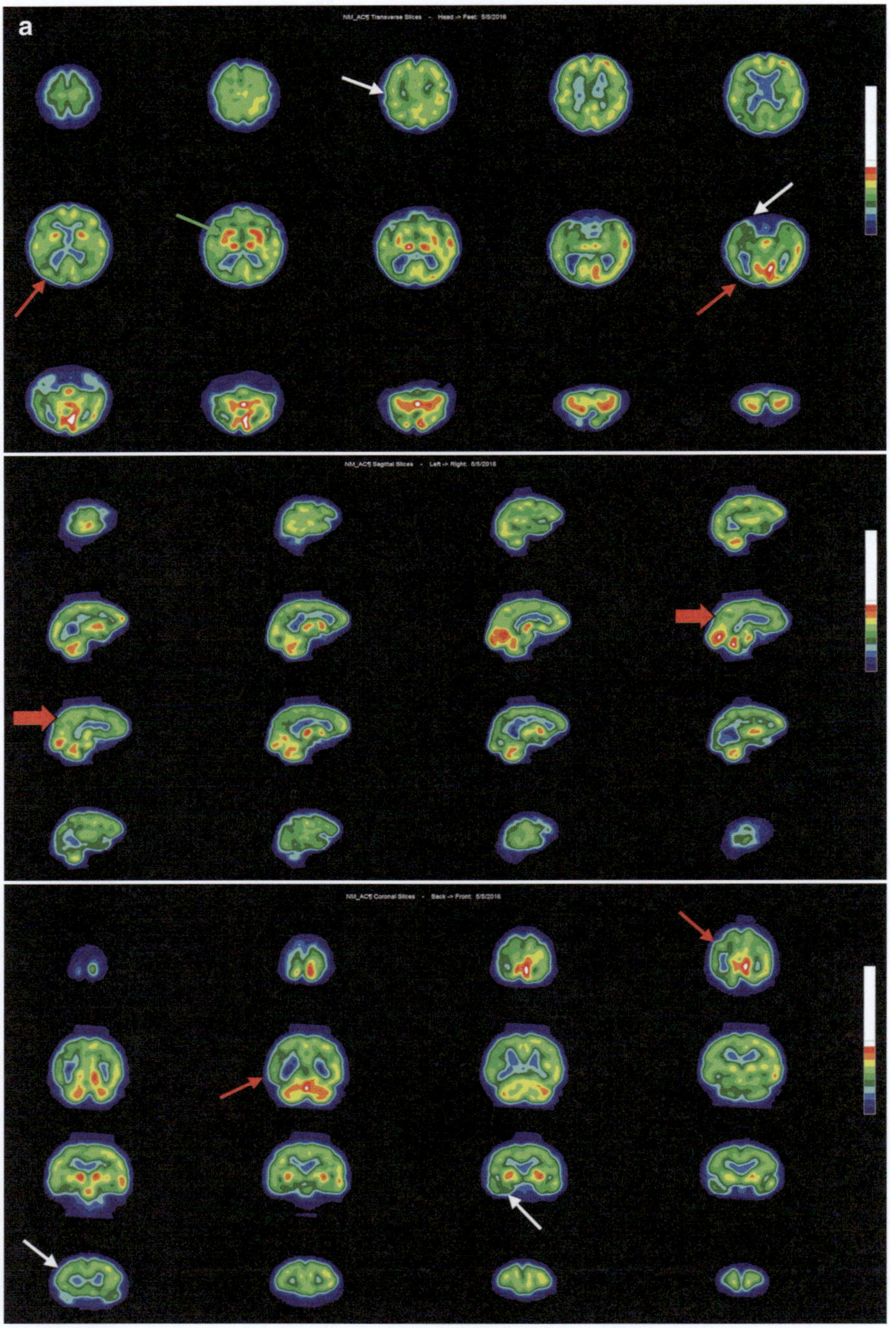

Fig. 2.10 (**a**) An 84-year-old female with possible posterior cortical atrophy (PCA) – a baseline study. (**b**) An 84-year-old female with possible posterior cortical atrophy (PCA) – a challenge study with Diamox

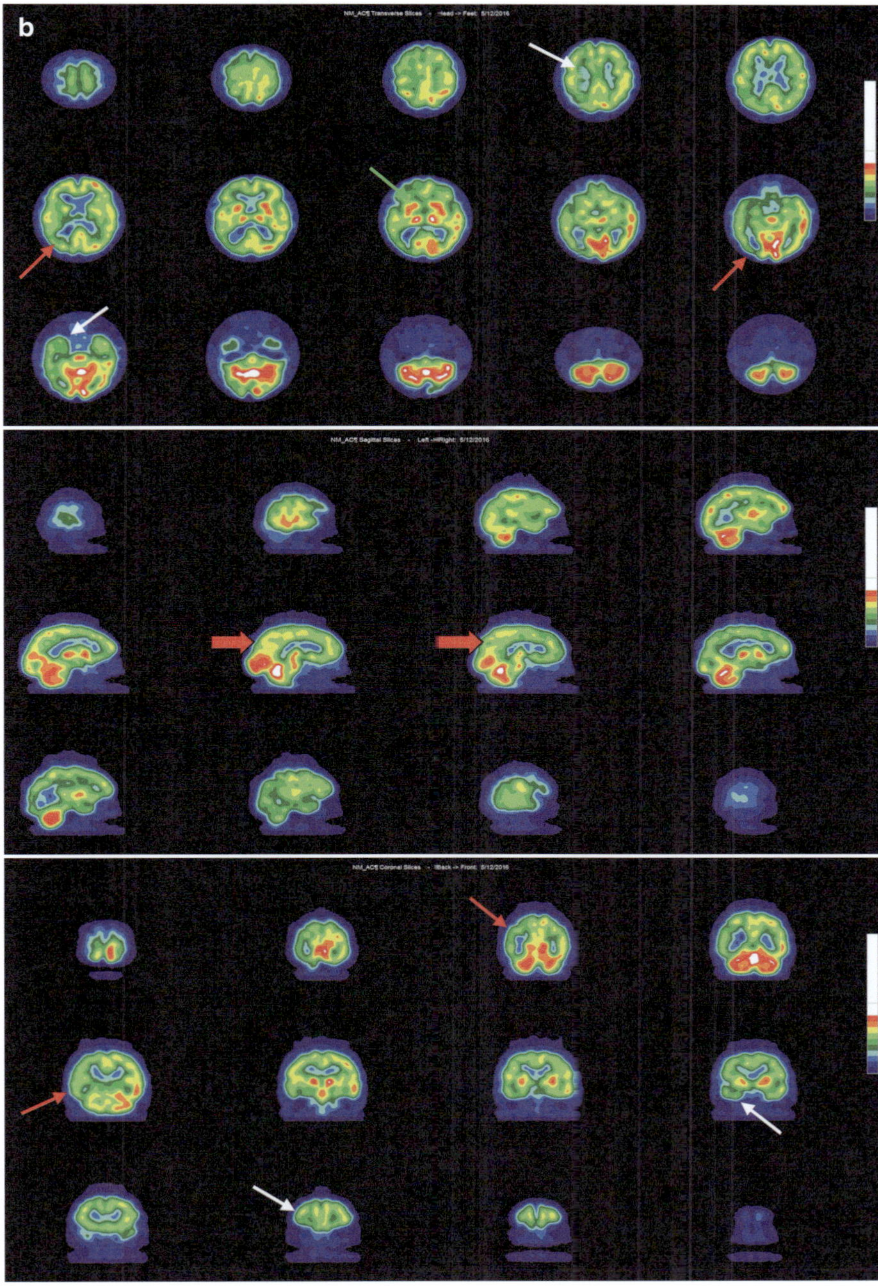

Fig. 2.10 (continued)

severe hypoperfusion or hypometabolism on SPECT or PET, respectively, in addition to predominant involvement of the occipital lobes (see Case 2.7 and or Case 1.10 for details). By contrast, the asymmetric pattern of hypoperfusion in this case is in favor of PCA [12]. Also, one of the typical clinical features associated with DLB is the presence of complex visual hallucination, but this did not occur in this patient.

Shortly after the brain SPECT perfusion studies, the patient began to take Aricept 10 mg daily. She tolerated the medication well and has achieved improvement in memory.

Case Summary

This case demonstrates functional neuroimaging characteristic of PCA, including asymmetric hypoperfusion involving the entire right hemispheric cortices, with predominance in the right occipitoparietal region. PCA is a rare neurodegenerative condition often associated with AD. The imaging diagnosis of probable PCA in this patient was supported by her good response to donepezil, a commonly prescribed central cholinesterase inhibitor commonly prescribed for the treatment of patients with AD.

References

1. Austin BP, Nair VA, Meier TB, Xu GF, Rowley HA, Carlsson CM, Johnsone SC, Prabhakaran V. Effects of hypoperfusion in Alzheimer's disease. J Alzheimers Dis. 2011;26(Suppl. 3):123–33.
2. Camargo EE. Brain SPECT in neurology and psychiatry. J Nucl Med. 2001;42:611–23.
3. Catafau AM. Brain SPECT in clinical practice. Part I: perfusion. J Nucl Med. 2001;42:259–71.
4. Davison CM, O'Brien JT. A comparison of FDG-PET and blood flow SPECT in the diagnosis of neurodegenerative dementias: a systematic review. Int J Geriatr Psychiatry. 2014;29(6):551–61.
5. Dougall NJ, Bruggink S, Ebmeier KP. Systematic review of the diagnostic accuracy of ^{99m}Tc-HMPAO-SPECT in dementia. Am J Geriatr Psychiatry. 2004;12:554–70.
6. Gorno-Tempini ML, Hillis AE, Weintraub S, et al. Classification of primary progressive aphasia and its variants. Neurology. 2011;76:1006–14.
7. Gupta A, Chazen JL, Hartman M, et al. Cerebrovascular reserve and stroke risk in patients with carotid stenosis or occlusion: a systematic review and meta-analysis. Stroke. 2012;43(11):2884–91.
8. Imabayashi E, Soma T, Sone D, Tsukamoto T, Kimura Y, Sato N, Murata M, Matsuda H. Validation of the cingulate island sign with optimized ratios for discriminating dementia with Lewy bodies from Alzheimer's disease using brain perfusion SPECT. Ann Nucl Med. 2017;31:536–43.
9. Rascovsky K, Hodges JR, Knopman D, et al. Sensitivity of revised diagnosis criteria for the behavioral variant of frontotemporal dementia. Brain. 2011;134(9):2456–77.
10. Tanaka F, Vines D, Tsuchida T, Freedman M, Ichise M. Normal patterns on 99mTc-ECD brain SPECT scans in adults. J Nucl Med. 2000;41:1456–64.
11. Tateno M, Kobayashi S, Saito T. Imaging improves diagnosis of dementia with Lewy bodies. Psychiatry Investig. 2009;6:233–40.
12. Whitwell JL, Graff-Radford J, Singh TD, Drubach DA, Senjem ML, Spychalla AJ, Tosakulwong N, Lowe VJ, Josephs KA. ^{18}F-FDGE PET in posterior cortical atrophy and dementia with Lewy bodies. J Nucl Med. 2017;58:632–8.

F-18 Fluorodeoxyglucose Positron Emission Tomography (FDG PET) in Epilepsies

3

Case 3.1 Negative FDG PET

Clinical Information

Chief Complaint *Having had intractable seizures for 3 years*

The patient is a 12-year-old right-handed female presenting with intractable seizures despite treatment with multiple antiepileptic medications. According to her parents, the seizures started at age 9 after she bumped her head. During seizures, which often occurred while awake, she would have behavioral arrest, eyes up and to either side, facial twitching (either side), and body slumping with subsequent tonic body stiffening. Postictal symptoms include headache and somnolence. The patient denies aura and has no history of prior traumatic head injury nor meningitis/encephalitis. Birth history and development are unremarkable. There is no family history of epilepsy.

Current medications include diazepam 20 mg prn, levetiracetam 1000 mg bid, and zonisamide 400 mg every night.

Past medical history is notable for obstructive sleep apnea (OSA), chronic headache, and obesity.

Brain MRI showed evidence of Chiari malformation, type I, with the cerebral tonsils down 6 mm, but no posterior fossa compression and no syrinx.

Several EEG studies were essentially unremarkable without consistent focal epileptiform activities.

The patient's blood glucose level was 94 mg/dL prior to FDG administration. There were no seizure activities during the EEG monitoring; therefore, the FDG PET scan was an interictal study.

FDG PET Imaging Findings (Fig. 3.1)

The images show symmetric brain hemispheres. Despite the MRI finding of Chiari malformation, there is no evidence of prominent or dilated ventricles. The conventional brain FDG PET color normalization using a 10-step color spectrum could not proceed for this case, due to symmetric hypometabolism in the basal ganglia, thalami, and cerebella (white arrows). Instead, the imaging colors are normalized with a reference to the frontal lobes where essentially symmetric normometabolism is seen. Mild to moderate hypometabolism is also noted in the bilateral temporal lobes, anterior and medial being more affected than the posterior and lateral (red arrows). Mildly decreased FDG activity is noted in the superior medial parietal lobes bilaterally (red triangles). Normometabolism is seen in the anterior cingulate (hatched green arrows) and posterior cingulate gyri (hatched red arrows), as well as the occipital lobes, especially the primary visual cortices.

D. Wu, *Clinical Nuclear Medicine Neuroimaging*, https://doi org/10.1007/978-3-030-40893-0_3

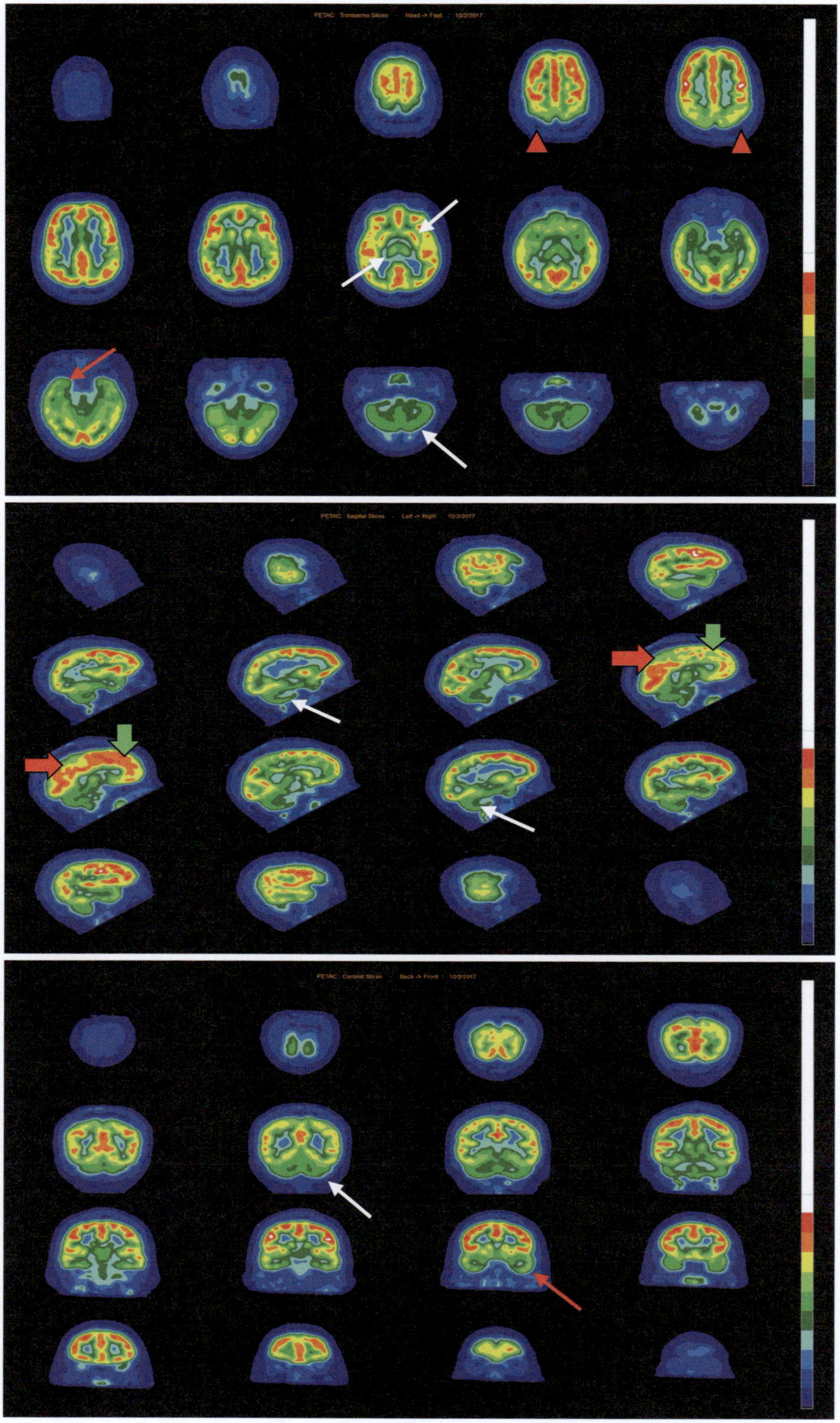

Fig. 3.1 A 12-year-old right-handed female without FDG PET evidence of an interictal epileptogenic focus/zone

Discussion and Follow-Up

Interpretation of FDG PET brain imaging in this patient is challenging due to multiple reasons, such as the lack of localized or lateralized findings in seizure semiology, unremarkable EEG and normal MRI, currently on multiple anti-seizure medications, and other comorbidities, to name a few. The mildly decreased FDG activity in the bilateral superior medial parietal lobes is suggestive of motion artifact due to difficulty in positioning. The conventional imaging color normalization using basal ganglia as a reference to red could not be applied due to symmetric hypometabolism involving bilateral basal ganglia, thalami, and cerebella. Although the mechanism underlying the multiple areas of hypometabolism is unknown, potential contributory factors include at least intractable seizures that started at early age and effects of multiple antiepileptic medications [9].

The mild to moderate hypometabolism in the temporal lobes is symmetric. The pattern of the anterior and medial portion being more affected than posterior and lateral aspect is suggestive of a normal variant rather than epileptogenic foci/zones. Therefore, the overall FDG PET findings are nonspecific, without definite evidence of an interictal epileptogenic focus/zone.

During the ensuring 1.5-year follow-up, repeat EEG studies were again unremarkable. Given the shifting lateralized seizure semiology, a working diagnosis of genetic generalized epilepsy (GGE) was proposed. Despite dosage adjustment for the patient's existing antiepileptic medications, she only achieved an incomplete seizure control.

Case Summary

This 12-year-old female patient has a 3-year history of drug-resistant epilepsy. EEG and MRI are unremarkable. FDG PET shows multiple regional hypometabolism involving the basal ganglia, thalami, and cerebella, in a symmetric pattern suggesting a nonspecific or non-epileptic feature, likely due to effects of multiple antiepileptic medications or due to developmental delay secondary to intractable seizures at an early age or both. Mild to moderate hypometabolism is noted in the bilateral temporal lobes, with a pattern suggestive of a normal variant. Therefore, the FDG PET study is essentially negative for an epileptogenic focus/zone, despite nonspecific abnormal findings. The imaging impression has been supported by clinical follow-up data.

Case 3.2 Surgically Proven Left Mesial Temporal Lobe Epilepsy (MTLE)

Clinical Information

Chief Complaint *Medically refractory seizures and abnormal MRI and EEGs*

The patient is a 21-year-old right-handed female with known complex partial epilepsy that started at age 2. She was treated at multiple institutions/hospitals with several antiepileptic medications; however, her seizures have been poorly controlled. The seizures are often preceded by a "rushing" sensation over her body, followed by impaired awareness and unresponsiveness, lasting approximately 30–60 seconds. No oral or manual automatisms are reported. Postictally, she often has trouble verbalizing or understanding speech for several minutes. In addition, she has a history of focal to bilateral tonic-clonic seizures.

The patient denies history of head injury, stroke, or meningitis/encephalitis. Family history is notable for seizures in her brother. Birth history and development are unremarkable.

Current medications include lacosamide 200 mg twice a day, lamotrigine 150 mg twice a day, and diazepam 20 mg PR Gel PRN.

Multiple EEG studies showed epileptogenic activity in the left temporal region.

Three recent MR imaging studies revealed "reduced volume and increased T2 FLAIR signal of the head, neck and body of the left hippocampal formation and blurring hypointense T2 signal at the associated white matter, consistent with left mesial temporal sclerosis."

The patient's blood glucose level was 87 mg/dL prior to FDG administration. There were no seizure activities during the EEG monitoring, indicating an interictal PET study.

FDG PET Imaging Findings (Fig. 3.2)

The images show diffuse hypometabolism involving the entire left temporal lobe, predominant in the medial/mesial portion (red arrows). Although there is mild hypometabolism in the bilateral superomedial parietal lobes (white arrows), normometabolism is overall seen the rest of the cerebral cortices. The left thalamus is smaller (green arrow) compared to the contralateral. Minimal hypometabolism is noted in the right cerebellum (hatched yellow arrows).

FDG activity in the bilateral basal ganglia, the right thalamus, and the left cerebellum is within normal limits.

Discussion and Follow-Up

This 21-year-old patient has a 19-year history of medically refractory epilepsy. Her seizures are often preceded by sensational auras, which is classic for seizures of temporal lobe origin [1]. The predominant hypometabolism in the medial/mesial left temporal lobe on FDG PET imaging is corresponding to the known left mesial temporal sclerosis on MR imaging, in line with the seizure semiology, highly suggestive of left mesial temporal lobe epilepsy (MTLE) [2, 5].

In addition to the predominant hypometabolism in the medial/mesial temporal lobe, mild to moderate hypometabolism is seen in the rest of the left temporal lobe, which is likely due to sequelae of intractable left MTLE. The diaschisis involving the left thalamus and right cerebellum is indirect imaging evidence of intractable left MTLE.

The FDG PET scan also demonstrates the integrity of glucose metabolism in the rest of the brain, except for mild to moderate hypometabolism in the superomedial parietal lobes. The underlying mechanism of the subtle parietal abnormality is unknown, but is unlikely epileptic in nature given the symmetric pattern.

One and a half years after the abnormal FDG brain PET study, the patient underwent left anterior temporal lobectomy. She has been seizure-free for nearly 2 years after the epilepsy surgery, and her anti-seizure medications have been tapered off as well.

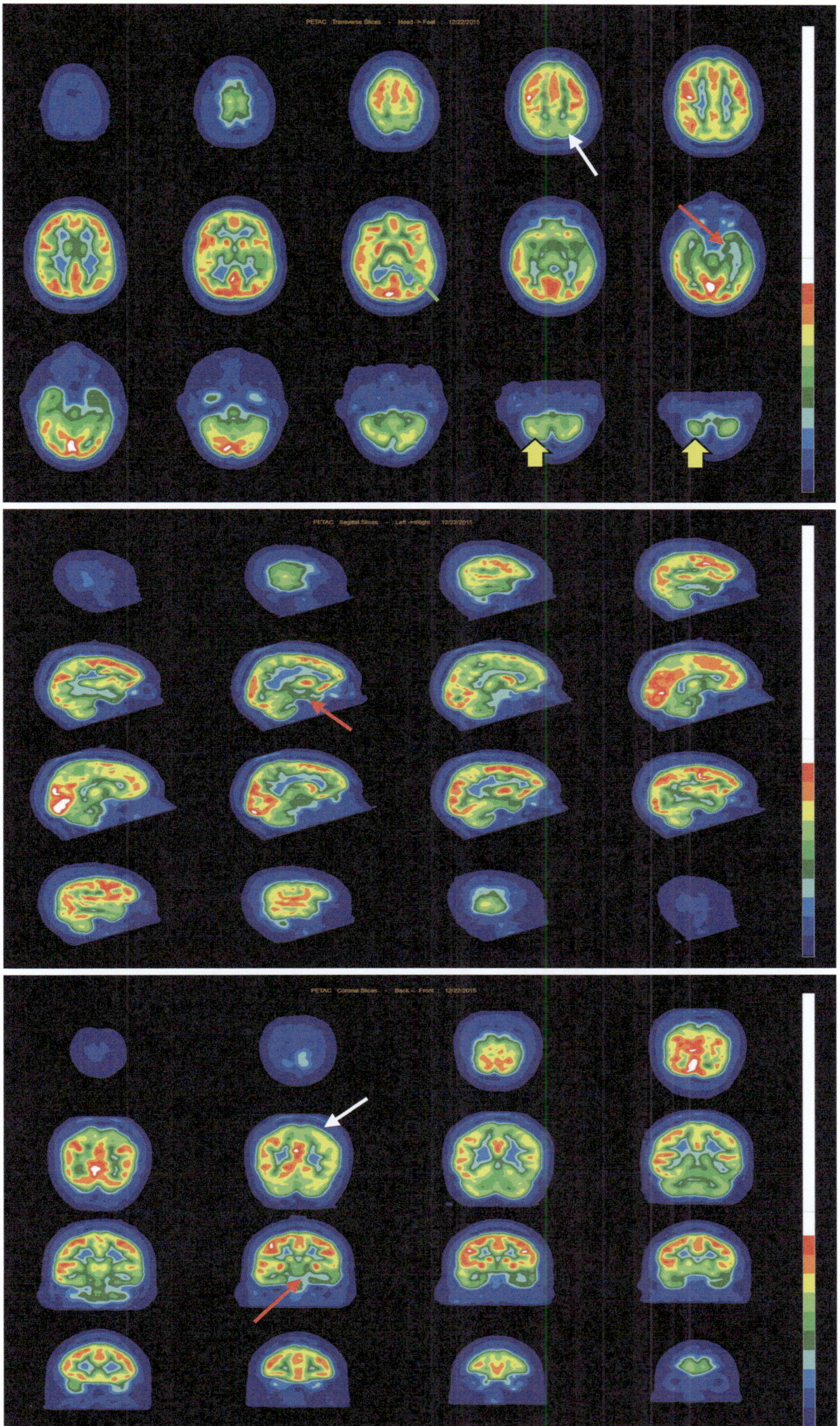

Fig. 3.2 A 21-year-old right-handed female with surgically proven left mesial temporal lobe epilepsy (MTLE)

Case Summary

Mesial temporal lobe epilepsy (MTLE) is the most commonly diagnosed epilepsy syndrome [1, 3, 6]. The clinical presentation shows typical features of MTLE in the form of intractable focal seizures associated with sensational auras. Prior MRI showed left mesial temporal/hippocampal sclerosis, and EEG results indicated epileptiform activities in the left temporal region. The FDG PET scan revealed predominant hypometabolism in the left mesial temporal region with less involvement of the rest of the left temporal lobe, and diaschisis in the left thalamus and the right cerebellum, highly suggestive of left MTLE. Further, the PET scan showed an overall integrity of glucose metabolism in the rest of the brain. The diagnosis of left MTLE in this patient was further supported by clinical follow-up data showing that the patient has so far been seizure-free 2 years after left anterior temporal lobectomy.

Case 3.3 Probable Right Lateral Temporal Lobe Epilepsy (LTLE)

Clinical Information

Chief Complaint *Medically refractory focal seizures with impairment of consciousness*

The patient is a 15-year-old right-handed male presenting with intractable focal epilepsy for 4 years despite being on antiepileptic medications. The seizures often occur in the afternoon from 2 to 5 pm, once a week, and usually last about 45 seconds to a few minutes. During the seizures, the patient reports seeing a dark curtain going down over his vision and feeling scared. The seizures involve chewing automatisms, copious drooling, eyes closed with slight left eye deviation, left upper extremity flexion at the elbow with dystonic hand contraction, and left lower extremity bicycling. The seizures are often preceded by auras including feeling "weird" and lightheaded and yelling "Dad," "Mom," and "I do not feel right."

There is no prior history of head injury, meningitis, encephalitis, or abnormal birth history/development.

Current medications include lamotrigine 125 mg in the morning, 125 mg in the afternoon, and 200 mg at night, oxcarbazepine 900 mg in the morning, 600 mg in the afternoon, and 900 mg at night.

Past medical history includes autism spectrum disorder, ADHD (attention deficit hyperactivity disorder)-combined type, and status epilepticus.

EEG studies showed right temporal intermittent rhythmic delta activity (TIRDA) > occipital intermittent rhythmic delta activity (OIRDA), focal epileptiform discharges independent right posterior temporal and right anteromedial temporal, with clear propagation pathway from right posterior temporal to right anteromedial temporal region.

Brain MRI with and without gadolinium was normal.

The patient's blood glucose level was 89 mg/dL prior to FDG administration. The FDG PET was performed without EEG monitoring due to a scheduling conflict.

FDG PET Imaging Findings (Fig. 3.3)

Predominant and diffuse hypometabolism is identified in the right lateral temporal lobe (red arrows). Additionally, mild to moderate hypometabolism is seen in the right occipital, frontoparietal lobes and the left temporal lobes (white arrows). Mild hypometabolism is noted in the right thalamus (green arrow) and the left cerebellum (hatched yellow arrows), consistent with diaschisis.

FDG activity in the bilateral basal ganglia, the left thalamus, or the right cerebellum is within normal limits.

Discussion and Follow-Up

The predominant hypometabolism involving the right temporal region, lateral > medial (mesial), in conjunction with the seizure semiology and abnormal EEG results, is suspicious for right lateral temporal lobe epilepsy (LTLE), although brain MRI was normal. The ipsilateral thalamic and crossed cerebrocerebellar diaschisis is indirect imaging evidence for an intractable right LTLE.

The mild to moderate hypometabolism in the right occipital, frontoparietal lobes and the left temporal lobe is likely due to sequelae of seizure propagations/expansions, which often occur in LTLE [10–12]. However, additional epileptogenic foci/zones cannot be excluded.

Following the abnormal FDG PET study, the patient has been on the antiepileptic medications, valproic acid and lamotrigine, with dosing adjustment for the past 1.5 years, and he has achieved better seizure control and improved high school performance.

Case Summary

This case demonstrates the value of FDG PET imaging in the evaluation of epileptogenic foci/zones in patients with unremarkable/normal MRI. The predominant hypometabolism involving the right temporal lobe, lateral > medial

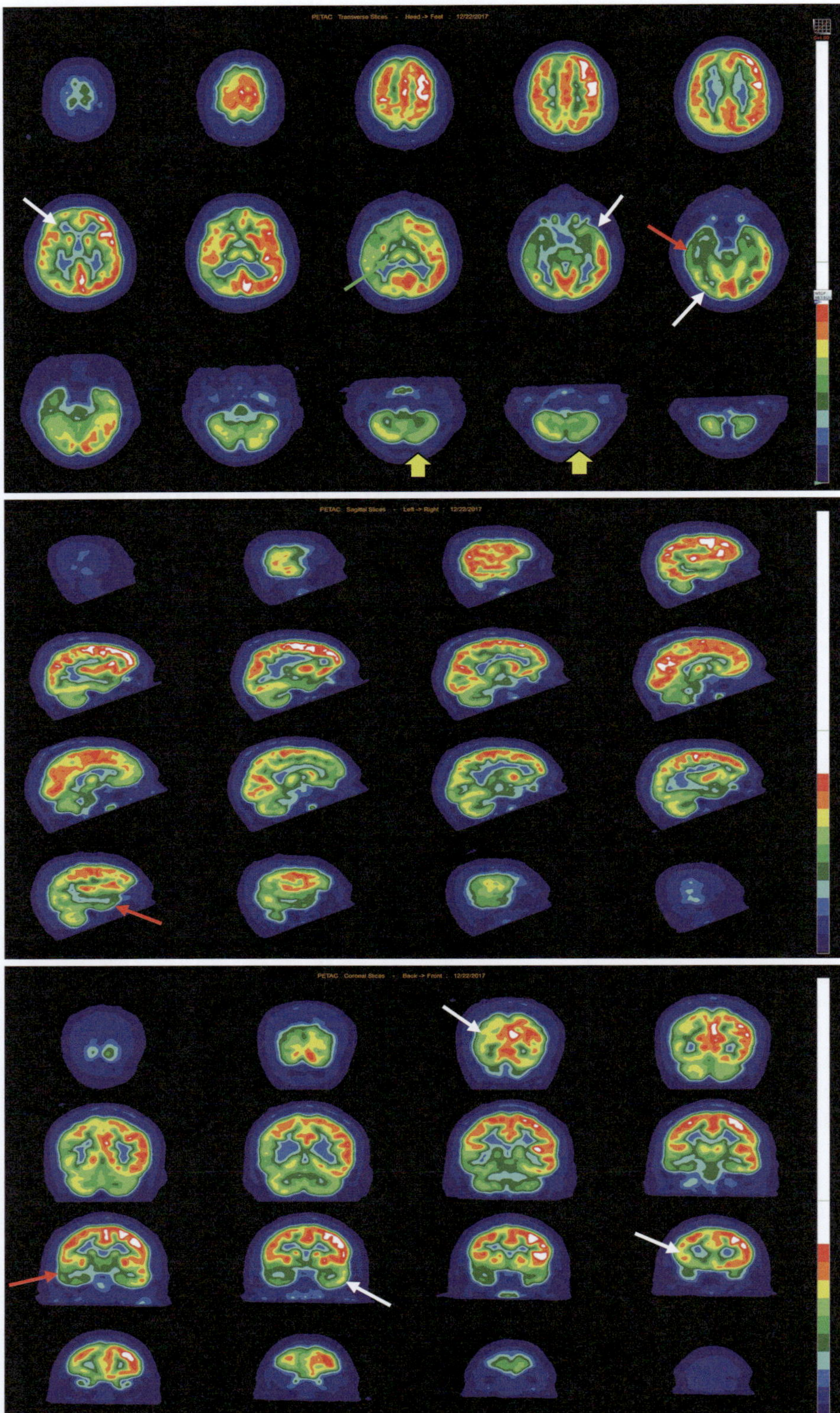

Fig. 3.3 A 15-year-old right-handed male with probable right lateral temporal lobe epilepsy (LTLE)

(mesial), in conjunction with the seizure semiology and abnormal EEG results, is suspicious for right LTLE, despite lack of an anatomic neuroimaging correlate. Additionally, the imaging finding of diaschisis involving the right thalamus and the left cerebellum is indirect evidence of intractable right TLE. Unlike MTLE that is often more localized and confined, seizure propagations/expansions often occur in LTLE. The mild to moderate hypometabolism in the rest of the right hemispheric cortices and the left temporal lobe is likely sequelae of seizure propagations or expansions. However, additional epileptogenic foci/zones cannot be excluded.

Case 3.4 Right Hemispheric Epilepsy

Clinical Information

Chief Complaint *Intractable focal seizures since 3 months of age*

The patient is a 9-year-old right-handed female presenting with intractable focal seizures with impaired consciousness that started approximately 8.5 years ago. The seizures occur randomly during the day, with frequency of 1–2 episodes a week, and often lasting about 10 seconds. During the seizures, the patient breathes fast, becomes pale, with left-sided stiffness and left arm shaking. Triggering factors for a seizure include low blood sugar, stress, and being tired. There is no aura reported nor visual disturbance.

In addition to seizures, the patient has an extensive neurological history, including global developmental delay, congenital hydrocephalus with VP shunting, left hemiparesis, macrocephaly, malformation of cortical development of the brain, cortical dysplasia and hypoplasia, and Dandy-Walker syndrome.

Current medications include lamotrigine 125 mg, twice a day; levetiracetam 800 mg, twice a day; diazepam 7.5 mg at night; and clonazepam 0.25 mg three tablets a day.

Brain MRI showed absence of a septum pellucidum and corpus callosum, a large posterior fossa cyst, hypoplastic inferior cerebellar vermis, small basal ganglia, and diffuse cortical hypoplasia, with a small portion of the remaining bilateral frontal and parietal cortices and subcortical white matter.

The patient's blood glucose level was 108 mg/dL prior to FDG administration. During the EEG monitoring, there were no seizure activities, indicating an interictal PET study.

FDG PET Imaging Findings (Fig. 3.4)

This is a technically limited study, due to difficulty positioning and multiple existing brain structural abnormalities.

Nevertheless, the FDG PET images confirm right macrocephaly and marked ventriculomegaly, consistent with known congenital hydrocephalus and cortical hypoplasia. Absent FDG activity is identified in the right parietal lobe, while moderate to severely decreased FDG activity is seen in the right frontal and occipital/parietal lobes (red arrows). Asymmetrically decreased FDG activity is noted in the right thalamus (white arrow) and the left cerebellum (hatched yellow arrows), suggestive of diaschisis.

FDG activity in the left hemispheric cortices is overall preserved, without discrete focal abnormalities. FDG activity in the basal ganglia bilaterally is symmetric and is within normal limits.

Discussion and Follow-Up

Despite technical limitations, the FDG PET scan showed dominant cerebral hypometabolism in the right hemisphere. The severe hypometabolism in the right parietal and occipital lobes is likely secondary to cerebral hypoplasia, known ventriculomegaly and hydrocephalus, as well as possible mass effects of a Dandy-Walker cyst in the posterior fossa.

The PET findings, given the diffuse hypometabolism involving the majority of the right brain, are suggestive of right hemispheric seizures. However, the regional moderate hypometabolism in the anterolateral portion of the right frontal lobe, in conjunction with the clinical left-sided ictal motor signs, is suggestive of right frontal lobe epilepsy.

The asymmetric, mild hypometabolism in the right thalamus and left cerebellum is consistent with diaschisis despite the presence of a Dandy-Walker malformation and MRI finding of a hypoplastic inferior cerebellar vermis.

Glucose metabolism in the left brain hemisphere is overall preserved, suggestive of relatively integrated left brain metabolic function.

During the follow-up for 2 years, EEG studies showed right frontal subclinical seizure activity during electrical status epilepticus in sleep (ESES). The patient is currently under review and being evaluated/considered for a modified right hemispherectomy.

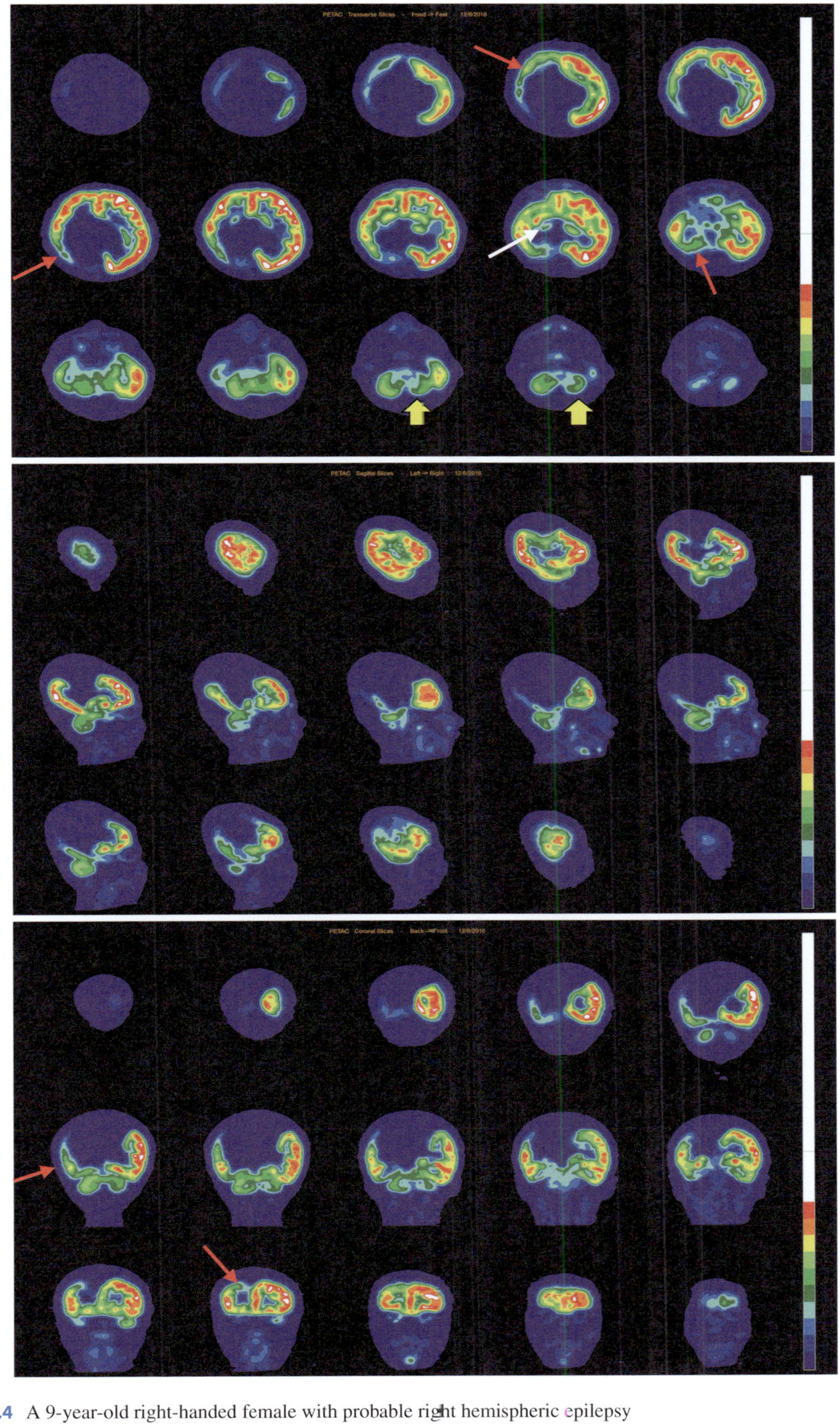

Fig. 3.4 A 9-year-old right-handed female with probable right hemispheric epilepsy

Case Summary

Interpretation of brain FDG PET scan in this patient is technically limited and challenging due to difficulty positioning and pre-existing complex brain structural abnormalities including macrocephaly, ventriculomegaly, cortical hypoplasia/dysplasia, and Dandy-Walker malformation. Despite these limitations, the diffuse and variable hypometabolism in the right parietofrontal and occipital lobes is suggestive of right hemispheric epilepsy, which is supported by seizure semiology and follow-up EEG data.

Case 3.5 Probable Multifocal Epilepsy

Clinical Information

Chief Complaint *Having had medically refractory seizures since a motor vehicle accident of 7 years ago*

The patient is a 16-year-old right-handed female with known multiform seizures (myotonic/tonic seizures, atypical absence, and partial seizures) that started after a motor vehicle accident (MVA) with traumatic head injury of 7 years ago. The seizures often occur when she is awake, occasionally during sleep, with frequency of 2–3 episodes a week, usually lasting 1–4 minutes. The seizures manifested as bilateral upper and lower extremity extension followed by jerking in the case of myotonic/tonic seizures or facial twitches during absence and/or partial seizures. Triggering factors include infection and fever, but there is no reported aura.

Current antiepileptic medications include clobazam 15 mg every bedtime, lacosamide 200 mg twice a day, and valproic acid 250 mg three times a day.

Past medical history is notable for left hemiparesis, spastic quadriparesis, developmental delay since the MVA, scoliosis of thoracolumbar spine, cognitive impairment, and Lennox-Gastaut syndrome.

A recent MRI of the brain showed chronic sequela of traumatic brain injury as evidenced by diffuse parenchymal volume loss, *ex vacuo* enlargement of the ventricular system, and atrophy of the corpus callosum and brainstem, in addition to chronic encephalomalacia involving the bilateral frontal lobes and the right temporo-occipital region.

EEG studies revealed "a multifocal interictal spike discharge (MISD) pattern."

The patient's blood glucose level was 80 mg/dL prior to FDG administration. There was no postinjection seizure activity during the EEG monitoring, consistent with an interictal PET.

FDG PET Imaging Findings (Fig. 3.5)

The PET images show diffuse cortical atrophy, *ex vacuo* ventriculomegaly, anterior horns > posterior horns (green arrow). In addition to global mild to moderate cortical hypometabolism, severe hypometabolism is identified in the left anterosuperior frontal and right lateroinferior occipital lobes (red arrows). Metabolic activity is preserved in the bilateral basal ganglia. In contrast, hypometabolism is noted in bilateral thalami (white arrow) and cerebella. Increased FDG activities are noted in the extracranial regions of the posterior nasopharyngeal regions and bilateral facial muscles (red triangles), suggestive of an inflammatory/reactive process and or muscle strain.

Discussion

Head trauma/brain injury is an important risk factor for epilepsy [1]. This patient's multiform seizures proceeded by MVA with severe head injury and intracranial damage. Consistent with the MRI findings of multifocal chronic encephalomalacia, FDG PET study reveals *ex vacuo* ventriculomegaly, anterior horns > posterior horns, most likely secondary to post-traumatic diffuse cortical atrophy. The predominant, severe cortical hypometabolism involving the left anterosuperior frontal lobe and the right lateroinferior occipital lobe in an opposite pattern suggests sequelae of direct and indirect impact brain injury, and suspicious for multifocal epileptogenic foci/zones.

The mechanism underlying the symmetric hypometabolism in the bilateral thalami and cerebella is unknown, but likely secondary to severe brain injury, effects of multiple antiepileptic medications, or combined.

Despite adjustment of antiepileptic medications, her multiform seizures were still poorly controlled. Approximately 1 year after the abnormal FDG PET study, the patient underwent VNS (vagus nerve stimulator) implant placement and achieved a better seizure control.

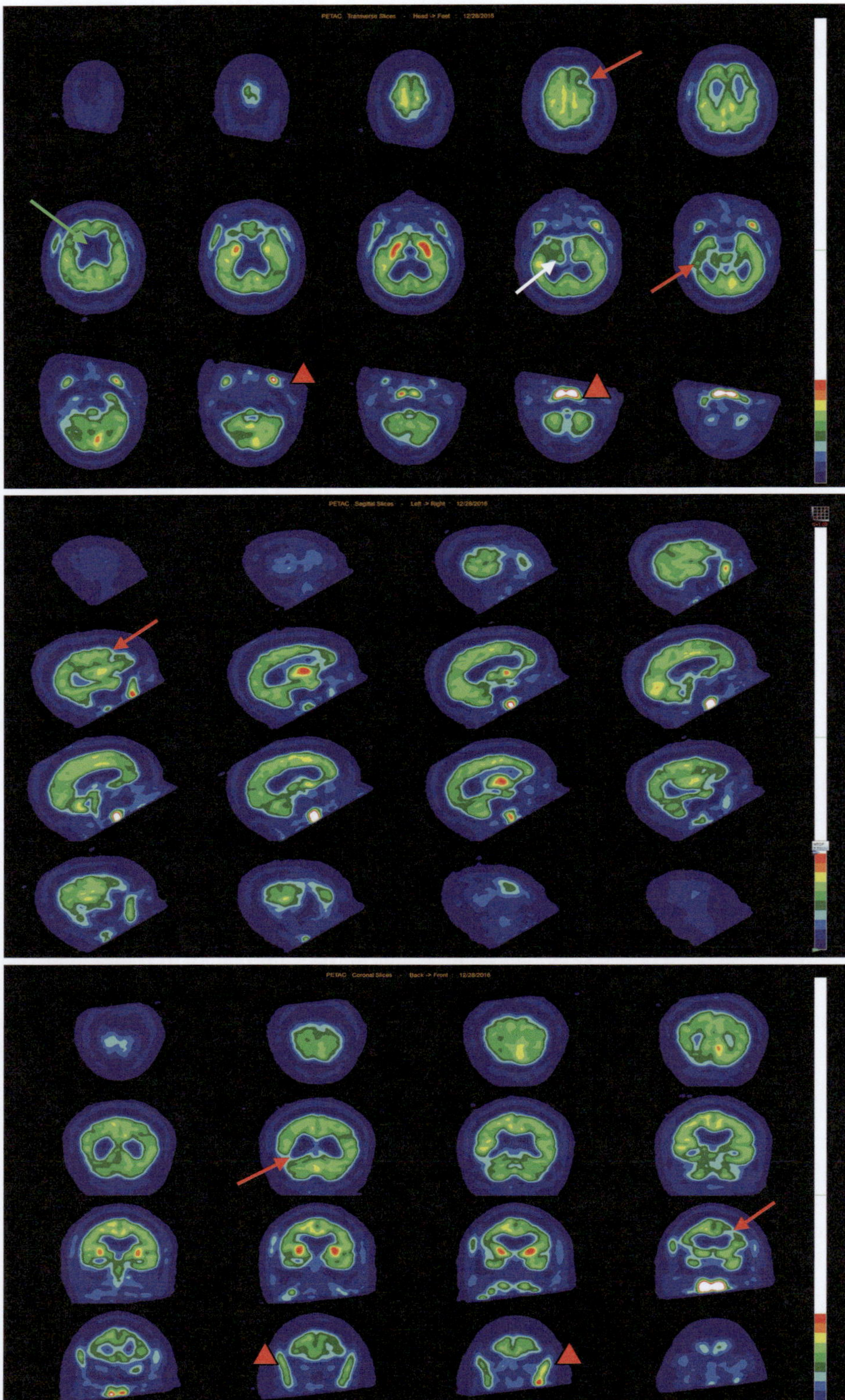

Fig. 3.5 A 16-year-old right-handed female with probable multifocal epilepsy

Case Summary

Consistent with MRI findings of bilateral/multiple chronic encephalomalacia, FDG PET study reveals diffuse cortical atrophy and associated *ex vacuo* ventriculomegaly. In addition, predominant cortical hypometabolism is identified in the left anterosuperior frontal lobe and the right lateroinferior occipital lobe, suggesting sequelae of direct and indirect impact brain injury. The concordant metabolic and anatomic neuroimaging findings, in conjunction with the seizure semiology (bilateral motor signs during seizures), are suggestive of multifocal epilepsy.

Case 3.6 Ictal FDG PET

Clinical Information

Chief Complaint *Medically refractory seizures since infancy*

The patient is a 9-year-old left-handed male presenting with medically refractory complex partial seizures that started 8 years ago. The seizures occur during awake, with frequency of 10–12 episodes per day, often lasting 10–40 seconds, during which the patient stares and experiences increased limb rigidity. There are no reported auras. In addition, the patient has a history of perinatal stroke, generalized tonic/clonic seizures, and status epilepticus. Prior neurological exam showed nystagmus.

There is no history of traumatic head injury, meningitis, nor encephalitis. There is no family history of epilepsy.

The patient has speech and language impairment and delayed motor skills, with borderline ataxia. He is part of a special needs program.

Current medications include levetiracetam, lamotrigine, and oxcarbazepine.

MRI of the brain was unremarkable.

EEG monitoring during the FDG PET scan showed frequent spikes and runs of spike and wave activity in the right occipital region, indicating an ictal FDG PET study.

FDG PET Imaging Findings (Fig. 3.6)

The PET images demonstrate a focus of intense FDG activity in the right occipitoparietal region (white arrows). Additionally, mild to moderately increased FDG activity is noted in bilateral frontal lobes (red arrows), right more prominent/diffuse than the left. In contrast, hypometabolism is seen in the left parietal region (red triangles) and the bilateral primary visual cortices (hatched red arrow). Metabolism in the left thalamus (green arrow) and the right cerebellum (hatched yellow arrows) is mildly decreased relative to the contralateral, indicating diaschisis.

Discussion and Follow-Up

This ictal FDG PET scan shows focal cortical hypermetabolism in the right occipitoparietal region, which is concordant with the monitoring EEG finding of "frequent spikes and runs of spike and wave activity in the right occipital region," suggestive of an ictal epileptogenic focus/zone [8]. The mild to moderate cortical hypermetabolism in bilateral frontal lobes is in a diffuse pattern, likely due to seizure propagation.

Regional cortical hypometabolism is identified in the left parietal lobe, for which an interictal epileptogenic focus/zone needs cannot be excluded. Additionally, asymmetric hypometabolism is present in the left thalamus and right cerebellum consistent with ipsilateral thalamic diaschisis and crossed cerebrocerebellar diaschisis, collectively suggestive of left brain intractable seizures.

The hypometabolism in bilateral primary visual cortices is severe and essentially symmetric. This abnormality, in conjunction with the known history of perinatal stroke and clinical presentation of nystagmus, is suggestive of prior ischemic insults.

During the follow-up, further workup revealed that the patient was deemed not a good candidate for epilepsy surgery due to the presence of multiform and multifocal/bilateral seizures. He was put on multiple antiepileptic medications, but still had a poor seizure control. Approximately 4 years after the ictal FDG PET study, the patient underwent a left vagus nerve stimulator (VNS) placement. He tolerated the implant well with stabilized and improved seizure activities. A follow-up MRI of the brain was performed, which showed "significant (brain) atrophy, encephalomalacia, and T2/FLAIR hyperintensity involving the parietal and occipital lobes bilaterally," likely related to prior ischemia or injury.

Case Summary

For a variety of reasons, an ictal FDG PET study is fortuitously and occasionally performed in

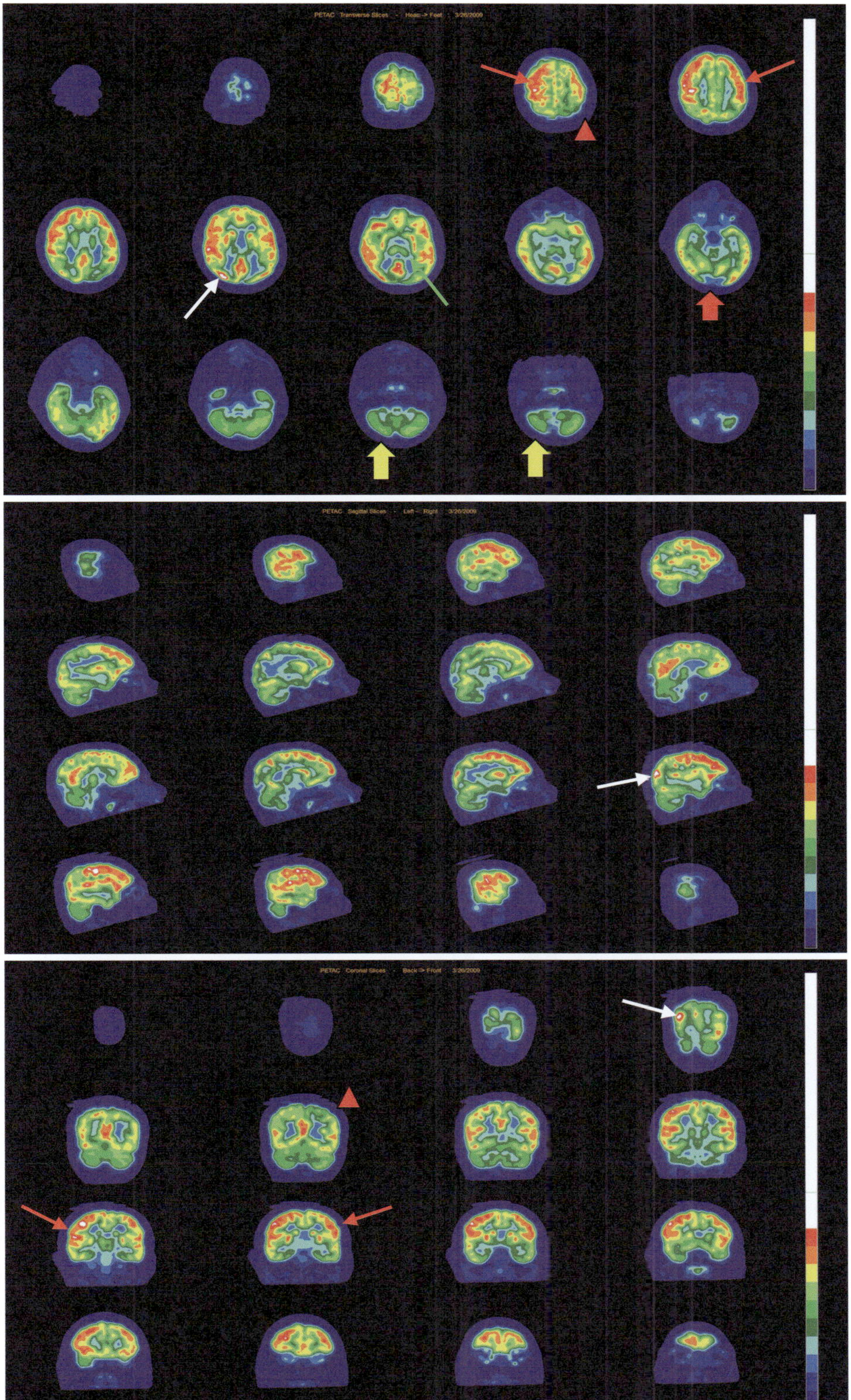

Fig. 3.6 A 9-year-old left-hand male with probable ictal right occipital epilepsy (OLE)

clinical services [3, 6]. This case exemplifies the value and limitations of an ictal brain FDG PET study in seizure workup. There is a focal cortical hypermetabolism in the right occipitoparietal region, concordant with the monitoring EEG finding of "frequent spikes and runs of spike and wave activity in the right occipital region," suggestive of an ictal right occipitoparietal epileptogenic focus/zone. However, there is diffuse cortical hypermetabolism involving the bilateral frontal lobes, likely representing seizure propagations, but the possibility of coexisting frontal lobe epilepsies with propagation to the contralateral side cannot be excluded. Additionally, regional hypometabolism is identified in the left parietal lobe, along with diaschisis in the left thalamus and the right cerebellum, collectively suggestive of intractable seizures originating from the left brain. The constellation of the FDG PET study findings, and the complex medical history as well as the seizure semiology, is suggestive of multifocal/bilateral seizures, an imaging impression that has been supported by the clinical and neuroimaging follow-up data.

Case 3.7 Surgically Proven Right Insular Lobe Epilepsy

Clinical Information

Chief Complaint *Medically refractory seizures for more than 2 years*

The patient is a 3-year-old right-handed female presenting with medically refractory seizures that started 2.5 years ago. During the first seizure, the patient's head and eyes were deviated to the right, followed by the loss of muscle tone. Despite antiepileptic treatment with two medications, the seizures continued with increasing bilateral extremity stiffness, now with more left upper extremity involvement at onset. The seizures occur randomly during the day, with frequency of a few episodes a day, and last 30–60 seconds. Postictal sleep was noted. No aura or trigger was observed, per mother.

There is no history of prior head injury or meningitis/encephalitis. Birth history was unremarkable, although global developmental delay is noted.

Current antiepileptic medications include diazepam 5 mg in the morning and 7.5 mg at night, and zonisamide 115 mg in the morning and 135 mg at night.

Initial EEGs were suspicious for left hemispheric seizures, but recent EEG studies showed a possible right central (or cingulate) versus right frontotemporal/insular seizure focus.

Recent CT of the head/brain was normal. Prior MRI of the brain was also unremarkable.

The patient's blood glucose level was 54 mg/dL prior to FDG administration for the brain PET scan. There were no postinjection seizure activities during the EEG monitoring, indicating an interictal PET study.

FDG PET Imaging Findings (Fig. 3.7)

The PET images show asymmetric hypometabolism in the right insular lobe (white arrows) and the right anterior cingulate gyrus (green arrows) when compared to the left. Additionally, mild to moderate hypometabolism is seen in the entire right frontotemporoparietal lobes (red arrows). Hypometabolism is noted in the thalami and cerebella bilaterally. Normometabolism is seen in the basal ganglia bilaterally, the right occipital lobe, and the entire left hemispheric cortices, with enhanced FDG activity in the bilateral primary visual cortices.

Discussion and Follow-Up

This patient has had drug-resistant seizures since infancy, although anatomic neuroimaging studies (CT and MRI) were unremarkable. Initial EEG examinations were suspicious for left hemispheric seizures, but recent EEG studies suggested seizure activities in the regions of the right insular and right cingulate gyrus. Concordant with the recent EEG results, the FDG PET study shows hypometabolism involving the right insular lobe and right anterior cingulate gyrus, suspicious for interictal epileptogenic foci/zones. Besides, mild-to-moderate hypometabolism is noted in the right anterotemporoparietal lobes likely due to sequelae of seizure expansion or propagation, however, additional epileptogenic foci/zones cannot be excluded.

The symmetric hypometabolism of bilateral thalami and cerebella is likely due to refractory seizures at an early age and effects of antiepileptic medications [3, 9].

Overall, glucose metabolism is preserved in the entire left brain hemisphere and in the right occipital lobe, indicating no neurosurgical contraindications.

After the FDG PET study, the patient underwent partial resection of the right parietal lobe at an outside institution. However, the patient had breakthrough seizures immediately following the surgery. The seizures persisted despite continued treatment with multiple antiepileptic medications.

Further workup including ictal and interictal SPECT brain perfusion studies confirmed right insular lobe epilepsy. Two years after, the patient had an epilepsy surgery in our hospital to resect the entire right frontal lobe including the anterior

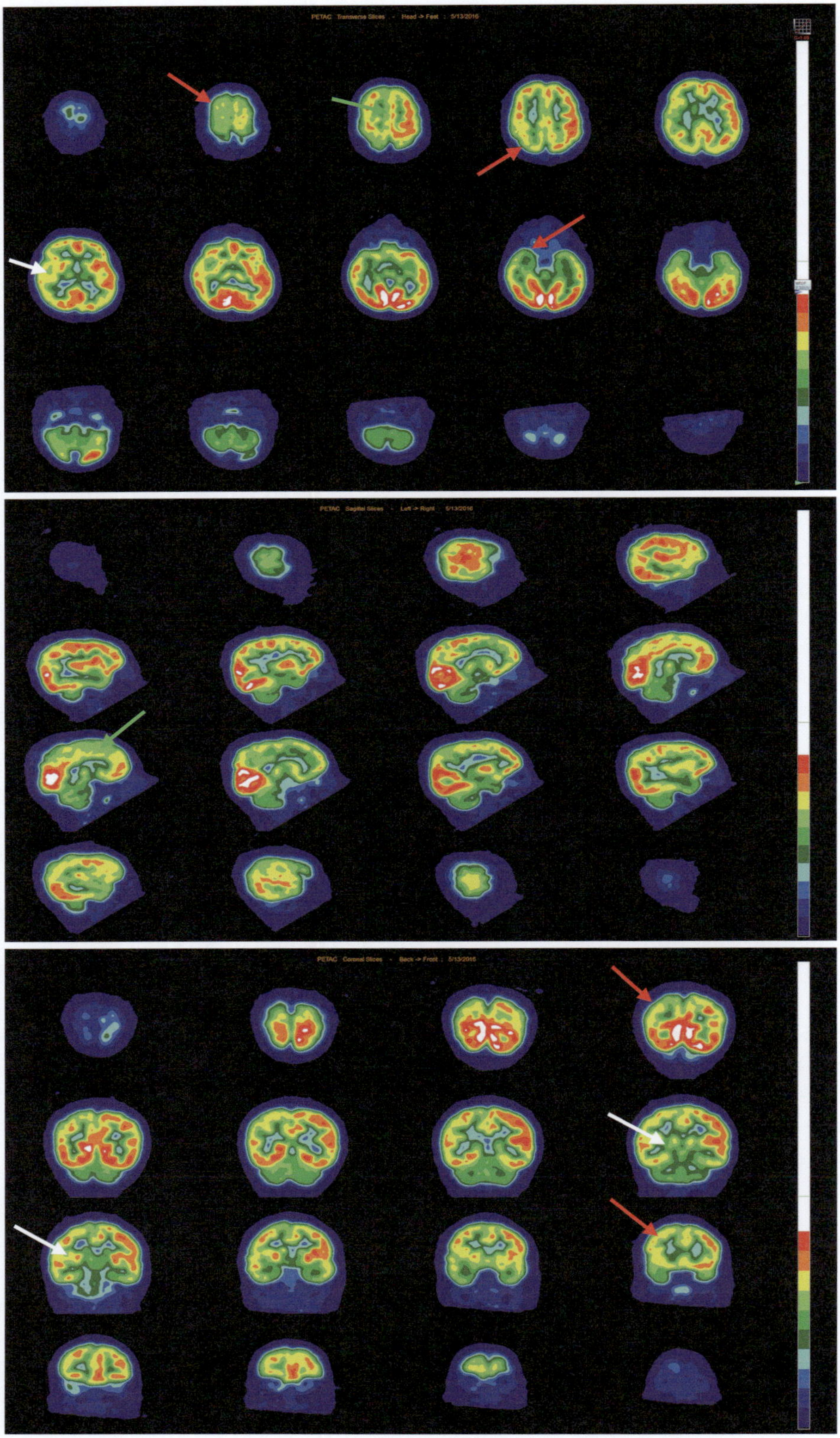

Fig. 3.7 A 3-year-old right-handed female with surgically proven right insular lobe epilepsy

cingulate gyrus and the right insular lobe. Pathology examination of the specimen revealed white matter heterotopia (white matter neurons) and focal cortical dysplasia (FCD). After the second surgery, the patient has been seizure-free for 8 months so far.

Case Summary

Insular lobe epilepsy is uncommon, and EEG localization of insular epileptic activity is extremely difficult due to its deep location and rapid seizure expansion and propagation [1]. In this case, FDG PET shows predominant hypometabolism in the right insular lobe, suspicious for an interictal epileptogenic focus/zone, with likely involvement of the adjacent right frontotemporoparietal lobes. Additionally, FDG PET also demonstrates the metabolic integrity of the left hemispheric brain and the right occipital lobe, indicating no neurosurgical contraindications. After surgical resection of the epileptogenic right insular lobe, the patient has achieved seizure-free for 8 months so far.

Case 3.8 Probable Right Frontal Lobe Epilepsy

Clinical Information

Chief Complaint *Having had different seizures for more than 30 years*

The patient is a 37-year-old right-handed female presenting with an extensive history of drug-resistant focal epilepsy that manifests as focal aware seizures and focal motor impaired awareness seizures for more than 30 years. Birth history was unremarkable and there is no history of head injury, meningitis, or encephalitis. Developmental history was also unremarkable until she was 5 years old when she experienced her first seizure which was presumed to be a secondarily generalized seizure. Her seizures often began with a focal aware seizure (aura), which consisted of a pulling sensation over her left face. There was no loss of awareness. Occasionally these would occur in isolation, but frequently would evolve into a focal motor impaired awareness seizure during which she would exhibit gasping or gasping vocalization. At times, clonic movements would occur in the right upper extremity and then progress to involve the left upper extremity and subsequently her bilateral lower extremities. Although she is unresponsive, she does not feel she completely loses awareness. These seizures often last 1–5 minutes in duration with postictal confusion for about 1 hour. The seizures occur randomly throughout the day without an early morning or nocturnal predilection.

She has been treated with multiple medications including phenytoin, carbamazepine, phenobarbital, clonazepam, topiramate, valproate, and gabapentin. However, she continues to experience frequent seizures (about five episodes a week). Because of the drug resistance, she has also been treated with vagus nerve stimulator (VNS) implantation with replacement of the internal pulse generator (IPG) twice.

In addition to seizure disorders, the patient has had developmental delay since age 5 when the seizures started, major depression, and cognitive dysfunction/dementia. She was placed in a special education program, but did not complete high school.

Current anti-seizure medications include clobazam 20 mg in the morning and 40 mg at bedtime, valproic acid 750 mg twice a day, lacosamide 40 mg twice a day, levetiracetam 2000 mg twice a day, and phenytoin 100 mg in the morning and 200 mg at bedtime. She tolerates these medications well without adverse reactions or side effects.

Previous multiple EEG studies have been suggestive of right lateralized seizures and a possible epileptogenic zone within the right frontal lobe.

CT of the head/brain and MRI of the brain were unremarkable.

Recent ictal and interictal SPECT brain perfusion studies showed subtle findings suggesting possible right medial temporal epilepsy.

The patient's blood glucose level was 90 mg/dL prior to FDG administration for the PET study. Monitoring EEG confirmed that the FDG PET was an interictal study.

FDG PET Imaging Findings (Fig. 3.8)

The PET images show an area of dominant hypometabolism in the posterior right frontal lobe (red arrows), likely in the supplementary motor area (SMA). Mild hypometabolism is also noted in the right orbitofrontal region and the mid-inferior frontal/insular area (white arrows). In addition, mild hypometabolism is seen in the right lateral temporal lobe (green arrows) relative to the left. Asymmetric, mild hypometabolism is noted in the left cerebellum, consistent with diaschisis (hatched yellow arrow).

FDG activity in the bilateral basal ganglia, thalami, the right occipital lobe, the entire left hemispheric cortices, and the right cerebellum is within normal limits.

Discussion and Follow-Up

Clinically this patient has two different types of seizure activity. However, the dominant motor features in the seizure semiology are suggestive of frontal lobe epilepsy. Consistent with the seizure

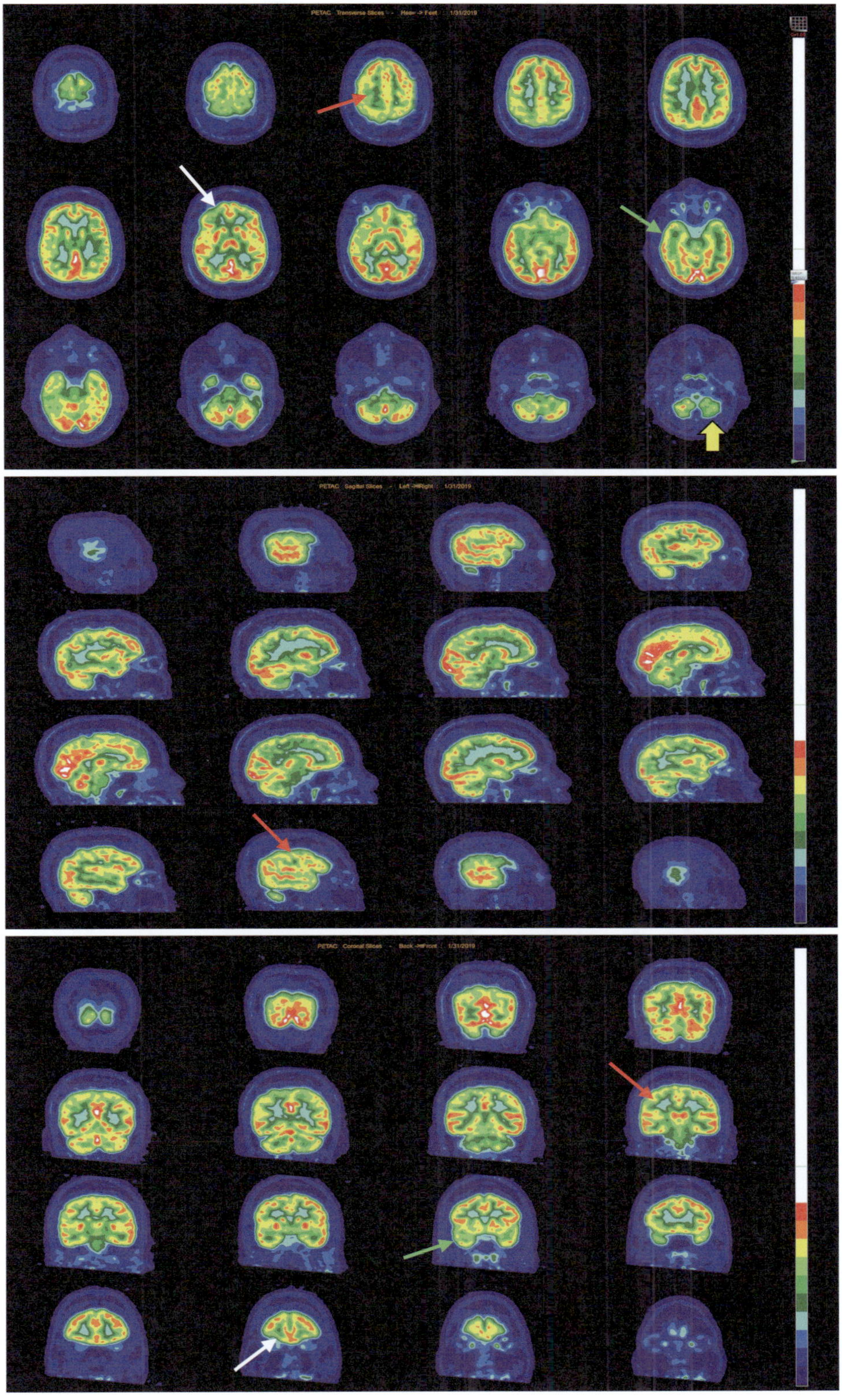

Fig. 3.8 A 37-year-old right-handed female with probable right frontal lobe epilepsy (FLE)

semiology, prior EEG results suggest right frontal epilepsies. The FDG PET scan also shows cortical hypometabolism in the posterior portion of the right frontal lobe, likely in the supplementary motor area (SMA). Mild hypometabolism is noted in the left cerebellum, suggestive of crossed cerebrocerebellar diaschisis. Constellation of the FDG PET findings, seizure semiology, and prior EEG results is suggestive of right frontal lobe epilepsy (FLE).

In addition, several areas of mild hypometabolism are noted, involving the right orbitofrontal lobe, the right mid-inferior frontal/insular region, and the right lateral temporal lobe. Since frontal lobe seizures tend to propagate [1], these findings raise concern for sequelae of seizure propagations versus additional interictal epileptogenic foci/zones, which require further workup.

The minimal hypometabolism in the bilateral superomedial parietal lobes is symmetric, given the known history of developmental delay, likely due to brain atrophy.

Despite the abnormalities in the right brain, glucose metabolism is preserved in the entire left brain hemisphere and in the right occipital lobe.

After the FDG PET study, the patient has been treated with five antiepileptic medications but still with frequent seizures (5–7 episodes per day). She is currently undergoing further presurgical evaluation including a stereo-EEG implantation for intracranial seizure monitoring.

Case Summary

Consistent with the seizure semiology and prior EEG results, the FDG PET finding of dominant hypometabolism in the posterior portion of the right frontal lobe (likely SMA), in conjunction with the crossed cerebrocerebellar diaschisis, is suggestive of right frontal lobe epilepsy (FLE). In addition, several areas of mild hypometabolism are noted in the right inferior frontal lobe and the right lateral temporal lobe, likely due to sequelae of seizure propagations. However, additional interictal epileptogenic foci/zones cannot be excluded. Thus, further workup such as intracranial seizure monitoring has been proposed.

Case 3.9 Seizures Due to Left Temporal Astrocytoma

Clinical Information

Chief Complaint *Having had recent onset of medically refractory seizures for 3 months*

The patient is a 59-year-old female who had a sudden onset of mental status change and grand mal seizure 3 months ago. MRI of the brain showed left temporal edema and abnormal signal suspicious for viral encephalitis. CSF studies were essentially unremarkable and CSF culture was negative. She received antiviral therapy (acyclovir) for potential herpes encephalitis, in addition to anti-seizure medication (levetiracetam). Despite the treatments, she developed recurrent seizures 3 months later. Family members stated that the patient would awake from sleep with a seizure, during which she would mumble words and have bilateral upper arm stiffening.

The patient is a non-smoker. She denies history of alcohol or drug abuse. Family history is negative for seizures.

Current medication is levetiracetam 500 mg twice a day.

Repeat CT of the head/brain showed persistent left temporal hypoattenuation, but no mass effect nor hemorrhage.

Repeat MRI of the brain revealed abnormal increased T2/FLAIR signal in the left mesial temporal lobe, stable over the last 3 months. There was no evidence of acute hemorrhage, mass effect, midline shift, or hydrocephalus.

The first brain FDG PET scan was performed with blood glucose level of 94 mg/dL. The follow-up brain FDG PET study, with approximately 2 months apart, was performed with blood glucose level of 96 mg/dL. Of note, the studies were requested by an infection specialist and a neuro-oncologist, respectively, both without arrangement for EEG monitoring.

FDG PET Imaging Findings

The first FDG PET images (Fig. 3.9a) show diffuse hypometabolism in the entire left temporal lobe (red arrows). In the posteromedial left temporal region, there is a focus of mild-to-moderate FDG activity (white arrows), which is not discernible or outstanding when compared to the contralateral side.

FDG activity in the bilateral basal ganglia, thalami, the remainder of the cerebral cortices, and the cerebella is within normal limits.

The follow-up FDG PET (Fig. 3.9b), which was performed 2 months later, reveals persistent hypometabolism in the entire left temporal lobe (red arrows), essentially unchanged from the initial scan. However, the previously noted mild-to-moderate FDG focus in the posteromedial left temporal lobe shows interval increased intensity (white arrows), with current maximal SUV (standardized uptake value) of 5.4, relative to the prior maximal SUV of 3.9, in retrospect. There is newly developed mild hypometabolism in the left thalamus (green arrow) when compared to the contralateral side.

Again, FDG in the remainder of the cerebral cortices is preserved with enhanced FDG activity in the bilateral primary visual cortices, likely due to physiological stimulation during FDG uptake period.

Discussion and Follow-Up

Brain tumors are a common cause of medically refractory seizures [1]. This patient's seizure semiology is atypical without lateralized symptoms from the initial to recurrent episodes. The MRI finding of left temporal edema is significant but nonspecific, which led to antiviral therapy for potential viral encephalitis initially. Despite the treatment, the patient developed recurrent seizures 3 months later.

The first FDG brain PET showed diffuse left temporal hypometabolism, which is indistinguishable from an interictal mesial temporal lobe epilepsy (MTLE) [2, 5, 8]. The focus of mild-to-moderate FDG activity in the posteromedial left temporal region is a subtle finding and is not discernible when compared to the contralateral side. Two months later, however, the follow-up FDG PET scan clearly shows interval increased FDG activity of the same focus in the posteromedial left temporal region, suspicious for a neoplastic process with a moderate metabolic rate. Therefore,

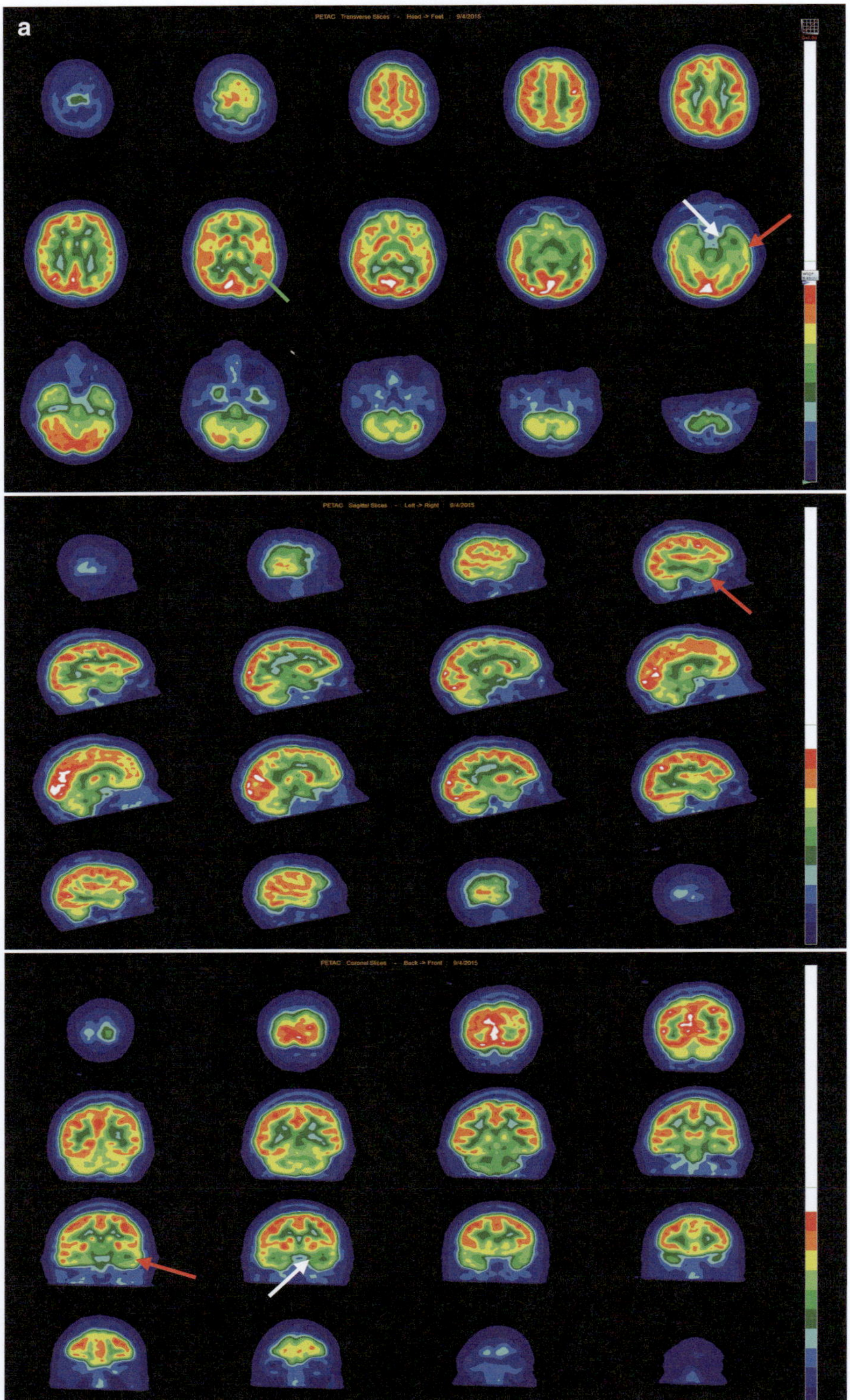

Fig. 3.9 (**a**) A 59-year-old female with seizures due to left temporal astrocytoma – the first brain FDG PET. (**b**) A 59-year-old female with seizures due to left temporal astrocytoma – a follow-up brain FDG PET with approximately 2 months apart

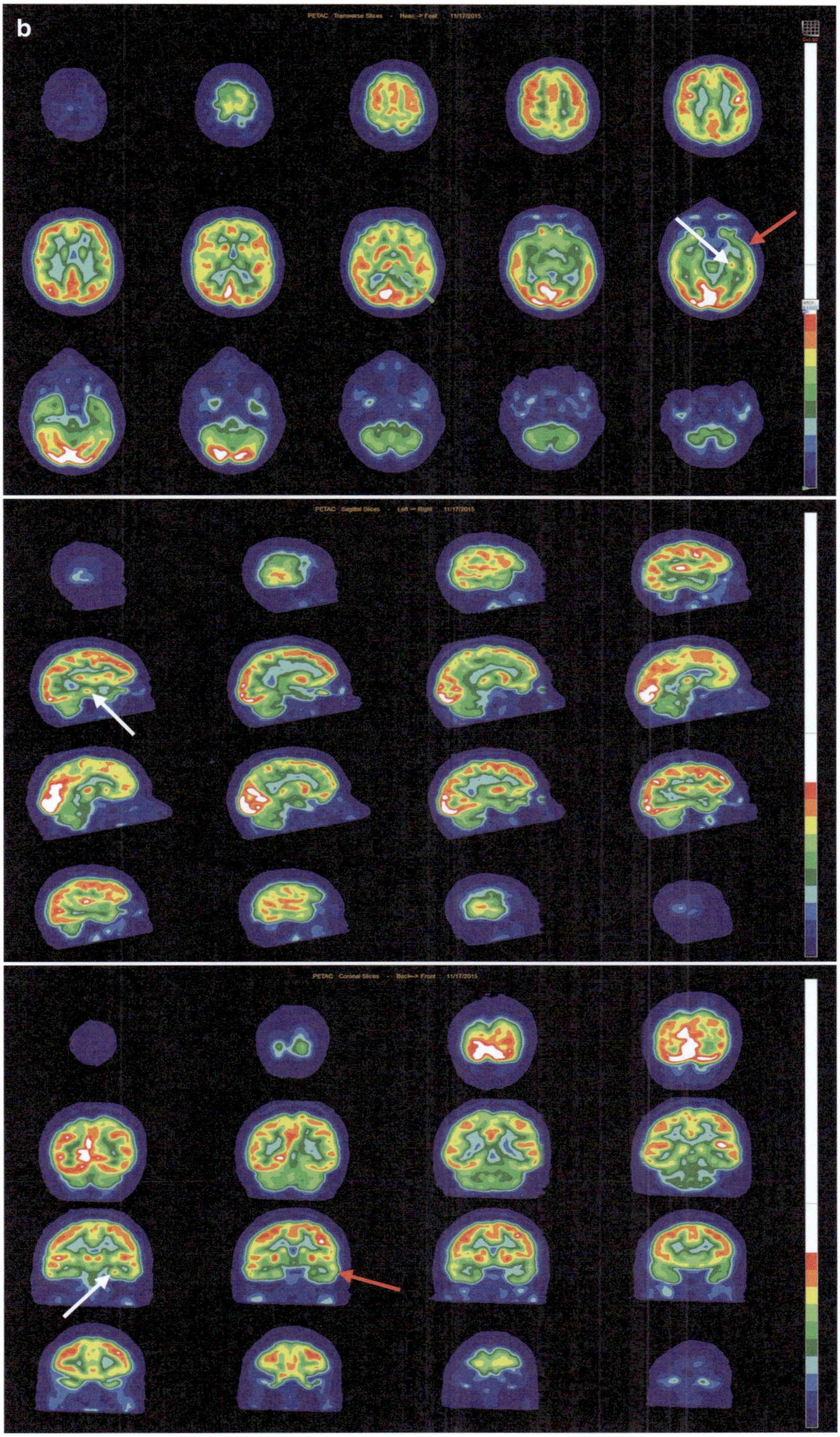

Fig. 3.9 (continued)

the persistent diffuse hypometabolism in the remainder of the temporal lobe is likely due to mass effect, tumor-associated vasogenic edema, or sequelae of seizure expansion/propagation, or combined. The mild hypometabolism in the adjacent left thalamus is likely due to mass effect or ipsilateral thalamic diaschisis.

Two months after the follow-up FDG PET scan, the patient underwent left craniostomy and biopsy of the posteromedial left temporal lesion which was positive for anaplastic astrocytoma, World Health Organization (WHO) grade 3, IDH1 (isocitrate dehydrogenase-1) mutant protein absent, with MIB (Ki-67) proliferation index 10%. Subsequently, she received radiation concurrently with eight cycles of adjuvant chemotherapy (temozolomide daily × 5 days, every 4 weeks).

Case Summary

Brain tumors are a common cause of medically refractory seizures. This case shows that one of the most common FDG PET findings for brain tumors is focal hypometabolism secondary to tumor-associated vasogenic edema, mass effect, or both. This can be disguised as an interictal epileptogenic focus/zone. The focal interval increased metabolic activity in the left mesial temporal lobe between the first and follow-up FDG PETs is suggestive of a neoplastic process rather than a conventional interictal seizure focus. After surgical resection, the lesion was positive for left temporal anaplastic astrocytoma, which is a rare malignant brain tumor leading to medically refractory seizures.

Case 3.10 Seizures Resulting from Cerebral Cavernous Malformations (CCMs)

Clinical Information

Chief Complaint *Recent onset of frequent seizures of variable duration*

The patient is a 16-year-old right-handed female presenting with frequent seizures that suddenly started 2 months ago. The seizures were often preceded by a self-reported "weird feeling," with frequency of two to three episodes a week, lasting about 2–15 minutes. During the seizures, the patient sits down, stops talking, and becomes confused. Postictally the patient has poor memory. The last episode occurred 1 day prior to presentation and became a generalized seizure refractory to phenytoin, which was finally resolved in the emergency department with levetiracetam loading.

The patient denies history of head injury, meningitis/encephalitis, or drug abuse. Birth history and development were unremarkable. Family history is notable for epilepsy in her sister.

Current medications include levetiracetam 750 mg twice a day and phenytoin 100 mg twice a day.

MRI of the brain showed a 17 × 15 × 14 mm lesion in the medial left temporal lobe with features suggesting a cavernous malformation (also called cavernous hemangioma), whereas MRA revealed no evidence of vascular malformation, aneurysm, or major branch occlusion.

EEG studies were suggestive of focal epileptogenic activities in the left anterior-mid temporal region.

The patient's blood glucose level was 84 mg/dL prior to FDG administration. EEG monitoring confirmed that the FDG PET scan was an interictal study.

FDG PET Imaging Findings (Fig. 3.10)

The images show focally decreased FDG activity in the left mesial temporal region (red arrows) when compared to the contralateral side. In addition, mildly decreased FDG activity is noted in the left thalamus (white arrow), suggestive of diaschisis.

FDG activity in the remainder of the cerebral cortices, bilateral basal ganglia, the right thalamus, and bilateral cerebella is preserved.

Discussion and Follow-Up

This interictal FDG PET shows focal hypometabolism in the left mesial temporal lobe corresponding to the MRI finding of a cavernous malformation that seems to be the underlying cause of epilepsy. The ipsilateral thalamic diaschisis is indirect evidence of intractable left brain epilepsy.

In addition, the FDG PET shows metabolic integrity of the rest of the brain, which is important in the assessment of the patient's neurosurgical candidacy.

Three months after the abnormal FDG brain PET study, the patient underwent left craniotomy and surgical resection of the known left mesial temporal cavernous hemangioma.

Postsurgically, the patient had been seizure-free for 3.5 years but recently developed breakthrough seizures.

Case Summary

Cerebral cavernous malformations (CCMs, also referred to as cavernous hemangiomas) and arteriovenous malformations (AVMs) are two neurovascular conditions that may cause epilepsies [1]. This case shows interictal FDG brain PET findings of focal cortical hypometabolism concordant with a CCM located in the left mesial temporal lobe as well as mild hypometabolism in the left thalamus indicating diaschisis. The glucose metabolism in the rest of the brain is unaffected, indicating no neurosurgical contraindications. Following the abnormal FDG PET study, the patient underwent surgical resection of the left mesial temporal cavernous hemangioma and has achieved seizure-free for 3.5 years.

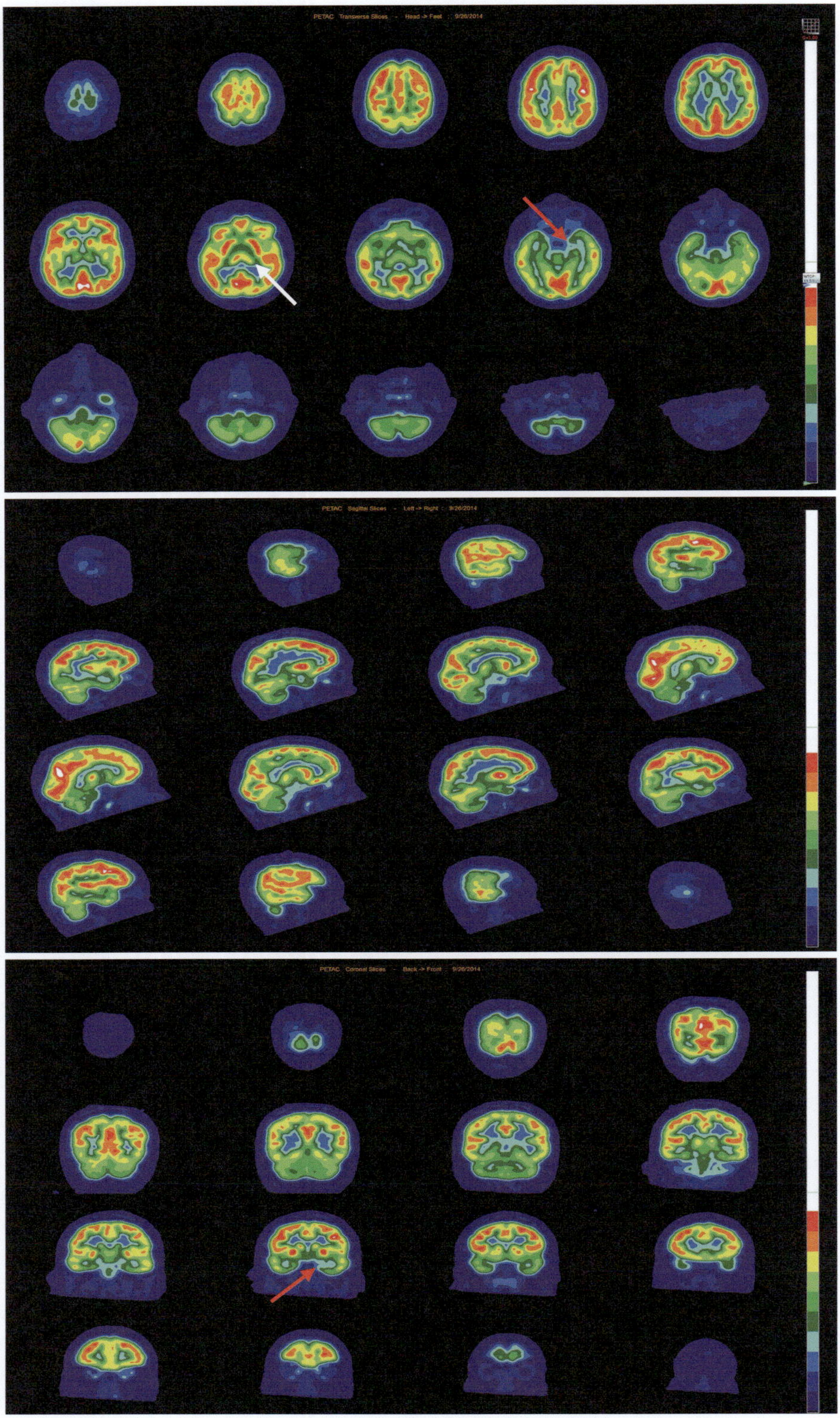

Fig. 3.10 A 16-year-old right-handed female with seizures resulting from left mesial temporal cerebral cavernous malformations (CCMs)

Case 3.11 Seizures Due to Tuberous Sclerosis (TS)

Clinical Information

Chief Complaint *Having had medically refractory seizures since early infancy*

The patient is a 3-year-old right-handed male with an extensive history of seizures that probably started from birth or early infancy according to his mother. He was treated with several antiepileptic medications, but has had a poor seizure control. The first type of seizure is described as staring off (with tendency to the left) and nostrils' flaring, followed by either rapid or slow breathing, and often lasts half to three minutes. The second type of seizure often occurs during sleep, with tremors, stiffening, staring off with eye rolling, and slight nystagmus.

The patient did not have a history of head injury, meningitis, or encephalitis. He was a full-term baby and was delivered through C-section without complications. However, global developmental delay has been observed.

Current antiepileptic medications include clobazam 20 mg twice a day, diazepam 2 mg by mouth PRN, divalproex 125 mg three times a day, and lacosamide 50 mg twice a day.

Past medical history is notable for known tuberous sclerosis and polycystic kidney disease. Family history is positive for seizures in a paternal aunt.

The patient's blood glucose level was 80 mg/dL prior to FDG administration. EEG monitoring confirmed that the FDG PET was an interictal study.

FDG PET Imaging Findings (Fig. 3.11)

The PET images show numerous cortical tubers of tiny or small sizes, all with decreased or absent FDG activity, involving at least the frontal, parietal, and temporal lobes bilaterally, the right occipital lobe, and even the right cerebellum (white arrows). In addition, diffusely decreased FDG activity is noted in the anterior cingulate gyri bilaterally, especially on the left (hatched red arrow). FDG activity in the left thalamus is minimally decreased (red arrow) relative to the right, despite slight head-tilting. FDG activity in the bilateral basal ganglia and the primary visual cortices is preserved, whereas FDG activity in the cerebella is diffusely decreased.

Discussion and Follow-Up

Tuberous sclerosis (TS) is a rare genetic multisystem disease characterized by formation of multiple benign tumors involving many organs including the brain leading to medically refractory seizures, global developmental delay, and behavioral problems [1, 6]. FDG PET findings are often confirmatory of multiple/numerous cortical tubers that are already detectable on brain MRI. The limitation of FDG PET imaging is that all the tubers show hypometabolism, without imaging features indicating their epileptogenicity. However, the mild left thalamic hypometabolism in this case is consistent with diaschisis, which is indirect evidence for intractable seizures originating from left brain. In addition to multiple cortical tubers, the diffusely decreased metabolic activity in bilateral cingulate gyri, left > right, is another significant finding, raising concerns for anterior cingulate epilepsy, especially on the left side, given the presence of ipsilateral thalamic diaschisis.

Following the FDG PET, EEG studies (ictal, interictal), in conjunction with clinical features, were suggestive of an epileptogenic region in the left anterior-mid cingulate cortex. Based on the results, the patient had Visualase laser ablation of the presumed left cingulate seizure focus. After the ablation, however, the seizures persisted despite reduced frequencies, indicating a partial response. Half a year later, the patient underwent left frontal lobectomy with left anterior insular resection. Since the surgery, there have been no reported seizures for nearly 5 months. According to his mother, the patient has improved eye contact with people, attention, and appetite.

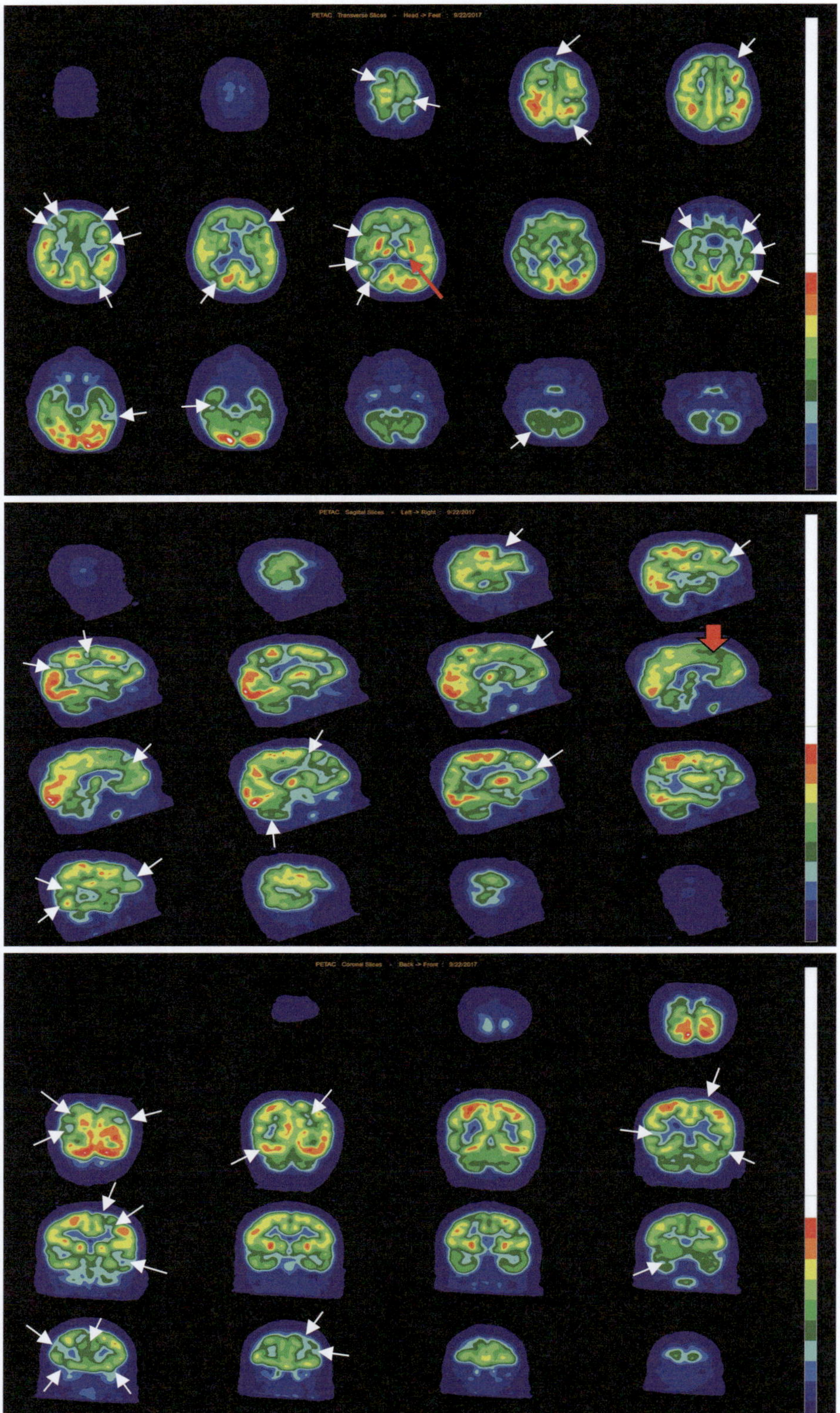

Fig. 3.11 A 3-year-old right-handed male with medically refractory seizures due to known multiple sclerosis (TS)

Case Summary

Tuberous sclerosis (TS) is a well-known underlying cause leading to medically refractory seizures [1, 6]. FDG PET often demonstrates the presence of multiple/numerous hypometabolic cortical tubers, without imaging features indicating their epileptogenicity, as shown in this case. However, additional FDG PET findings, such as left thalamic diaschisis and diffuse left cingulate hypometabolism, helped localize epileptogenic foci/zones into the left frontal lobe. This was supported or confirmed by further workup including ictal/interictal SPECT brain perfusion scans and EEG monitoring, leading to effective Visualase laser ablation and surgical resection of the left frontal epileptogenic cortex.

Case 3.12 Seizures Due to Intrauterine Stroke

Clinical Information

Chief Complaint *Intractable seizures and history of intrauterine stroke*

The patient is a 4-year-old left-handed girl who was born at 37-week gestation as twin B in a pregnancy complicated by intrauterine stroke. Within 2 days after birth, she had seizure-like activity according to her parents. Starting at 6 months of age, her movements were sporadic throughout the day, with jerking that was symmetrical on both sides. These would occur while awake and during sleep. She often would lose her balance and would fall. In addition, she was noticed to have staring spells. She was treated with sabril, levetiracetam, and phenobarbital for infantile spasms and myoclonic seizures. However, she continued to have seizures. Further workup showed electrical status epilepticus of sleep (ESES).

In addition to her seizure disorder, she has global developmental delay with disproportionate language (expressive > receptive) delay and right hemiparesis.

Current antiepileptic medications include levetiracetam 500 mg twice a day and clobazam 10 mg twice a day.

There is no history of traumatic head injury or meningitis/encephalitis. Family history is negative for seizure or epilepsy.

MRI of the brain showed "extensive cystic encephalomalacia of the left cerebral hemisphere, *ex vacuo* dilatation of the left lateral ventricle and evidence of left-sided Wallerian degeneration."

The patient's blood glucose level was 82 mg/dL prior to FDG administration for the PET scan. EEG monitoring confirmed that the FDG PET was an interictal study.

FDG PET Imaging Findings (Fig. 3.12)

The images show a large area of absent FDG activity that appears in the left middle cerebral artery territory, including the majority of the left frontotempoparietal and occipital cortices and the left basal ganglia and thalamus. In contrast, small portions of the left forefrontal lobe and superior left parietal lobe are noted with preserved FDG activity. FDG activity in the left inferomedial temporal lobe and the left inferolateral occipital lobes is moderate to severely decreased (red arrows).

FDG activity in the entire right brain hemispheric cortices is within normal limits, whereas diffusely decreased FDG activity is noted in the right basal ganglia and thalamus (white arrow) as well as the cerebella bilaterally. Slight further decreased FDG activity is noted in the right cerebellum (hatched yellow arrows) relative to the left, indicating crossed cerebrocerebellar diaschisis.

Discussion and Follow-Up

Given the history of intrauterine stroke, the FDG PET findings are essentially confirmatory of MRI results, consistent with a large infarct in the left middle cerebral artery (MCA) territory. FDG activity in the para-infarct tissues such as the left medial forefrontal lobe and left superior parietal lobe is well preserved, suggesting intact or preserved blood supply from the left anterior and posterior cerebral arteries. Although the majority of the infarct area shows absent FDG activity, some residual FDG activity is noted in the left inferolateral occipital lobe and the left inferomedial temporal lobe, raising concerns for interictal epileptogenic foci/zones.

FDG activity in the entire right brain hemispheric cortices is preserved, indicating intact glucose metabolism despite a massive left brain stroke. In contrast, FDG activity in the right basal ganglia and thalamus and the cerebella bilaterally is diffusely decreased. Additionally, slight further decreased FDG activity is seen in the right cerebellum relative to the left, indicating cerebrocerebellar diaschisis.

Following extensive workup including EEG monitoring, the patient underwent a comprehensive epilepsy surgery including left hemispherectomy, left insular hemispherotomy, left temporal

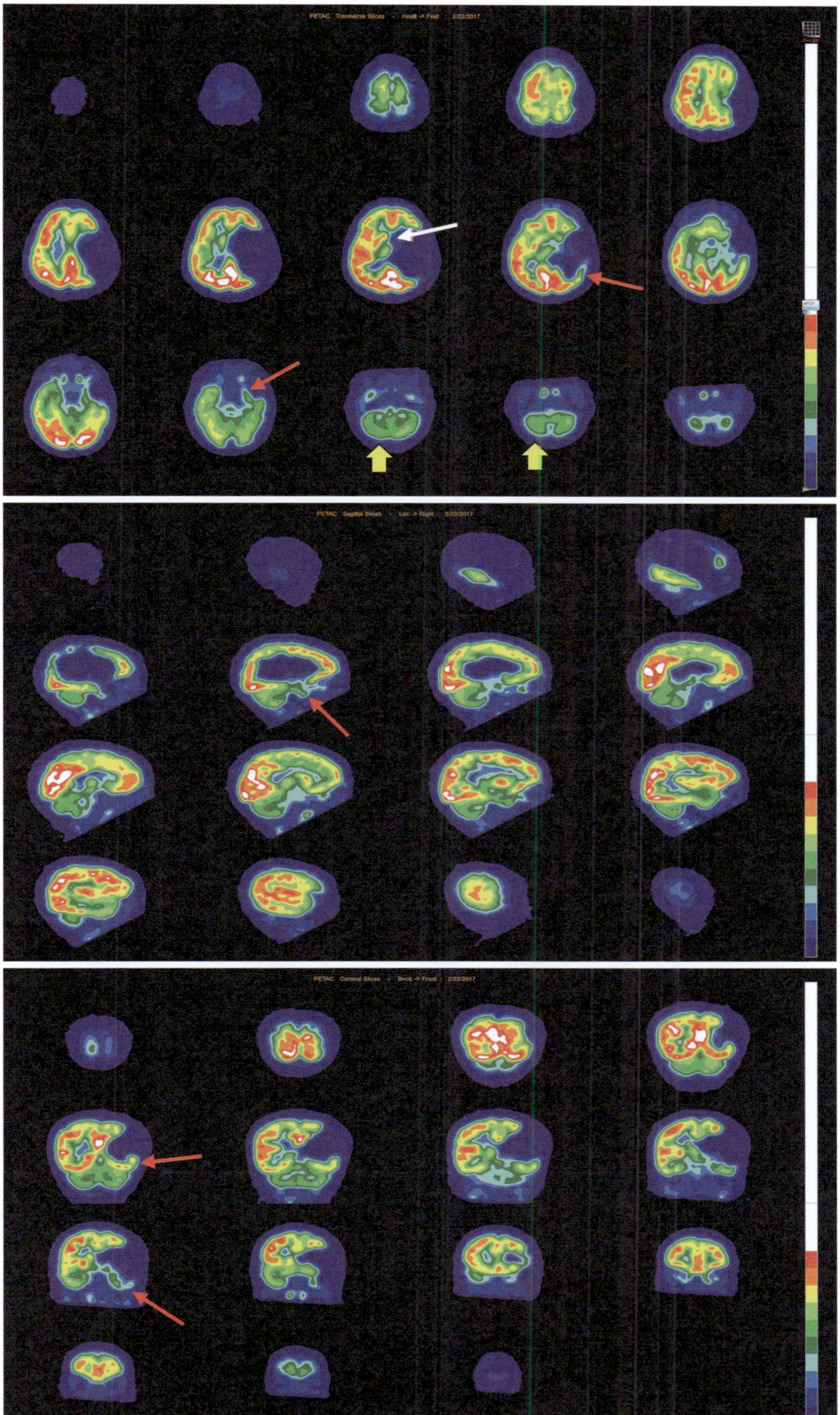

Fig. 3.12 A 4-year-old left-handed female with intractable seizures due to left intrauterine stroke

lobectomy, resection of amygdala and hippocampus, ligation of choroid plexus, corpus callosotomy, and frontal basal disconnection. Pathology examination revealed "foci of cortical dysplasia (International League Against Epilepsy type Ic)" in the resected left temporal lobe. Post-surgically, she has been doing well, without clinically overt seizures for half a year. Her development has been progressing, with improvement in language, comprehension, motion, and social interaction.

Case Summary

Stroke is a common cause of seizures [1]. The value of FDG PET in the evaluation of stroke-related medically refractory seizures as described in this case is at least twofold: (1) to identify potential epileptogenic foci/zones that likely emanate from para-infarct/residual tissues, in conjunction with seizure semiology and EEG results, and (2) to evaluate glucose metabolic integrity of the rest of the brain to rule out neurosurgical contraindications. Following extensive workup, the patient underwent a comprehensive epilepsy surgery. Post-surgically, pathology confirmed foci of cortical dysplasia in the resected left temporal lobe. Limited follow-up data shows that the patient is seizure-free with improved development and functions of daily life.

Case 3.13 Recurrent Seizures After Hemispherectomy

Clinical Information

Chief Complaint *Having had recurrent seizures after right hemispherectomy of 10 years ago*

The patient is a 19-year-old right-handed male with a complex neurological history including spastic cerebral palsy, hemimegalencephaly, and medical refractory focal epilepsy. His recurrent seizures started at 6 weeks of age. The seizure semiology includes eye deviation, head turning, unresponsiveness, and generalized convulsion. He was treated with several antiepileptic medications (phenobarbital, topiramate, phenytoin, and carbamazepine), still with a poor seizure control. MRI of the brain in the past revealed right hemimegalencephaly. Subsequently, he underwent a modified right hemispherectomy at an outside institution in 2001 when he was 19 months old. After the procedure, he was seizure-free for about 10 years until 2011 when seizures returned, with increasing frequency. The recurrent seizures are very short in duration (<10 seconds), so his parents have never directly observed them. The patient reports that he experiences some tingling, symptoms of an aura, prior to seizure onset. During seizures the patient describes left arm flexing. There is no head or eye deviation.

Current antiepileptic medications include levetiracetam 1000 mg twice a day and clonazepam PRN for focal seizure control.

EEG study was suggestive of a deep hemispheric epileptogenic source, likely in the right frontocentrotemporal or insular region.

Subsequent MRI of the brain showed "resection of most of the right cerebral hemisphere with edema and/or gliosis of the residual right frontal and occipital cortex." The presence of the right basal ganglia is noted.

The patient's blood glucose level was 89 mg/dL prior to FDG administration. EEG monitoring confirmed that the FDG PET was an interictal study.

FDG PET Imaging Findings (Fig. 3.13)

Extensive postsurgical changes are present in the right brain hemisphere, with visible midline shift to the right. There are only small areas of mild FDG activity noted in the right inferior frontal lobe (red arrows) and the right inferomedial occipital lobe (white arrows), suggesting residual cortical tissues with hypometabolism. In line with the MRI finding, a small area of mild FDG activity is noted in the right basal ganglia region (green arrow). Adjacent to this, there is a smaller area of mild FDG activity (orange arrow, the lower panel), likely representing a small amount of right insular tissue. Relative to the left cerebellum, FDG activity in the right cerebellum is diffusely decreased (hatched yellow arrows), indicating Wallerian degeneration.

FDG activity in the entire left cerebral cortices, the left basal ganglia and thalamus, and the left cerebellum is within normal limits.

Discussion and Follow-Up

The PET findings in this case are confirmatory of post-surgical changes from the prior right hemispherectomy. In addition to a large surgical cavity as evidenced with absent metabolic activity, there are small areas of residual tissue with hypometabolism in the in the right inferior frontal lobe, the right inferomedial occipital lobe, and the right insular region, in conjunction with the EEG findings, suspicious for interictal epileptogenic foci/zones.

The hypometabolism in the right basal ganglia and cerebellum is likely secondary to Wallerian degeneration and/or diaschisis.

In contrast, FDG activity in the entire left hemisphere including the left cerebellum is well preserved without discrete global or focal abnormalities. The metabolic integrity of the left brain effectively rules out contraindications for further surgical treatment of potential epileptogenic foci/zones in the right hemisphere.

Epilepsy surgery is an effective treatment for patients with pharmacoresistant focal seizures [7].

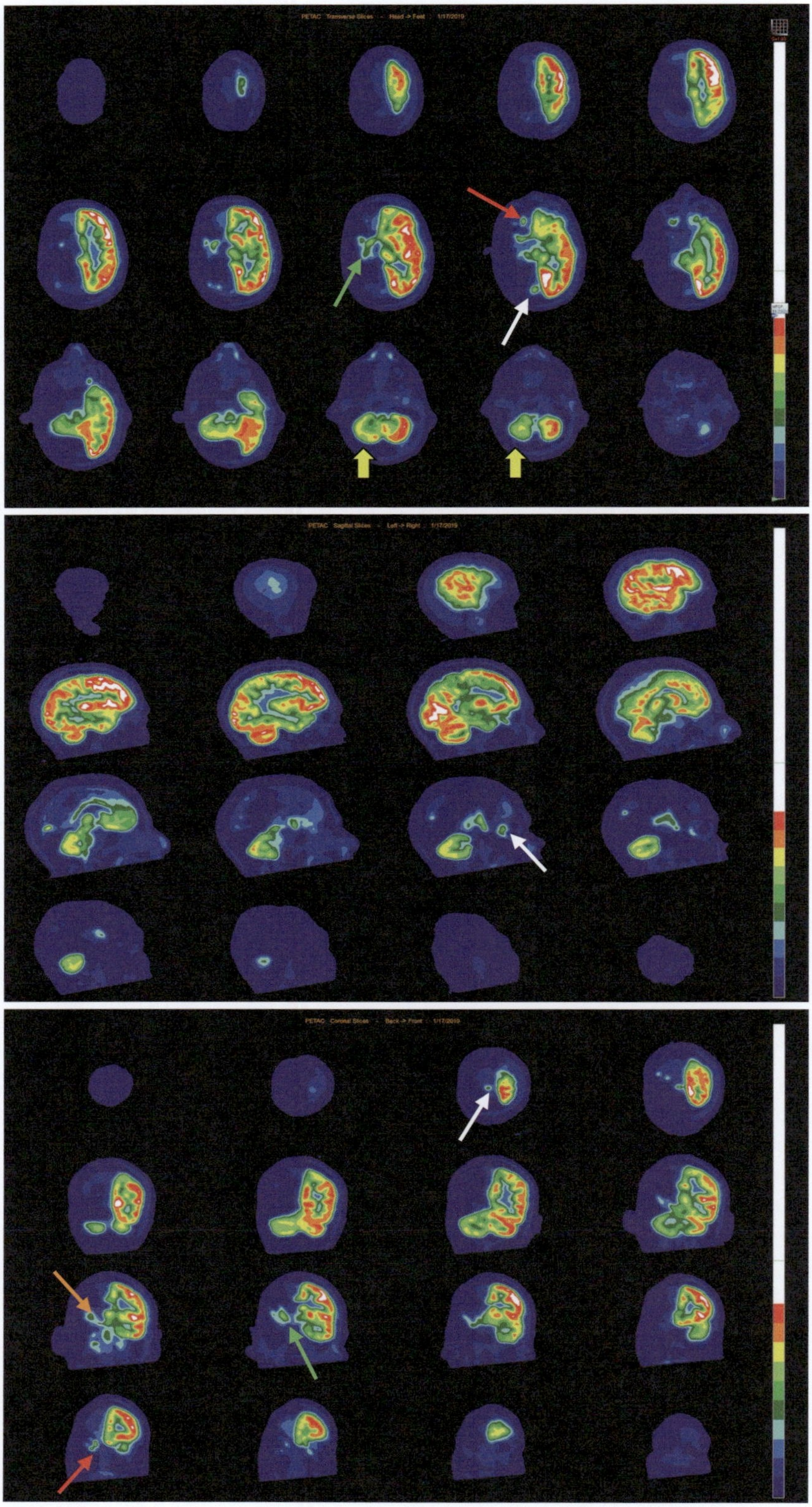

Fig. 3.13 A 19-year-old right-handed male with recurrent seizures after right hemispherectomy of 10 years ago

However, only 47% of the patients remain seizure-free 10 years after surgery [4]. This patient achieved 10-year seizure-free but developed breakthrough seizures after that. Following the abnormal FDG PET study, the patient underwent video EEG monitoring, which confirmed right insular epilepsy, leading to a new recommendation for surgical completion of the previous right hemispherectomy.

Case Summary

This patient had a successful epilepsy surgery in the past, but developed recurrent seizure after achieving seizure-free for 10 years. FDG PET scan not only shows residual tissues with hypometabolism suspicious for epileptogenic foci/zones in the right brain but also provides evidence of glucose metabolic integrity of the entire left brain, indicating that there is no surgical contraindication for a complete right brain surgery from an imaging point of view. The FDG PET findings, in conjunction with the recurrent seizure semiology and the MRI and EEG results, lay a strong foundation for the recommendation for surgical completion of the previous right hemispherectomy.

References

1. Abou-Khalil BW, Gallagher MJ, Macdonald RL. Epilepsies. In: Daroff R, Jankonic J, Mazziotta J, Pemerony S, editors. Bradley's neurology in clinical practice. London: Elsevier; 2016. p. 1563–614.
2. Cendes F, Theodore WH, Brinkmann BH, et al. Neuroimaging of epilepsy. Handb Clin Neurol. 2016;136:985–1014.
3. Gaillard WD. Nuclear imaging (PET, SPECT). In: Wyllie E, editor. Wyllie's treatment of epilepsy: principles and practice. 5th ed. Philadelphia: Wolters Kluwer; 2011. p. 860–8.
4. Hirsch LJ. Long-term outcome after epilepsy surgery: relapsing, remitting disorder? Epilepsy Curr. 2012;12(4):140–2.
5. Kumar A, Chugani HT. The role of radionuclide imaging in epilepsy, part 1: sporadic temporal and extratemporal lobe epilepsy. J Nucl Med Technol. 2017;45(1):14–21.
6. Kumar A, Chugani HT. Application of PET and SPECT in pediatric epilepsy surgery. In: Cataltepe O, Jallo GI, editors. Pediatric epilepsy surgery: preoperative assessment and surgical treatment. New York: Thieme; 2010. p. 82–98.
7. Rathore C, Dickson JC, Teotonio R, et al. The utility of 18F-fluorodeoxyglucose PET (FDG PET) in epilepsy surgery. Epilepsy Res. 2014;108:1306–14.
8. Sarikaya I. PET studies in epilepsy. Am J Nucl Med Mol Imaging. 2015;5(5):416–30.
9. Seitz RJ, Piel S, Arnold S, et al. Cerebellar hypometabolism in focal epilepsy is related to age of onset and drug intoxication. Epilepsia. 1996;37(12):1194–9.
10. Vaugier L, Aubert S, McGonigal A, et al. Neural networks underlying hyperkinetic seizures of "temporal lobe" origin. Epilepsy Res. 2009;86(2):200–8.
11. Wang ZI, Jin K, Kakisaka Y, et al. Interconnections in superior temporal cortex revealed by musicogenic seizure propagation. J Neurol. 2012;259(10):2251–4.
12. Yu T, Zhang G-J, Wang Y-P, et al. Surgical treatment of hypermotor seizures originating from the temporal lobe. Seizure. 2013;22(10):862–6.

4 Single Photon Emission Computed Tomography (SPECT) in Epilepsies

Case 4.1 Probable Right Lateral Temporal Lobe Epilepsy (LTLE)

Clinical Information

Chief Complaint *Having had intractable seizures for 10 years*

The patient is a 16-year-old right-handed female presenting with intractable seizures that started 10 years ago. During her seizures, she became pale and had glazed eyes and decreased speech with left-sided deviation of her head and eyes. She has been treated in the past with multiple antiepileptic medications but continued to have a poor seizure control. Her last seizure was 2 months ago and lasted about 1 minute in duration. After the seizure, she had slurred speech and felt sleepy.

Birth history was unremarkable, but she had a history of developmental delay in gross motor, fine motor/visual, language/comprehension, and social capacity. There is no history of head injury, meningitis, or encephalitis.

Current medications include levetiracetam 2000 mg twice a day, oxcarbazepine 900 mg in the morning and 1050 mg at night, zonisamide 200 mg at night, and sertraline 25 mg at night.

Several EEG studies showed focal seizures with somatosensory aura (touching lip, throat/chest), and regional seizure activities in the right frontotemporal area.

The patient underwent an ictal brain perfusion SPECT study, with radioactive tracer injected at 23 seconds after ictal EEG onset. Clinically, the focal seizure lasted for 82 seconds.

On the next day, the patient had an interictal brain perfusion study, followed by a SISCOM analysis.

SPECT and SISCOM Findings

The ictal perfusion images (Fig. 4.1a) show predominant hyperperfusion in the right lateral temporal lobe (red arrows). Additionally, mild to moderate hyperperfusion is noted in the right orbitofrontal lobe, the posteromedial portion of the right parietal lobe, the right thalamus, the right primary visual cortex, the left insular region, and the left cerebellum (white arrows). Tracer activity in the remainder of the cerebral cortices, bilateral basal ganglia, the left thalamus, and the right cerebellum is within normal limits.

The interictal perfusion images (Fig. 4.1b), however, show overall normoperfusion in the right lateral temporal lobe (red arrows). The prior ictal SPECT findings of hyperperfusion in the right orbitofrontal lobe, right posteromedial parietal lobe, right thalamus, right primary visual cortices, left insular region, and left cerebellum are not evident on this interictal study. Minimal to mild hypoperfusion is noted in the parietal

D. Wu, *Clinical Nuclear Medicine Neuroimaging*, https://doi.org/10.1007/978-3-030-40893-0_4

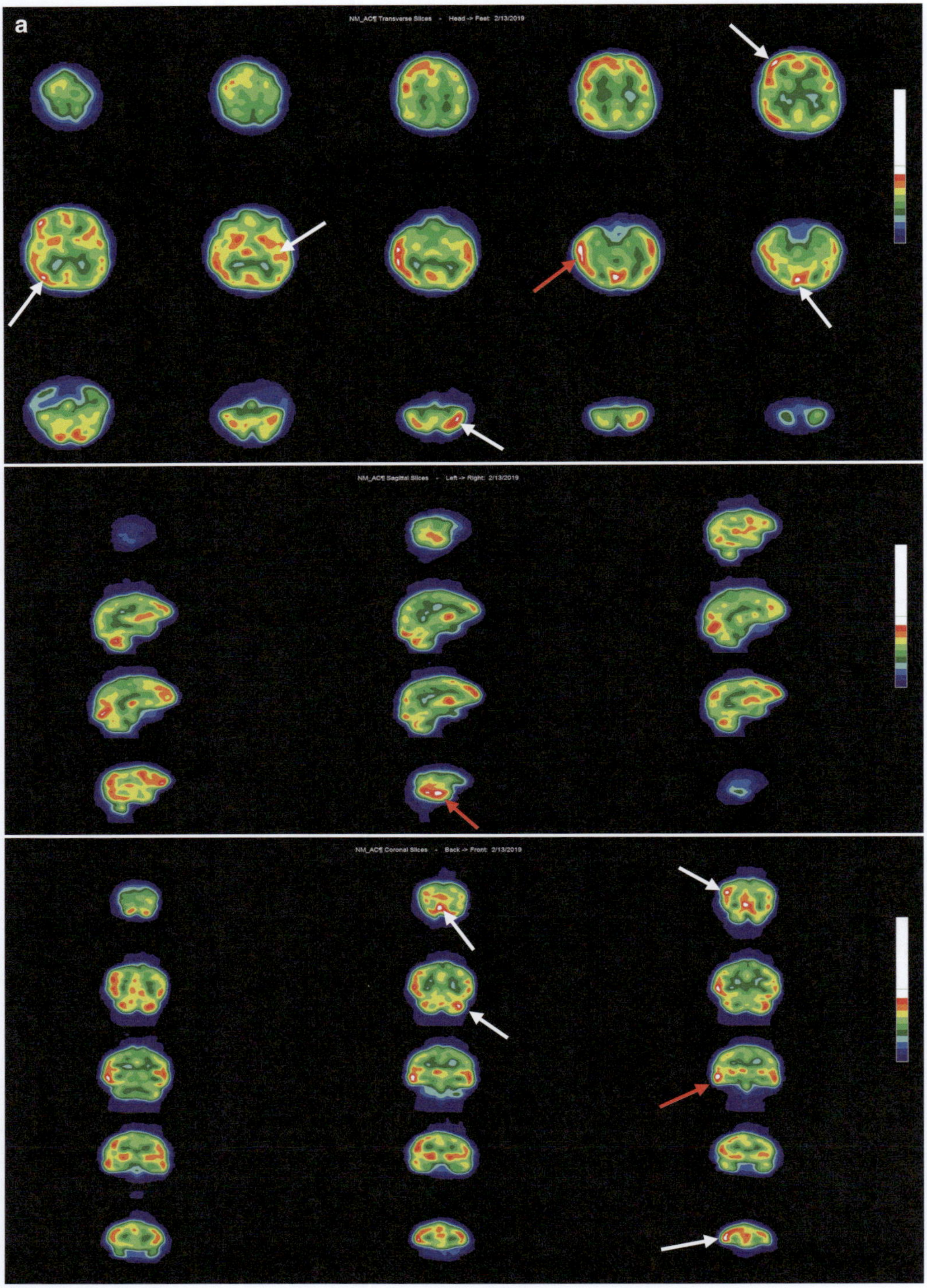

Fig. 4.1 (**a**) A 16-year-old right-handed female with probable right lateral temporal lobe epilepsy (LTLE) – an ictal brain perfusion SPECT. (**b**) A 16-year-old right-handed female with probable right lateral temporal lobe epilepsy (LTLE) – an interictal brain perfusion SPECT. (**c**) A 16-year-old right-handed female with probable right lateral temporal lobe epilepsy (LTLE) – SISCOM analysis. Top Panel: Upper row – Interictal study transaxial slides; Middle row – Ictal study transaxial slides; Lower row – Delta results. Bottom Panel: Top row – T_2 MR images; Bottom row – Delta results coregistered to the brain MRI

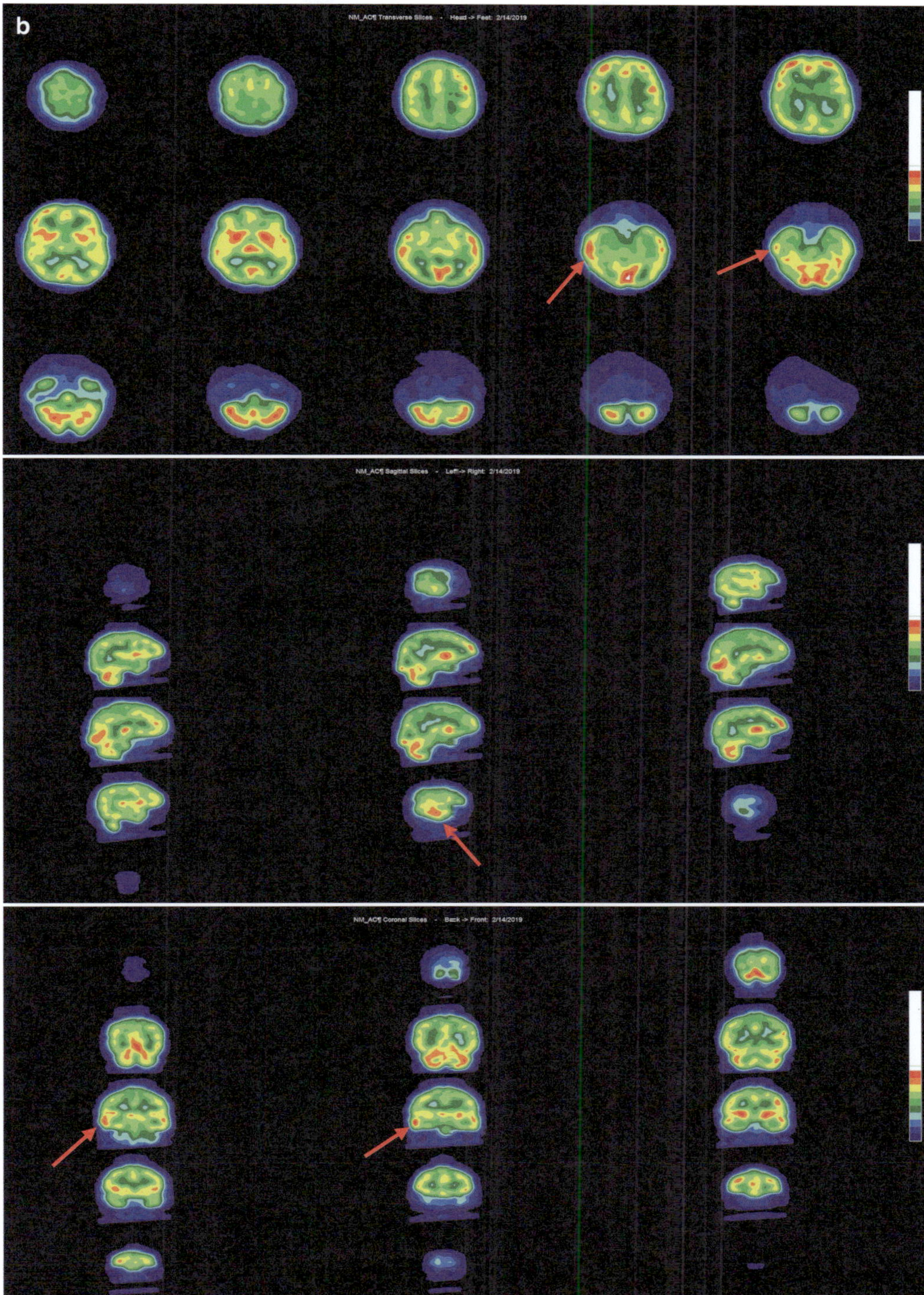

Fig. 4.1 (continued)

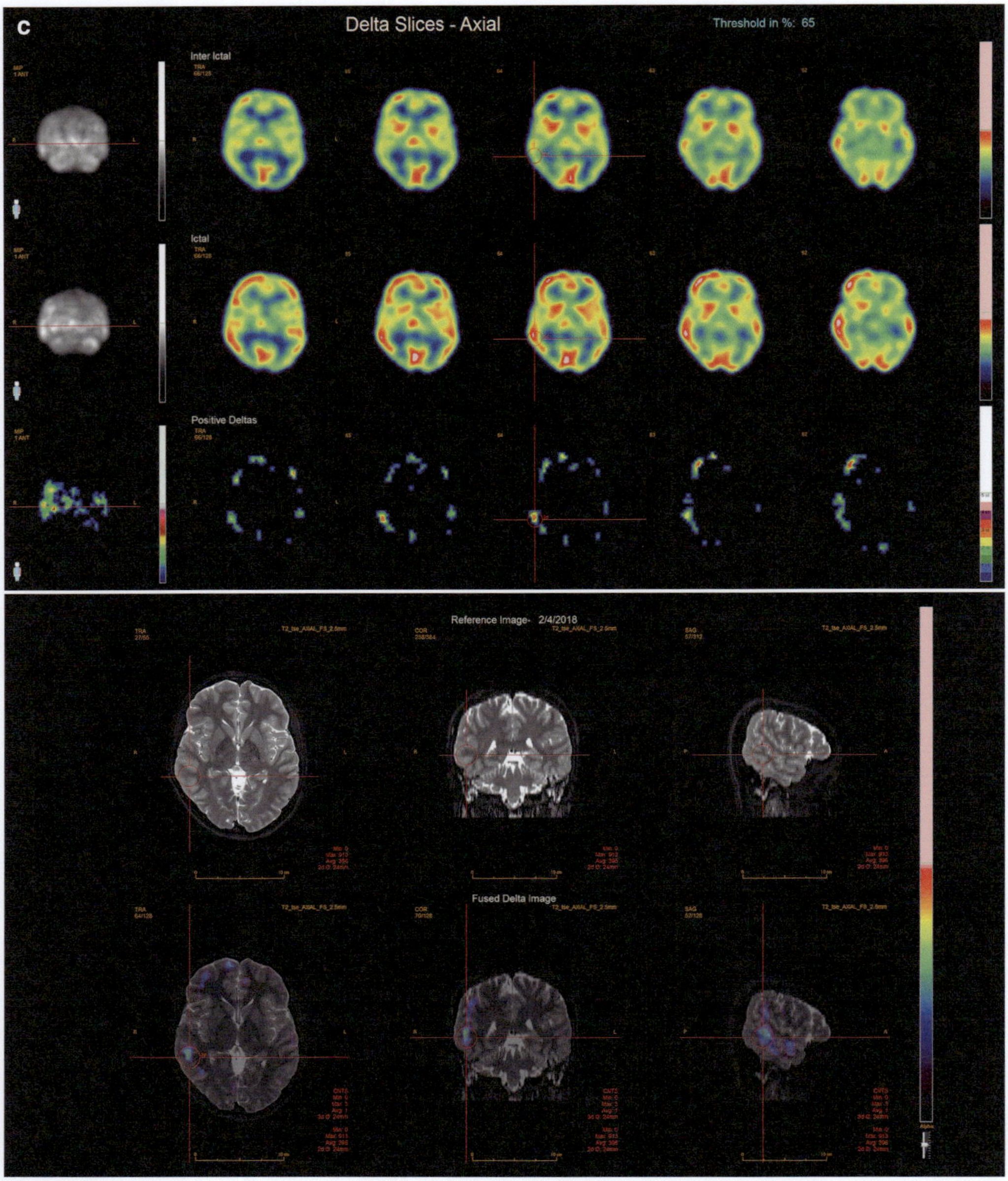

Fig. 4.1 (continued)

lobes, with a bilateral pattern suggestive of a non-epileptogenic nature.

The SISCOM analysis (Fig. 4.1c) demonstrates a dominant positive focus (crosshairs in the lower row of the top panel) in red color, which is coregistered to the lateral posterosuperior portion of the right temporal lobe (crosshairs in the bottom panel) on the patient's T2 MRI sequence, suspicious for an epileptogenic focus/zone. This is adjacent to the right temporo-parieto-occipital (TPO) junction region. A moderate focus is seen in the right orbitofrontal lobe, likely due to seizure propagation, whereas there are no delta positive findings after subtraction in the right thalamus and right primary visual cortex due to similar tracer intensities on both ictal and interictal SPECT scans.

Discussion and Follow-Up

Lateral TLE (LTLE) is less common when compared to mesial/medial TLE (MTLE) [1]. Semiology of LTLE often manifests focal motor seizures, as shown in this case, likely due to rapid seizure propagation into the frontal lobe(s). In this case, prior EEG studies already suggest regional seizure activities in the right frontotemporal area. Although the ictal SPECT images show a predominant cortical hyperperfusion in the lateral right temporal lobe, the involvement is diffuse, indicating local expansion. Additionally several areas of hyperperfusion are noted involving the right orbitofrontal lobe, the posteromedial portion of the right parietal lobe, the right thalamus, the right primary visual cortices, the left insular region, and the left cerebellum, suggestive of seizure propagation. The interictal SPECT images, however, show overall normoperfusion in the lateral right temporal lobe. Also, the several areas of hyperperfusion on the ictal study likely due to seizure propagation are not evident. The mild hypoperfusion in parietal lobes is suggestive of a non-epileptic nature, given the bilateral and symmetric pattern.

The SISCOM analysis reveals a dominant focus coregistered to the lateral posterosuperior portion of the right temporal lobe, suspicious for an epileptogenic focus/zone. Additionally, there is a moderate focus in the right orbitofrontal lobe, suggestive of seizure propagation, but another epileptogenic focus/zone cannot be excluded. Due to the uncertainty, the patient is currently under further workup for potential epilepsy surgery.

Case Summary

Lateral temporal lobe epilepsies (LTLEs) are much less common when compared to mesial temporal epilepsies (MTLEs). Clinical workup of lateral LTEs is a challenge due to rapid seizure propagation. In this case, ictal brain perfusion SPECT study showed focal hyperperfusion in the lateral right temporal lobe, but the localization value is limited due to local expansion and likely propagation to several distal locations. Although interictal SPECT is falsely negative in the lateral right temporal region, SISCOM analysis confirms a dominant focus superimposed in the lateral posterosuperior portion of the right temporal lobe on the patient's MRI, suspicious for an epileptogenic focus/zone.

Case 4.2 Probable Left Occipitoparietal Epilepsy

Clinical Information

Chief Complaint *Having had seizures, memory loss, and functional decline since a head injury 3 years ago*

The patient is a 63-year-old right-handed male presenting with drug-resistant seizures that started shortly after a closed head injury 3 years ago. The seizures manifest as tongue biting, extremity jerking, and loss of consciousness.

In addition to seizures, the patient has been found to have functional decline with increasing difficulty at his work as a public library director. He reports difficulty in decision-making and typing on computer with his right hand. He denies tremor and has no changes in spelling or comprehension. During the visit, his gait was normal and no significant behavioral symptoms were noted.

Past medical history is notable for depression (with two remote episodes of suicidal ideation), sleep apnea, hypertension, hyperlipidemia, hypothyroidism, and coronary artery disease with known myocardial infarction.

Current medications include levothyroxine 75 mcg daily, divalproex 500 mg twice a day, duloxetine 60 mg at night, carvedilol 6.25 mg twice a day, aspirin 81 mg daily, ranitidine 150 mg twice a day, aripiprazole 5 mg daily, clopidogrel 75 mg daily, and atorvastatin 40 mg daily.

MRI of the brain showed age-disproportionate general cortical atrophy, more prominent in the parietal regions. In addition, there were advanced chronic white matter ischemic changes.

SPECT Findings (Fig. 4.2)

The SPECT images show prominent lateral ventricles, posterior horns being more affected than the anterior horns, left > right, consistent with the prior MRI finding of brain atrophy.

There is overall global, minimal to mild hypoperfusion in nearly the entire left hemisphere cerebral cortices. In addition, moderate to severe hypoperfusion is identified in the anteroinferior portion of the left parietal lobe and the posteromedial portion of the left occipital lobe (red arrows). Mild hypoperfusion is also noted in the left thalamus (white arrow) compared to the right.

Radiotracer activity in the remainder of the right hemisphere cerebral cortices, bilateral basal ganglia, right thalamus, and bilateral cerebella is overall within normal limits.

Discussion and Follow-Up

Interpretation of this patient's brain perfusion SPECT study is difficult due to lack of epileptology evaluation and no EEG results for correlation. Given the history of closed head injury which is a common cause of seizures, the brain perfusion SPECT findings are suspicious for at least two interictal epileptogenic foci/zones involving the posteromedial portion of the left occipital and the anteroinferior portion of the left parietal lobe. The left thalamic hypoperfusion is consistent with diaschisis – further imaging evidence of intractable left brain epilepsy.

The left-sided mild global cerebral hypoperfusion has unknown etiology. However, this may be secondary to ischemic vascular disease, given the MRI finding of age-disproportionate advanced chronic white matter ischemic changes. Additional possible etiologies for this finding include sequelae of closed head injury and/or seizure expansion/propagation.

Clinically, the patient was suspected to have corticobasal degeneration (CBD) given the function decline and right-hand typing difficulty. However, the brain perfusion SPECT study shows no defect in basal ganglia. Subsequently, there was clinical concern for Parkinson's plus syndrome, for which a DaTscan was performed and was read as normal. The patient continues to take divalproex, 500 mg twice a day, with a good seizure control.

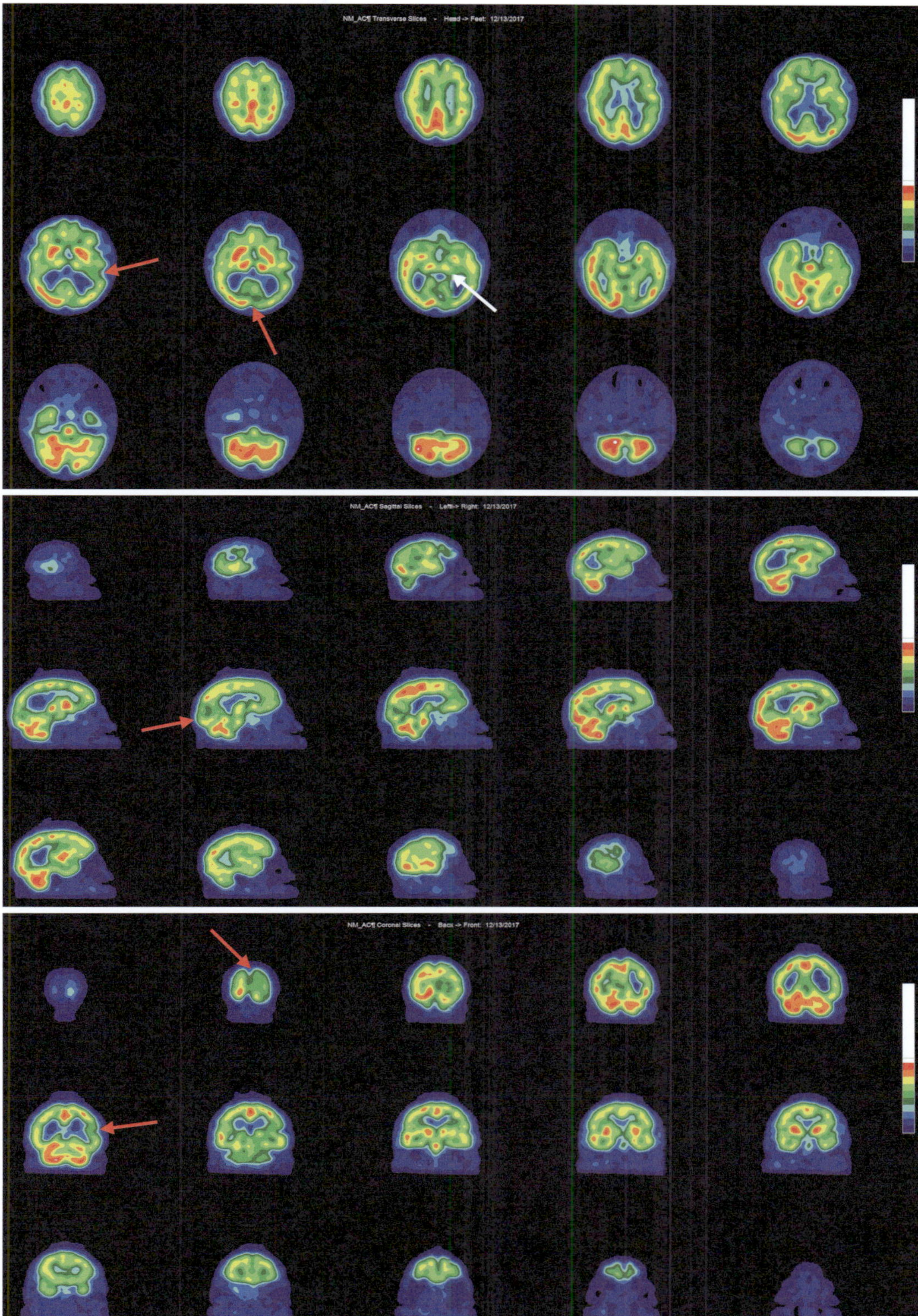

Fig. 4.2 A 63-year-old right-handed male with probable left occipitoparietal lobe epilepsy

Case Summary

Post-traumatic head injury is a common cause for seizures [1, 3]. Interictal SPECT brain study is valuable to detect focal cortical hypoperfusion that may represent an epileptogenic focus/zone for further workup. In this case, the SPECT images show two distinct areas of moderate to severe hypoperfusion involving the posteromedial portion of the left occipital lobe and the anteroinferior portion of the left parietal lobe, suspicious for left parieto-occipital epilepsy with diaschisis involving the left thalamus.

The underlying mechanism of additional mild global hypoperfusion in the nearly entire left hemispheric cerebral cortices is unknown, but likely multifactorial, including possible ischemic vascular disease, sequelae of closed head injury, or seizure expansion/propagation.

Case 4.3 Probable Left Temporal Lobe Epilepsy (TLE)

Clinical Information

Chief Complaint *Medically refractory seizures prior to and after excision of a left brain tumor*

The patient is a 33-year-old right-handed female with history of partial complex seizures and known left insular anaplastic astrocytoma, status post surgical excision 7 years ago followed by adjuvant radiation and chemotherapy. Despite the surgery and therapies, she continues to have seizures, with frequency of twice a week. Her seizures manifest as right arm and leg tingling/stiffening, word-finding difficulty, increased lacrimation/salivation, and intermittent diplopia or blurred vision but no loss of consciousness.

There is no history of head injury, meningitis, or encephalitis.

Current medications include lacosamide 100 mg twice a day, lamotrigine 250 mg daily, and levetiracetam 1500 mg twice a day.

A recent MRI of the brain was stable compared to prior studies and continued to show postoperative changes with a large mixed cystic and solid lesion with inhomogeneous contrast involving the left temporal lobe, left frontal operculum, and left basal ganglia.

SPECT Findings (Fig. 4.3)

The images show a cortical defect in the left inferior frontal lobe, consistent with a surgical cavity (white arrow). Decreased radiotracer activity is identified in the entire left temporal lobe, more prominent in the anterior and inferior portions (red arrows). Tracer activity in the left basal ganglion and thalamus is moderately decreased (green arrow) compared to the contralateral.

Tracer activity in the remainder of the cerebral cortices, the right basal ganglion/thalamus, and the bilateral cerebella is within normal limits, indicating normoperfusion.

Discussion and Follow-Up

This patient's initial (pre-surgical) partial complex seizures were likely secondary to or related to known left insular anaplastic astrocytoma. After the surgical resection and adjuvant chemoradiation, however, she continues to have drug-resistant seizures. The SPECT images show postsurgical changes in the inferior lateral frontal lobe and diffuse hypoperfusion in the entire left temporal lobe, more prominent in the anterior and inferior portions, which, in conjunction with the seizure semiology, is suspicious for left TLE. However, given the abnormal MRI finding, left temporal recurrent low-grade brain tumor or post-radiation necrosis cannot be excluded. The mild hypoperfusion in the left thalamus and asymmetric hypoperfusion in the left basal ganglion may represent diaschisis, although this could also be sequelae of post-surgical/treatment changes.

After the brain perfusion SPECT study, the patient had a follow-up visit with her radiation oncologist and underwent a repeat MRI of the brain, which was stable. Therefore, there was no clinical and radiographic evidence of brain tumor progression. She had been treated with three antiepileptic medications (lamotrigine, levetiracetam, and lacosamide) with reduced seizure frequency.

Case Summary

This patient's history of left insular anaplastic astrocytoma and post-surgical persistent seizures raised concerns for a recurrent brain tumor. Brain perfusion SPECT shows post-surgical changes in the left inferior frontal lobe and diffuse hypoperfusion in the entire left temporal lobe with involvement of the ipsilateral basal ganglia and thalamus. In conjunction with the patient's seizure semiology, these findings are suspicious for TLE, although left temporal low-grade tumor or post-radiation necrosis cannot be excluded. This imaging impression was supported by limited clinical follow-up data.

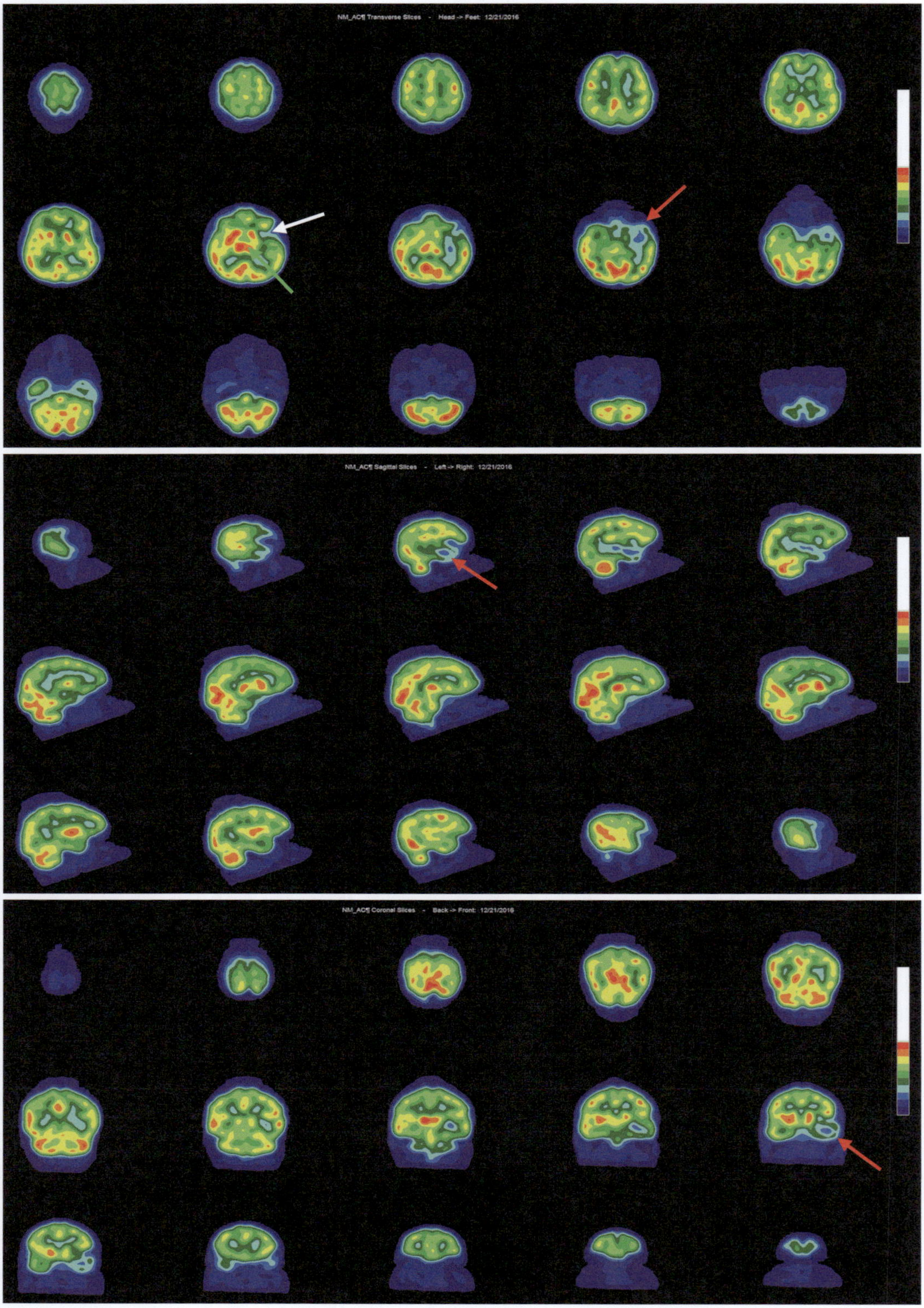

Fig. 4.3 A 33-year-old right-handed female with probable left TLE

Case 4.4 Surgically Proven Right Parietal Lobe Epilepsy (PLE) Due to Focal Cortical Dysplasia (FCD)

Clinical Information

Chief Complaint *Having had frequent refractory seizures since age of 5 months*

The patient is a 3-year-old ambidextrous-handed (right > left) girl presenting with medically refractory focal motor seizures and infantile spasms that started when she was 5 months old. Past treatments included steroids, ACTH, and multiple antiepileptic medications.

The seizures occur at variable times, but mostly in the mornings, and are triggered by sun exposure without accompanying aura. The seizures manifest as brief events during which she would have a blank stare with fluttering eyelids and shaking upper extremities. The duration of the seizures was often a few seconds but sometimes lasted 20–25 seconds. If the patient was standing when the seizure occurred, she would fall forward. She would return to her baseline state shortly after the seizures.

The patient does not have a history of head injury, meningitis, or encephalitis. Birth history was unremarkable. Development history is notable for expressive speech delay. Family history is negative for seizures or epilepsy but is notable for ADHD in her siblings.

Current medications include trileptal 360 mg twice a day, clobazam 25 mg at night, diazepam 2.5 mg rectal gel PRN, and topiramate 100 mg twice a day.

Several prior MRI studies of the brain were unremarkable.

Brain FDG PET with EEG monitoring demonstrated a region of local cortical hypometabolism in the anterosuperolateral portion of the right occipital lobe, suspicious for an interictal epileptogenic focus/zone.

EEG studies consistently showed focal epileptiform discharges from right parietal/posterior temporal/centrotemporal region.

An ictal SPECT perfusion study was performed, with radiotracer injection at 4-second ictal onset, and flush completed prior to seizure generalization at 16 seconds. Clinical observation and EEG study showed that this was a typical seizure while awake shortly after provoked arousal from sleep.

Afterward, an interictal SPECT perfusion study was performed, and followed by a SISCOM analysis.

SPECT and SISCOM Findings

The ictal brain perfusion SPECT (Fig. 4.4a) shows an area of cortical hyperperfusion in the posterior and posterolateral portion of the right parietal/occipital lobes (red arrows), suspicious for an ictal epileptogenic focus with local expansion. Hyperperfusion is also noted in the bilateral insular regions (white arrows), with unknown etiology. Tracer activity in the remainder of the cerebral cortices, bilateral basal ganglia, thalami, and cerebella is within normal limits, indicating normoperfusion.

In contrast, the interictal SPECT study (Fig. 4.4b) reveals focal hypoperfusion in the posterior and posterolateral portion of the right parietal/occipital lobes (red arrows), suspicious for an interictal epileptic focus/zone. Again, symmetric hyperperfusion is noted in the bilateral insular regions (white arrows).

The SISCOM analysis (Fig. 4.4c, top panel) confirms a dominant delta focus in red color indicating that the difference is more than 3 standardized deviations (SD), which coregisters in the right posterior parietal cortex on the patient's MRI (Fig. 4.4c, bottom panel). This is suspicious for an epileptogenic focus/zone. Two foci in orange-red color (>2 SD) are noted in the right basal ganglia/thalamus region and left frontal lobe, suggestive of seizure propagation.

Discussion and Follow-Up

This case highlights the value of nuclear medicine neuroimaging studies for MRI-normal patients with intractable epilepsies due to focal cortical dysplasia (FCD) [3, 7]. The patient

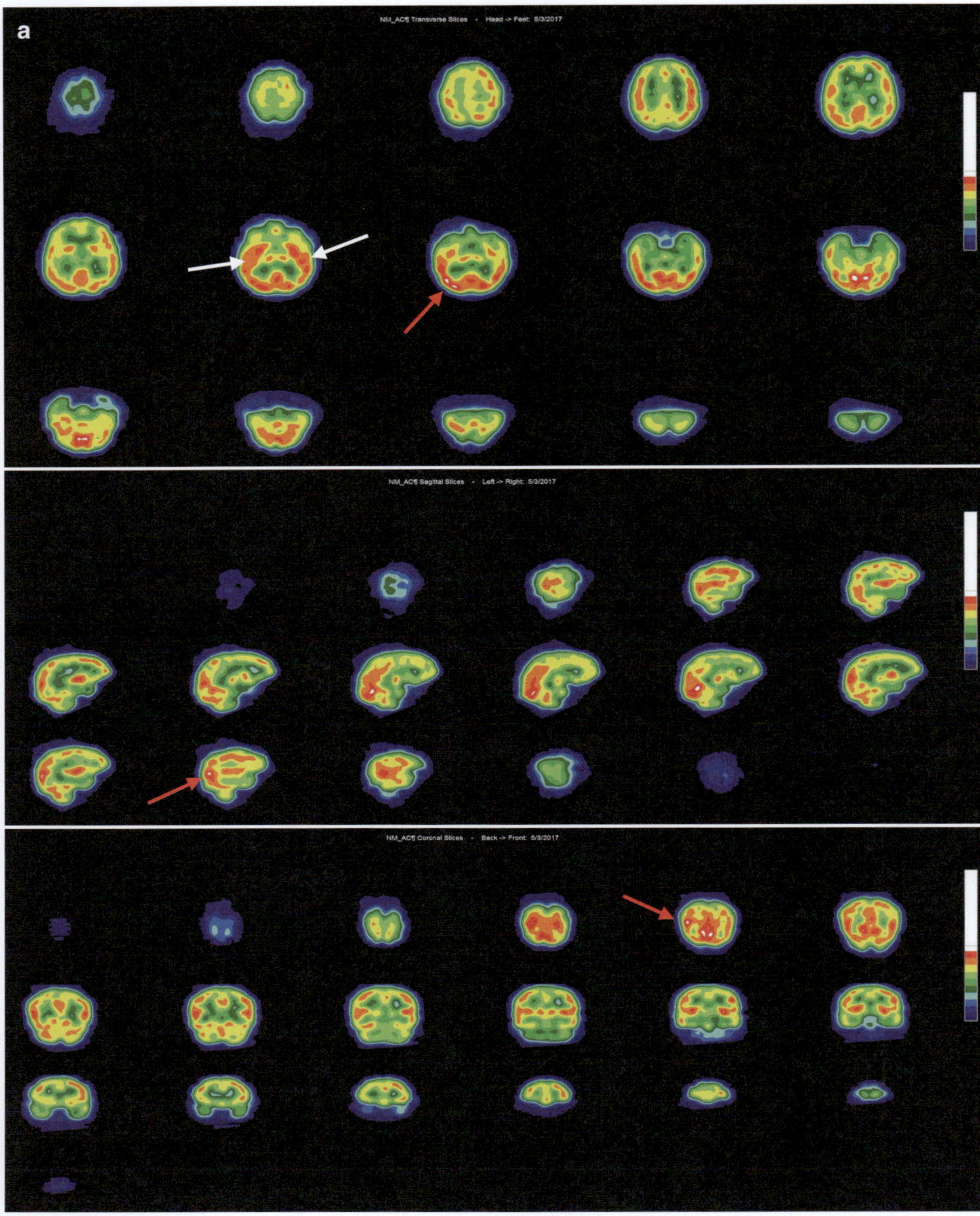

Fig. 4.4 (**a**) A 3-year-old ambidextrous-handed female with surgically proven right parietal lobe epilepsy (PLE) secondary to focal cortical dysplasia (FCD) – *an ictal study* (**b**) A 3-year-old ambidextrous-handed female with surgically proven right parietal lobe epilepsy (PLE) secondary to focal cortical dysplasia (FCD) – *an interictal study* (**c**) A 3-year-old ambidextrous-handed female with surgically proven right parietal lobe epilepsy (PLE) secondary to focal cortical dysplasia (FCD) – *SISCOM analysis*

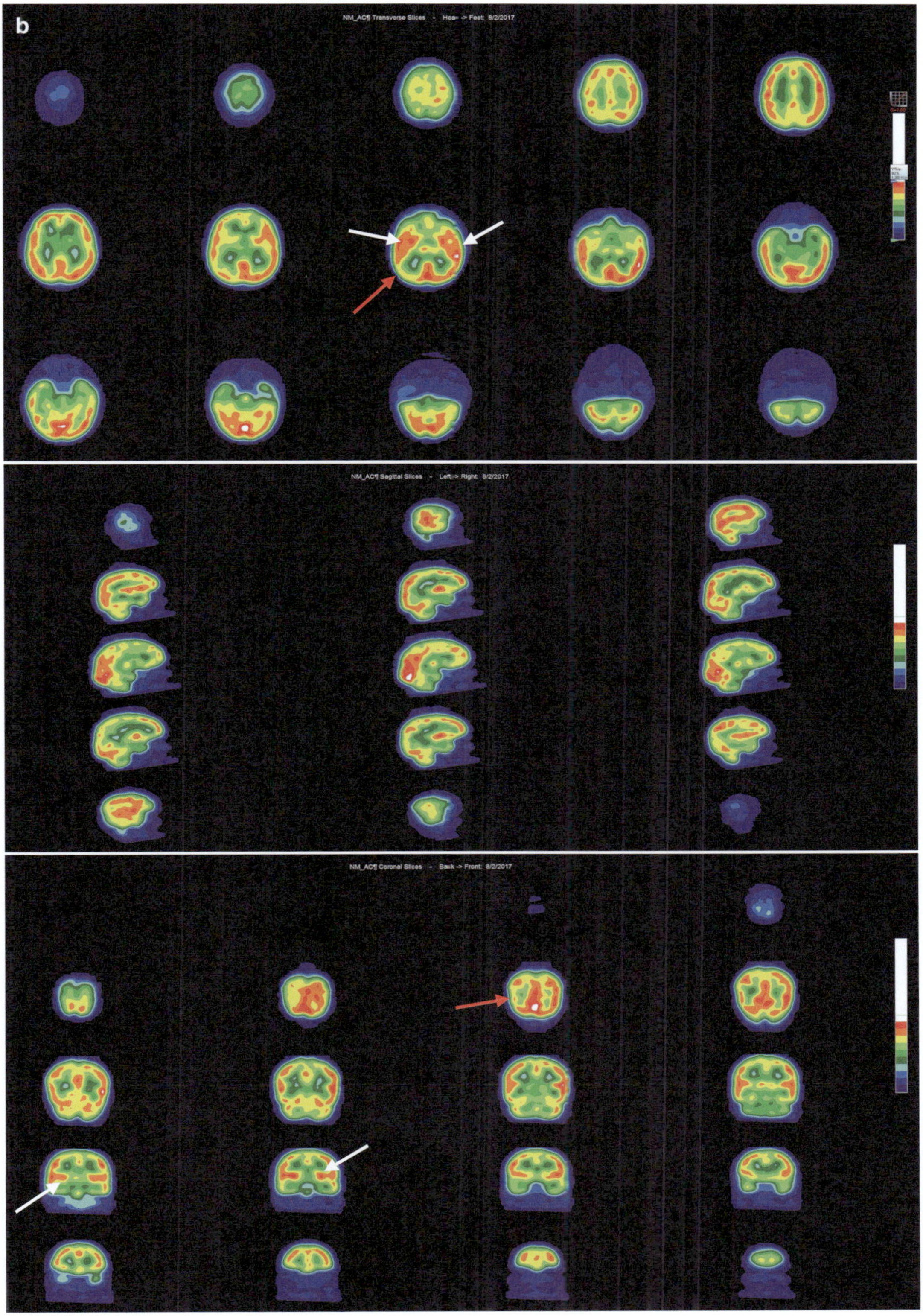

Fig. 4.4 (continued)

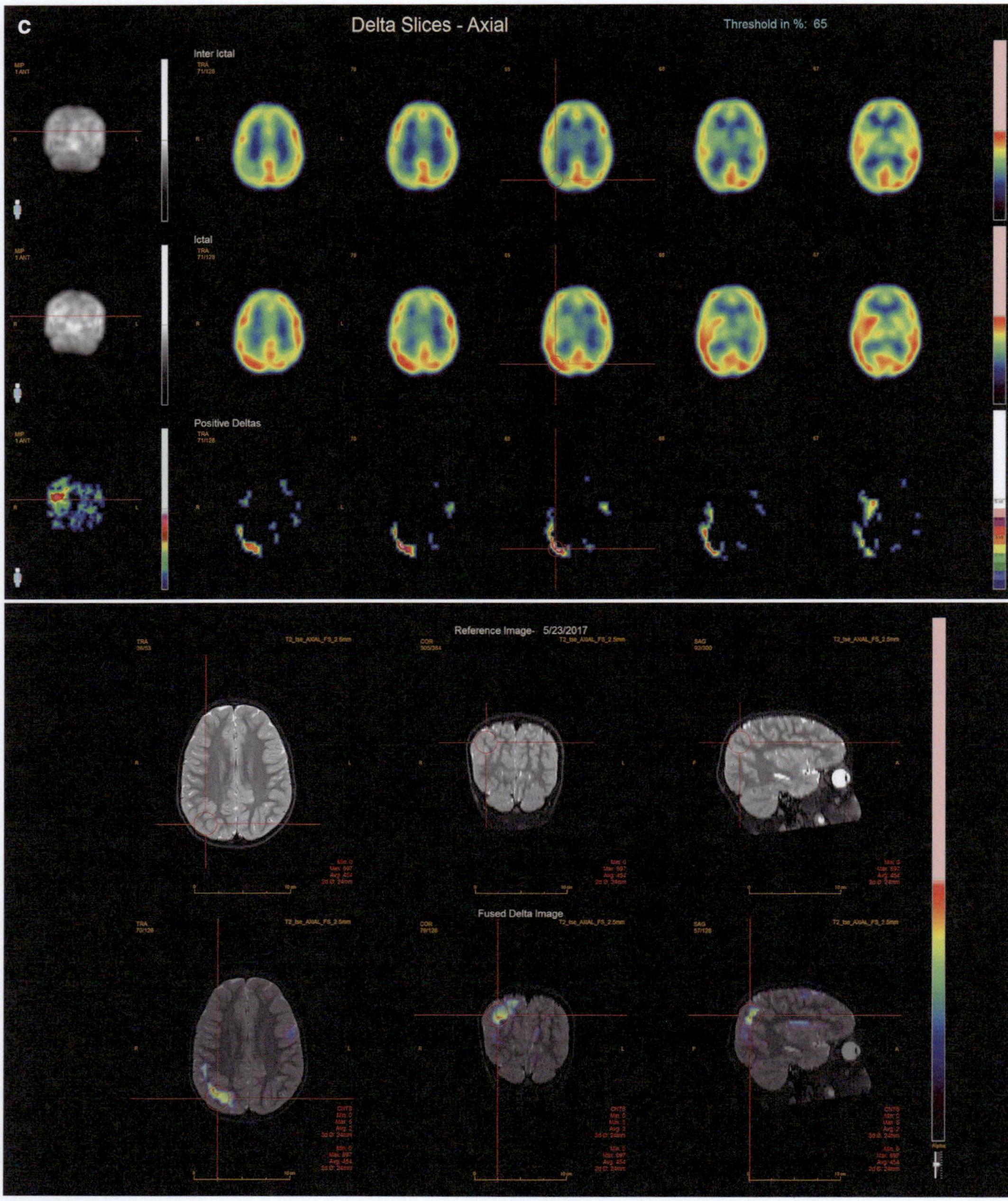

Fig. 4.4 (continued)

underwent brain MRI prior to and after a positive ictal SPECT brain perfusion scan; all the MRI studies were read as unremarkable.

In line with the prior FDG brain PET findings, ictal and interictal SPECT brain perfusion studies in this case consistently show cortical perfusion abnormalities in the right posterior parietal lobe. The SISCOM analysis further reveals a dominant delta focus superimposed in the right posterior parietal cortex on the patient's MRI. The color of the dominant focus is red, indicating the difference of tracer intensity in this region between the interictal and ictal SPECT scans is more than 3 SD, suspicious for an epileptogenic focus/zone. In addition, there is a focus in orange-red (more than 2 SD) in the right basal ganglia/thalamus and left frontal regions, suggestive of seizure propagation. The focal hyperperfusion in the bilateral insular regions has unknown etiology and uncertain clinical significance (likely non-epileptic in nature), given the symmetric pattern, the similar tracer intensity on both ictal and interictal SPECT studies, and the negative delta results on SISCOM analysis.

After the SPECT studies, an elective stereo-EEG implantation study was completed, which confirmed an epileptogenic origin in this patient's posteroinferior portion of the parietal region.

The patient then underwent elective parieto-occipital craniotomy for surgical resection of the epileptic posterior right parietal cortex. Just prior to the surgery, the patient had a Stealth MRI of the brain with gadolinium, which was still read unremarkable for the area suspicious for cortical dysplasia. However, pathology was consistent with focal cortical dysplasia with dysmorphic neurons (International League Against Epilepsy type IIa) [5].

The patient has been seizure-free for 1 year after the epilepsy surgery, even off antiepileptic medication, with improving developmental and cognitive functions.

Case Summary

This case shows the value of a combined nuclear medicine neuroimaging approach including ictal and interictal SPECT scans as well as subsequent SISCOM analysis. This comprehensive approach plays a crucial rule in the pre-surgical evaluation of an MRI-normal patient with focal cortical dysplasia (FCD) that is highly epileptogenic and often drug-resistant [1, 5]. Prior FDG PET was also informative but less accurate in localization as shown in this case. Constellation of the clinical semiology, EEG results, and clinical nuclear medicine neuroimaging studies (FDG PET, ictal/interictal SPECTs and SISCOM analysis) is highly suggestive of right posterior parietal lobe epilepsy, which was surgically proven with FCD being the underlying cause. The patient has achieved 1 year of seizure-free after epilepsy surgery.

Case 4.5 Surgically Proven Left Lateral Temporal Lobe Epilepsy (LTLE)

Clinical Information

Chief Complaint *Having had medically refractory seizures since traumatic brain injury 2 years ago*

The patient is a 19-year-old right-handed male presenting with severe medically refractory epilepsy for 2 years. His seizures started 2 years ago, for which he was treated with levetiracetam. The initial seizure type was reported to be grand mal. One month after the initial seizure onset, he had a motor vehicle accident (MVA) with traumatic brain injury (TBI). Over the last 2 years, he was treated with increased dose of levetiracetam but still had poor seizure control. Recently he has been on valproate, clobazam, and zonisamide; however, breakthrough seizures still occurred 2–6 times per month. His seizures manifest as a blank stare with no response to voice or touch, left head deviation, mouth automatisms, forced laugh, and nonsensical speech. The seizures occur while awake and during sleep and usually last 1–2 minutes, without apparent aura or trigger.

There is no prior history of meningitis or encephalitis. Birth history and development are unremarkable. Family history is also unremarkable.

Current medications include clobazam 40 mg at night, divalproex 500 mg twice a day, zonisamide 600 mg at night, and diazepam rectal gel 15 mg PRN.

Initial EEG studies 2 years before this presentation showed left hemispheric epileptic activities. Recent EEGs confirmed the early finding and further showed evidence of two different seizure types, both in the left hemisphere.

Brain FDG PET study showed focal hypometabolism in left parietal region, suspicious for an interictal epileptogenic focus/zone.

CT of the head/brain following the MVA/TBI revealed pneumocephalus and subarachnoid hemorrhage, which have now improved or resolved.

Prior MRI of the brain was initially read as normal. However, image review, in conjunction with the abnormal FDG PET study, shows a focal cortical dysplasia in the left parietal region.

Three brain perfusion SPECT studies were then performed in the following order:

- An ictal SPECT perfusion was performed for his typical dialeptic seizure which appeared to be more consistent with an epileptic spasm. The radioactive tracer was injected at 5-second seizure onset and flush completed at 8 seconds into the seizure.
- Another ictal SPECT perfusion was carried out for his typical asymmetric tonic seizure. The radioactive tracer was injected at 10-second seizure onset and flush completed at 12 seconds into the seizure.
- An interictal SPECT perfusion was then performed for SISCOM analysis.

SPECT and SISCOM Findings

The first ictal SPECT study (Fig. 4.5a) demonstrates focally increased tracer activity in the posterosuperior portion of the left temporal lobe (red arrows), indicating cortical hyperperfusion. In contrast, tracer activity in the left thalamus (white arrow) is minimally to mildly decreased, suggestive of diaschisis.

The second ictal SPECT study (Fig. 4.5b), however, only shows a small focus of mild tracer activity in the left forefrontal lobe (red arrow, the top panel), which is not evident or confirmatory on other views. The previously noted focal hyperperfusion in the posterosuperior portion of the left temporal lobe is not evident, although persistent minimal to mild hypoperfusion is noted in the left thalamus (white arrow). The asymmetric tracer activity in the bilateral forefrontal lobes (red arrow, the bottom panel) is likely due to asymmetric and diffuse hypoperfusion to the left forefrontal lobe.

The interictal SPECT study (Fig. 4.5c) shows asymmetric, mild to moderately decreased tracer activity in the left superolateral temporal region (red arrows). Despite head-tilting and heterogeneity, tracer activity in the remainder of the cerebral cortices, bilateral basal ganglia, thalami, and cerebella is within normal limits.

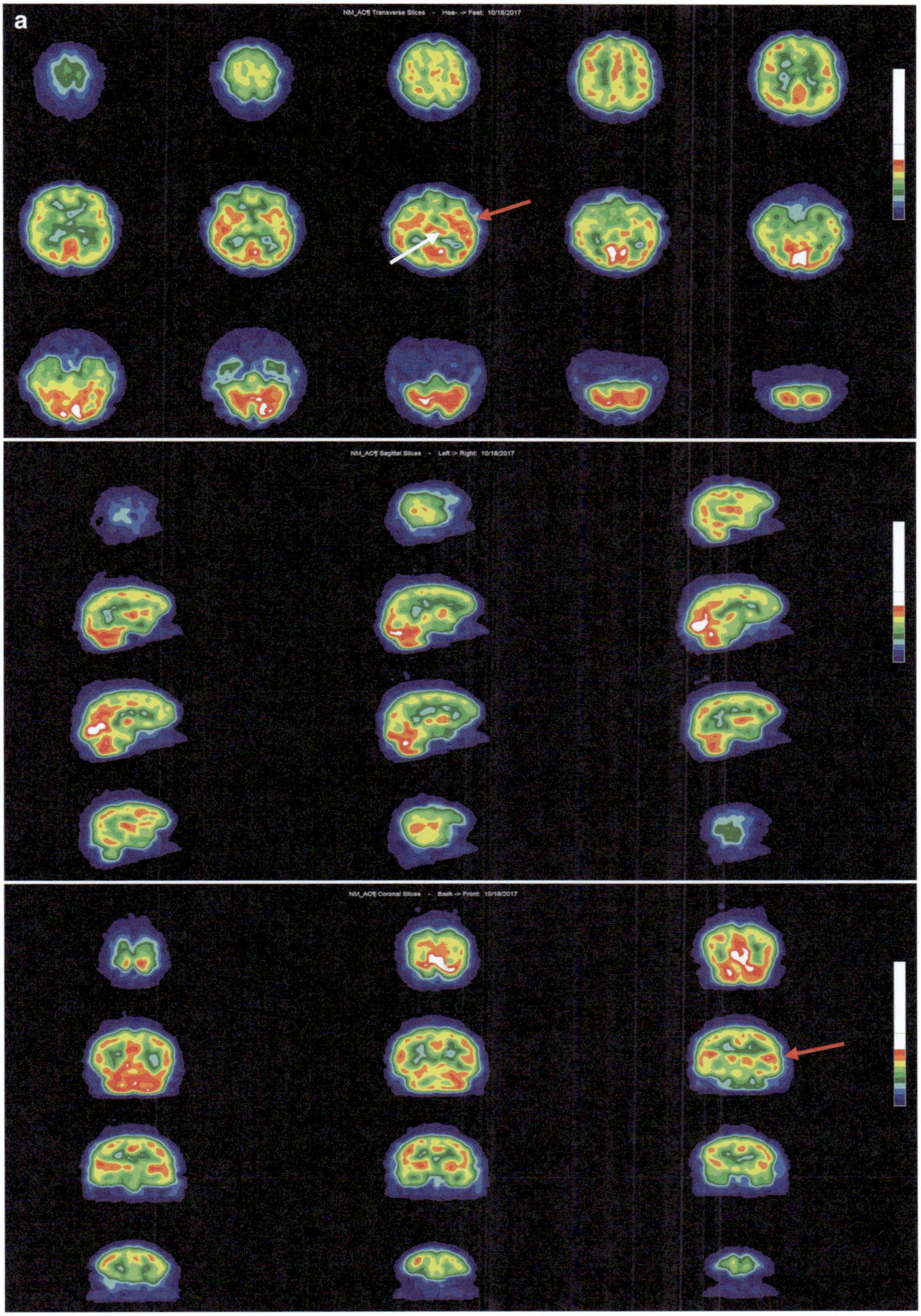

Fig. 4.5 (**a**) A 19-year-old right-handed male with surgically proven left lateral temporal lobe epilepsy (LTLE) – the first ictal study. (**b**) A 19-year-old right-handed male with surgically proven left lateral temporal lobe epilepsy (LTLE) – the second ictal study. (**c**) A 19-year-old right-handed male with surgically proven left lateral temporal lobe epilepsy (LTLE) – the interictal study. (**d**) A 19-year-old right-handed male with surgically proven left lateral temporal lobe epilepsy (LTLE) – the first SISCOM analysis. (**e**) A 19-year-old right-handed male with surgically proven left lateral temporal lobe epilepsy (LTLE) – the second SISCOM analysis

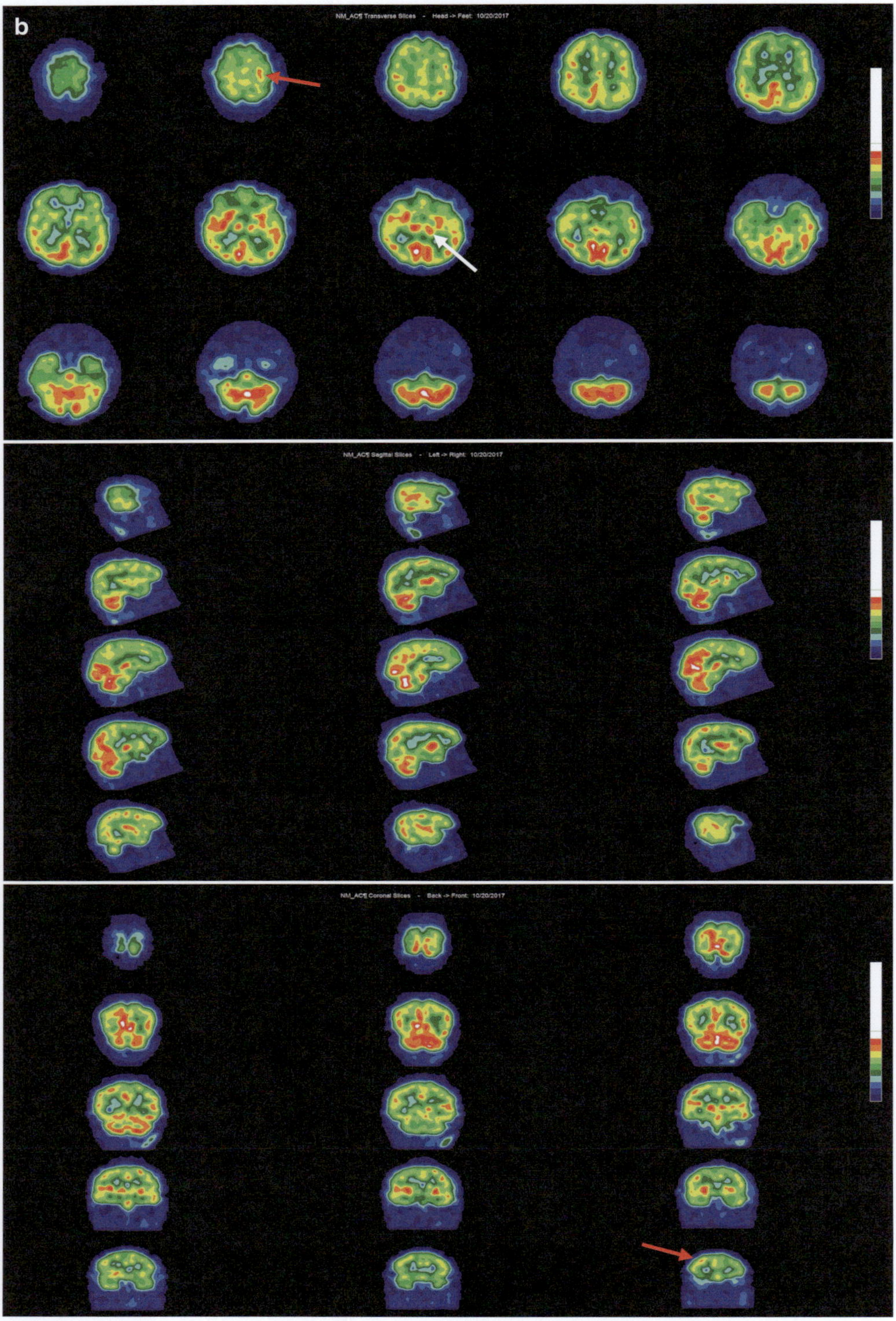

Fig. 4.5 (continued)

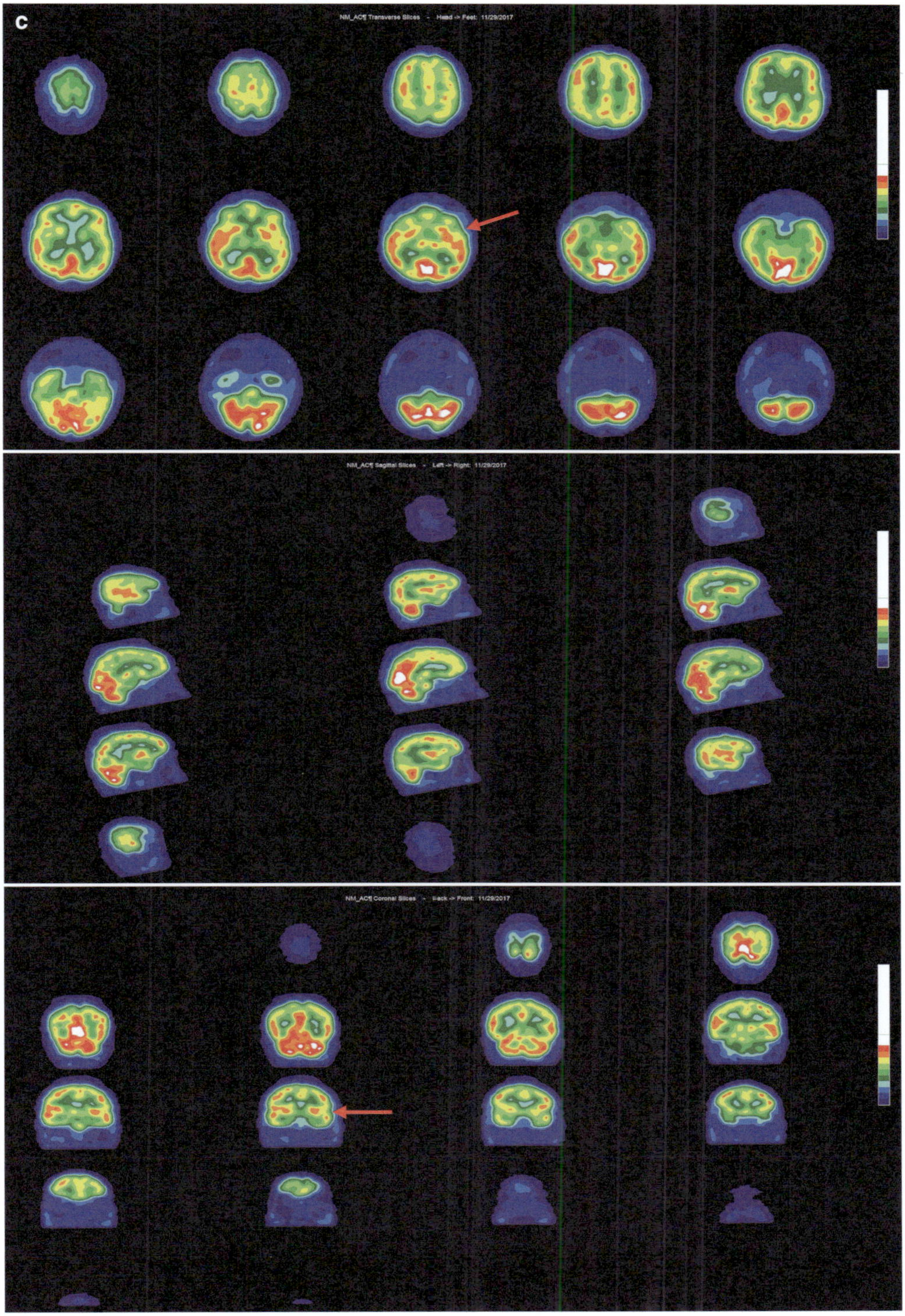

Fig. 4.5 (continued)

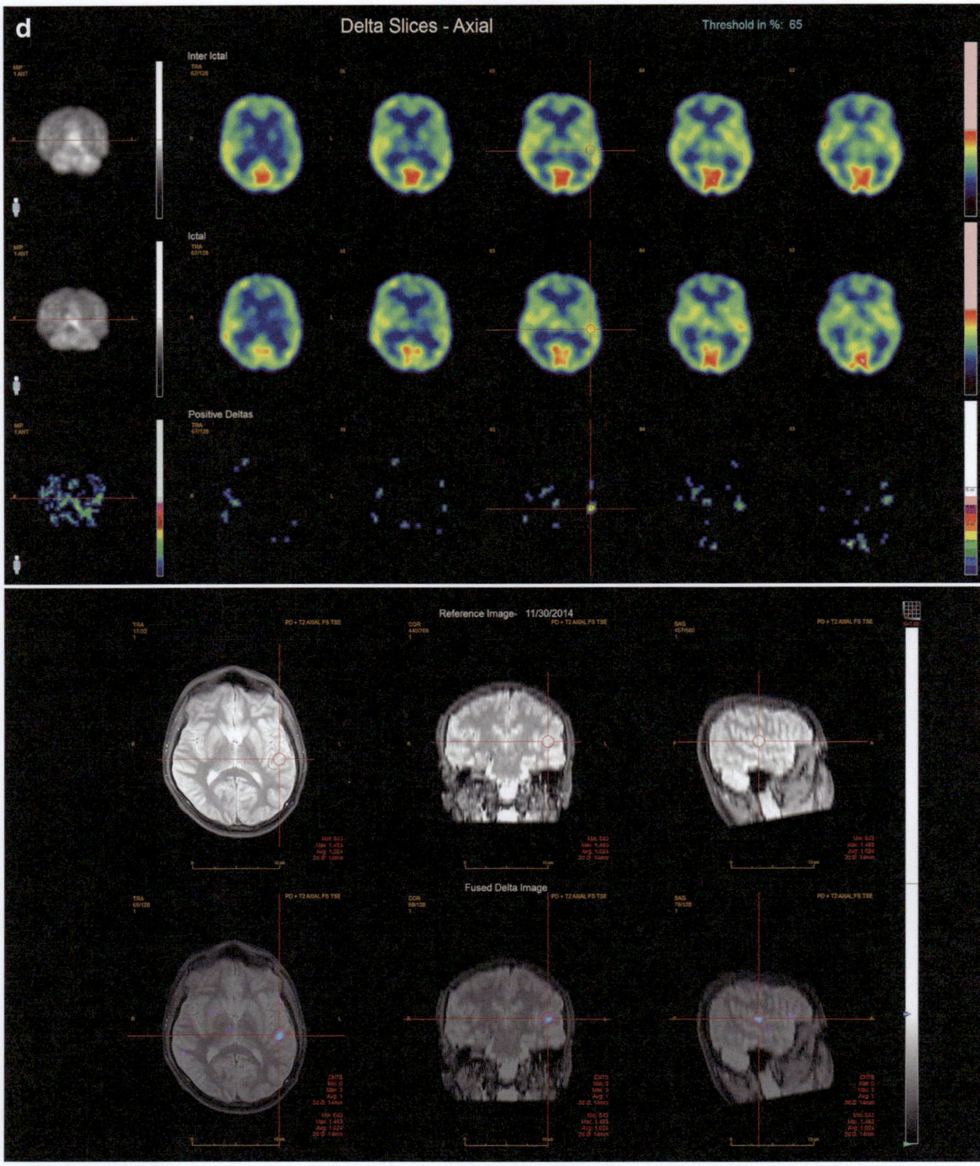

Fig. 4.5 (continued)

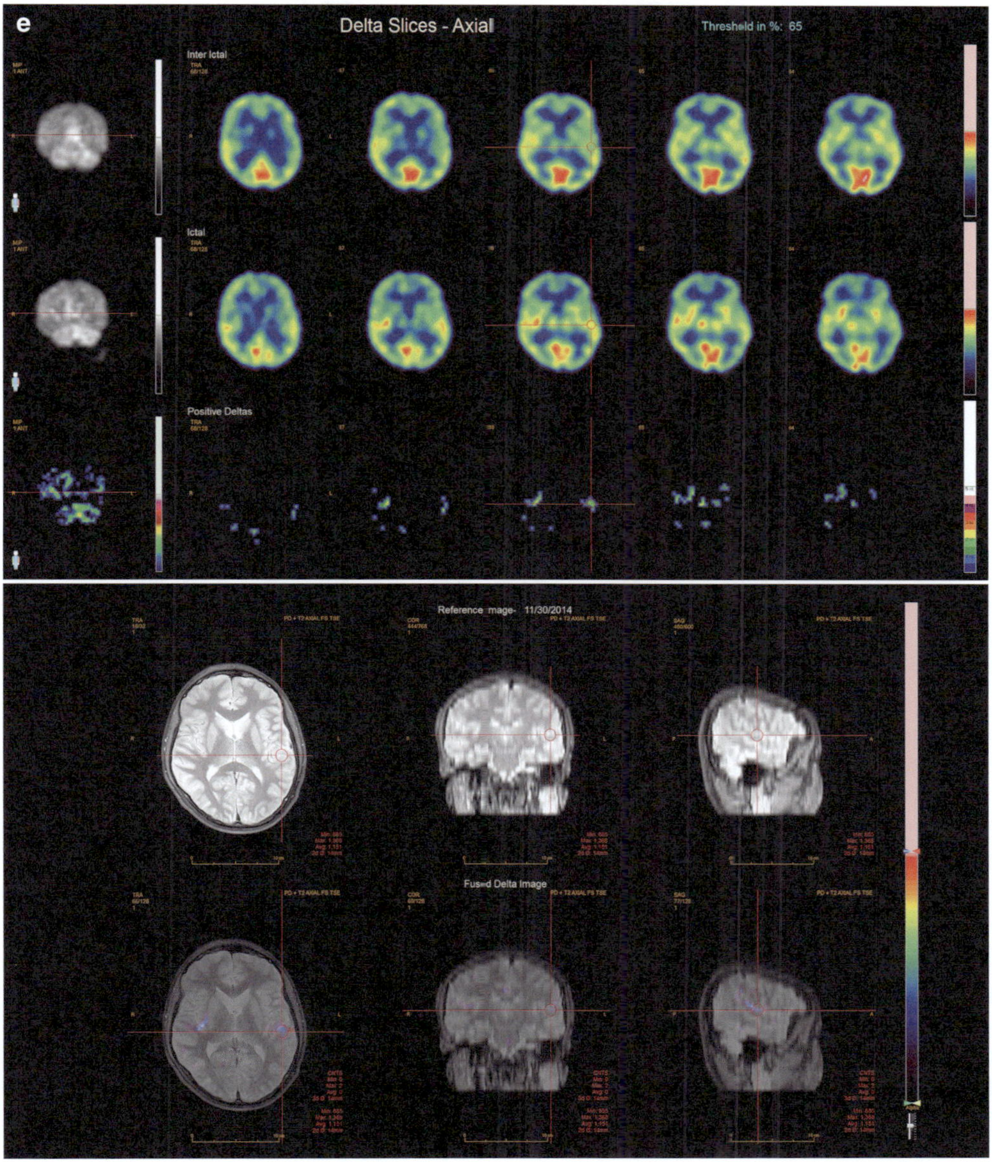

Fig. 4.5 (continued)

SISCOM analysis (Fig. 4.5d) of the first ictal study versus the interictal study demonstrates a delta focus with the difference being >2 SD, corresponding to the left superolateral temporal cortex on MRI, suspicious for left LTLE.

The SISCOM analysis of the second ictal study versus the same interictal study (Fig. 4.5e), however, shows a small focus in blue color indicating the difference being <2 SD in the posterosuperior portion of the left temporal lobe of uncertain significance. In contrast, there is a focus in red-orange indicating the difference being >2 SD in the right insular region, suggestive of seizure propagation. There are no appreciable foci after subtraction in the frontal lobes, with a special reference to the left. Therefore, there is no convincing evidence of an epileptogenic focus/zone in the anticipated left frontal lobe.

Discussion and Follow-Up

This patient has a complex seizure semiology including at least dialeptic seizures and asymmetric tonic seizures. Although the prior FDG PET and MRI show findings suspicious for left parietal lobe epilepsy, the first ictal brain perfusion study, targeted for the typical dialeptic seizure in the patient, shows focal robust hyperperfusion in the posterosuperior portion of the left temporal lobe, suspicious for an ictal epileptic focus/zone. The second ictal study targeted the asymmetric tonic seizure only shows mild and questionable hyperperfusion in the left frontal lobe where another epileptic focus was clinically suspected. Nevertheless, there is persistent, minimal to mild hypoperfusion on both ictal studies in the left thalamus, consistent with diaschisis, which is indirect evidence of intractable left brain epilepsy. The interictal SPECT study showed hypoperfusion to the left temporal lobe as expected. The SISCOM analysis of the first ictal and the interictal SPECT studies confirms an epileptogenic focus/zone in the superior lateral portion of the left temporal lobe. In contrast, the SISCOM analysis of the second ictal study versus the interictal study shows no convincing epileptogenic focus/zone. Instead, there is evidence of seizure propagation to the right insular region.

Extensive further workup, including stereo-EEG monitoring, was confirmatory for left TLE. The patient then underwent subtotal left temporal lobectomy, with a final pathology diagnosis of focal white matter neuronal heterotopia, which is a neurological condition often causing intractable seizures [1]. During the follow-up, the patient has been seizure-free for 1 month after the epilepsy surgery, compared to four to five seizure episodes a day prior to the surgery.

Summary

Although prior FDG PET and MRI results suggest left parietal lobe epilepsy in this patient, ictal and interictal brain perfusion studies in conjunction with SISCOM analysis consistently revealed an epileptogenic focus/zone coregistered in the superolateral portion of the left temporal cortex on the patient's MRI. The second ictal SPECT, in conjunction with SISCOM analysis, helped to rule out additional epileptic focus/zone. The scintigraphic diagnosis was further confirmed by stereo-EEG monitoring. The patient underwent a subtotal left temporal lobectomy and has been seizure-free for 1 month since the surgery.

Case 4.6 Probable Left Insular Epilepsy

Clinical Information

Chief Complaint *Having had medically refractory nocturnal focal seizures since childhood*

The patient is a 38-year-old right-handed male presenting with focal to bilateral tonic-clonic seizures (FBTCS) that started at the age of 5. Despite anti-seizure treatment with multiple medications including phenobarbital, phenytoin, valproate, carbamazepine, and levetiracetam, his seizures have persisted. He reports that these seizures always begin with a "hard-to-describe" sensation that occurs as a wave over his body. He then loses consciousness and starts convulsing, but no lateralizing signs that have been reported. There is no history of head trauma or incontinence. The seizure duration is not entirely clear. Postictally, he returns to his baseline status within seconds to minutes. Although all the prior seizures were reported to occur exclusively during sleep, there were two recent seizure episodes that occurred during the daytime.

He has an unremarkable birth history and no history of developmental delay. Medical history is notable for Crohn's disease and osteoporosis, but there was no history of head injury, meningitis, or encephalitis. Family history is negative for seizures or epilepsy.

Current antiepileptic medications include levetiracetam, 2000 mg twice a day, and carbamazepine 600 mg three times a day.

A 24-hour video-EEG recording was normal during wakefulness and drowsiness.

Prior brain MRI was reported normal. A recent CT of the head/brain was also unremarkable.

The patient had an ictal SPECT with radioactive tracer injection at 12-second ictal onset and flush completed 19 seconds into the seizure.

Afterward, he underwent an interictal SPECT for SISCOM analysis.

SPECT and SISCOM Findings

The ictal SPECT perfusion images (Fig. 4.6a) show focally increased radioactive tracer activity in the left insular region (red arrows), to a lesser degree in the left lateral temporal lobe (white arrows). Radioactive tracer activity in the remainder of the cerebral cortices, bilateral basal ganglia, thalami, and cerebella is essentially symmetric and within normal limits.

In contrast, the interictal brain perfusion SPECT study (Fig. 4.6b) only shows mildly increased tracer activity or normointensity in the left posterior insular region (red arrows), whereas the previously increased tracer activity seen in the left lateral temporal lobe is no longer evident. Instead, minimal to mildly decreased tracer activity is noted in the left frontal lobe and the superomedial portion of the left parietal lobe (white arrows).

As expected, SISCOM analysis (Fig. 4.6c, top panel) reveals a dominant delta focus in red color indicating the difference being >3 SD in the left insular region, suspicious for an epileptogenic focus/zone (red arrow). Also, two small foci in red-orange color indicating the difference being >2 SD are noted in the right basal ganglia (white arrow) and the lateral left temporal lobe (green arrow), suggestive of seizure propagation. There is no discrete focus in the left frontal lobe. After coregistration, the suspected epileptogenic focus/zone appears to reside in the posterior left insular cortex on the patient's MRI (Fig. 4.6c, bottom panel).

Discussion and Follow-Up

In this case, although the clinical semiology is suggestive of seizures arising from the insula or frontal cortex, anatomic neuroimaging studies (CT and MRI) were unremarkable, and EEG monitoring was normal without lateralized findings. The ictal brain perfusion SPECT, however, demonstrates dominant and focal cortical hyperperfusion, diffusely involving the entire left insular region, which is suspicious for an ictal epileptic focus/zone. Also, moderate hyperperfusion is noted in the lateral left temporal lobe, suspicious for seizure propagation. Normoperfusion is seen in the remainder of the cerebral cortices, basal ganglia, thalami, and cerebella, without evidence of diaschisis. In contrast, the interictal study only reveals mild hyperperfusion in the left posterior insular region without evidence of left

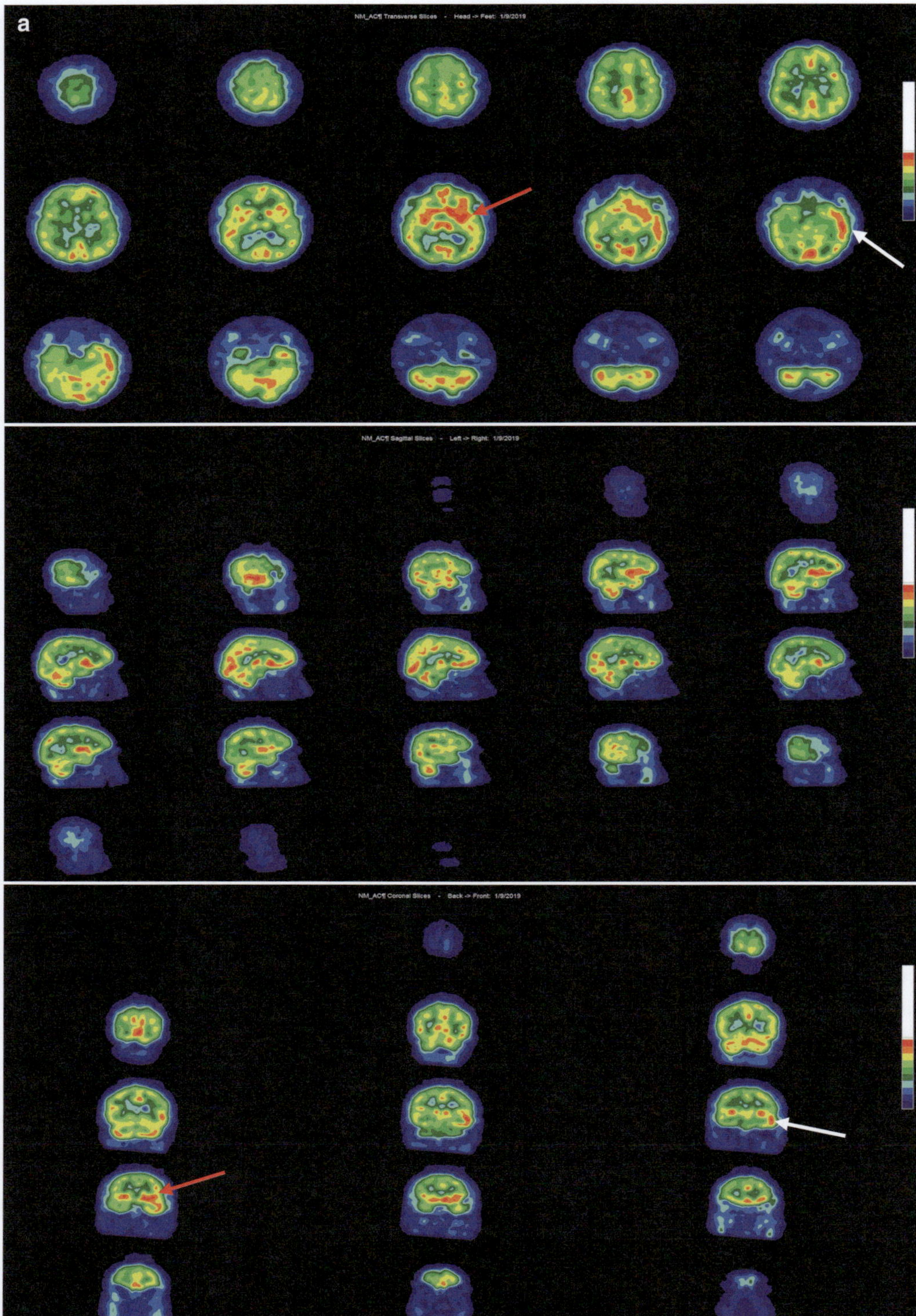

Fig. 4.6 (**a**) A 38-year-old right-handed male with probable left insular lobe epilepsy (ILE) – an ictal study (**b**) A 38-year-old right-handed male with probable left insular lobe epilepsy (ILE) – an interictal study. (**c**) A 38-year-old right-handed male with probable left insular lobe epilepsy (ILE) – SISCOM analysis

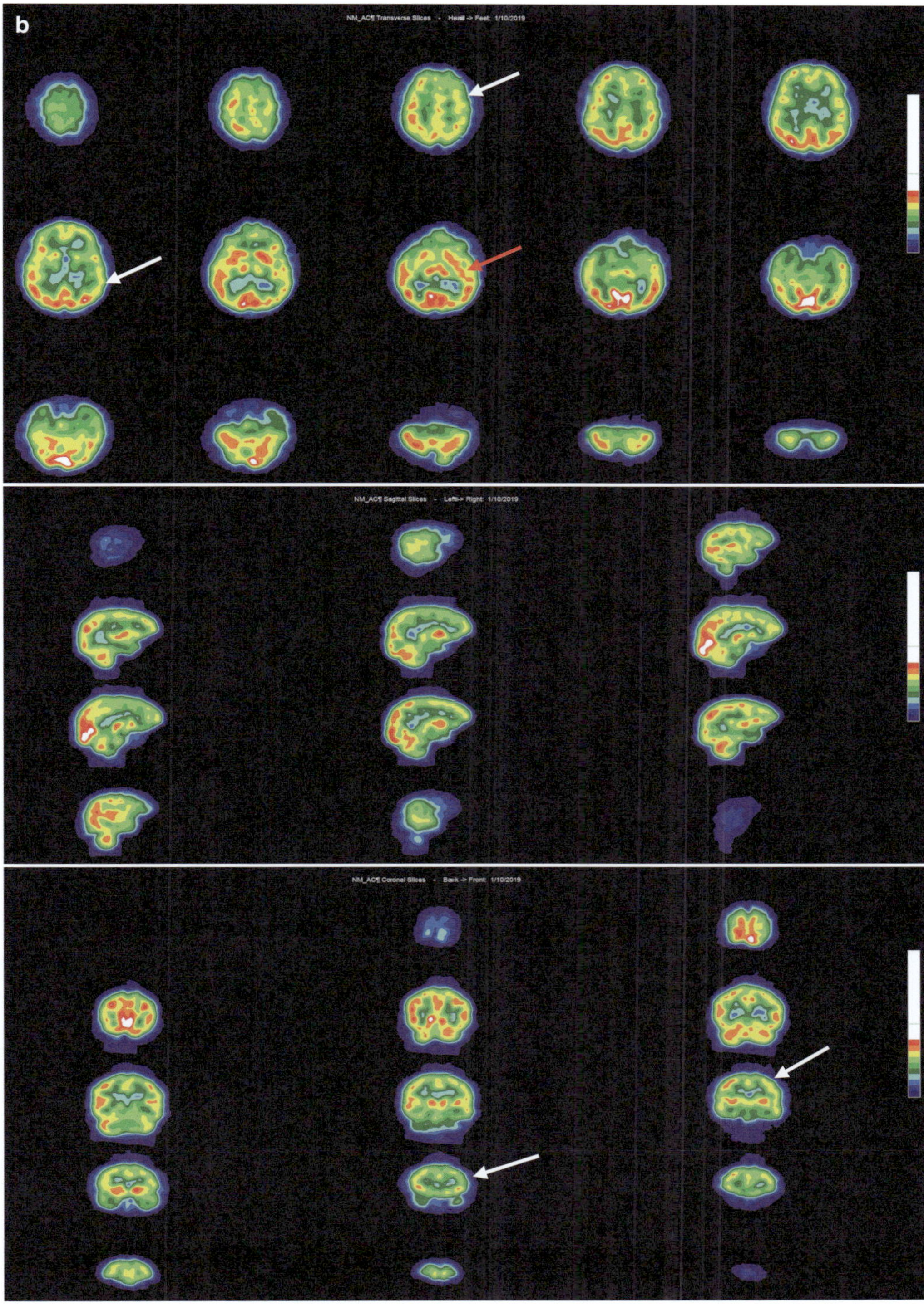

Fig. 4.6 (continued)

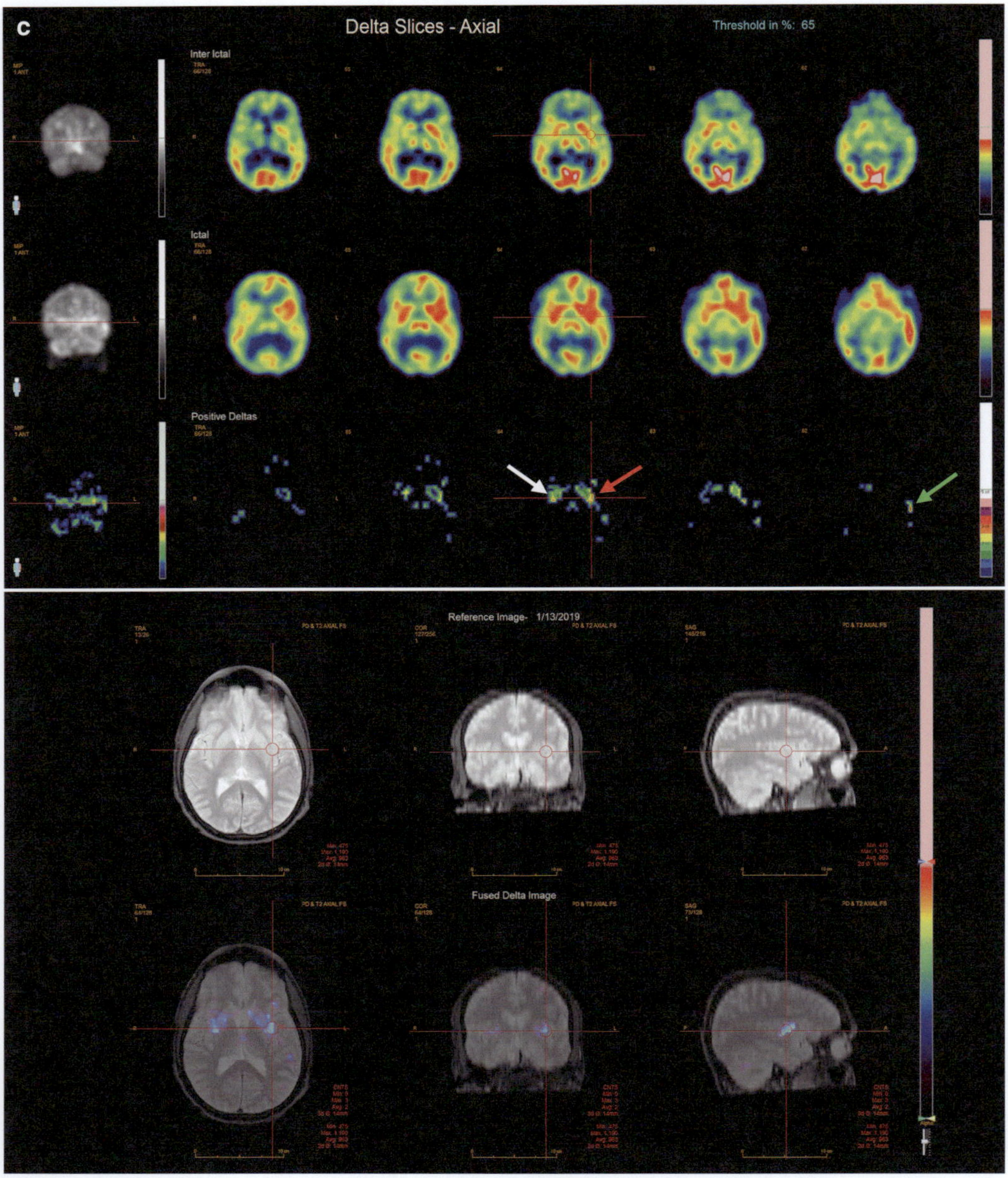

Fig. 4.6 (continued)

temporal hyperperfusion. Without comparison to the ictal study, the findings on the interictal study as described could lead to a false impression of left frontal lobe epilepsy.

As expected, the SISCOM analysis reveals a dominant focus with the difference being >3 SD, which appears to reside in the posterior left insular cortex, suspicious for an epileptogenic focus/zone. To a lesser degree, there are two small foci with moderate intensity superimposed in the lateral left temporal cortex and the right basal ganglia, suggestive of seizure propagation [8, 9].

Afterward, the patient underwent an FDG brain PET which showed left insular hypometabolism, which was consistent with the SPECT findings and suspicious for left insular epilepsy. Also, there is hypometabolism in the left frontal lobe, and this is in line with the interictal SPECT finding of hypoperfusion in the same region, suggestive of sequelae of intractable left insular epilepsy, though additional epileptogenic foci/zones cannot be excluded.

During the follow-up for 8 months, the seizures have persisted despite dose adjustment for his antiepileptic medications and addition of another antiepileptic medicine (eslicarbazepine). He does not tolerate the medications well. Therefore, the patient is currently still under further workup for potential epilepsy surgical treatment.

Case Summary

Insular epilepsies are uncommon [1]. EEG studies could be falsely normal, as shown in this case, due to the inability to record directly from the insula with scalp electrodes. Ictal SPECT in this case shows strong evidence of left hemispheric epilepsy, but seizure expansion and propagation make it difficult for further localization. Interictal study reveals areas of hypoperfusion suggestive of diaschisis or sequelae of intractable left brain seizures. SISCOM analysis not only localizes an epileptogenic focus/zone in the posterior left insular cortex but also shows findings suggestive of seizure propagation to the lateral left temporal lobe and the right basal ganglia.

Case 4.7 Probable Left Frontal Lobe Epilepsy (FLE)

Clinical Information

Chief Complaint *Having had intractable seizures for 3 years*

The patient is a right-handed 5-year-old boy with unremarkable birth history and age-appropriate developmental milestones. He had his first seizure at age of 2, which manifested as a staring episode without response to voice for a few seconds. Over time, the seizures began to include left eye twitching and left hand/arm jerking. During the seizures he retained posture and could continue simple motor tasks such as chewing or walking but did not respond to voice. The seizures occurred primarily in the evening and while falling asleep, often lasting 10–40 seconds. There were no apparent auras or triggering factors.

The patient has no history of head injury, meningitis, or encephalitis. Family history is negative for seizures or epilepsy, headache, learning difficulties, ADD/ADHD, muscular dystrophy, mitochondrial or genetic disorders, autoimmune disease, or stroke.

Current antiepileptic medications include oxcarbazepine 45 mg/kg/day and levetiracetam 32 mg/kg/day.

Recent MRI of the brain studies were unremarkable.

Multiple EEG studies were suggestive of left frontotemporal seizures.

The patient underwent an ictal SPECT study, with radioactive tracer injection at the 20-second ictal onset, and subsequent classic focal motor seizure lasted for 97 seconds prior to offsetting.

Subsequently, the patient had an interictal SPECT for comparison to the ictal study and for SISCOM analysis.

SPECT and SISCOM Findings

The ictal brain perfection study (Fig. 4.7a) shows focal cortical hyperperfusion in the LEFT lateral frontal lobe (red arrows). Additional focal hyperperfusion is noted in the RIGHT insular lobe (white arrows). Minimally decreased perfusion is noted in the RIGHT cerebellum (hatched yellow arrows), suggestive of crossed cerebrocerebellar diaschisis.

In contrast, the interictal study (Fig. 4.7b) reveals normal or minimally decreased perfusion in the LEFT lateral frontal region (red arrows) relative to the contralateral. Tracer activity in the remainder of the cerebral cortices, bilateral basal ganglia, and thalami, as well as the cerebella, is overall symmetric and within normal limits. The previously noted focal hyperperfusion on the ictal study is again seen in the right insular region (white arrow). Again, minimal hypoperfusion is noted in the right cerebellum, consistent with diaschisis.

The SISCOM analysis (Fig. 4.7c) reveals a positive focus after subtraction, coregistered to the lateroinferior portion of the left frontal cortex (red arrow). Several additional positive foci are noted, and they are scattered in the right orbitofrontal lobe, the right insula, and the posterosuperior portion of the right temporal lobe (white arrows), suggestive of seizure propagation, though additional epileptogenic foci/zones cannot be excluded.

Discussion and Follow-Up

This patient's seizure semiology, brain FDG PET, and EEG studies are consistently suggestive of LEFT frontotemporal seizures. The ictal/interictal brain perfusion studies, in conjunction with SISCOM analysis show essentially concordant findings further suggestive of an epileptogenic focus/zone in the lateroinferior portion of the LEFT frontal cortex. This finding is important not only for further workup but also explaining rapid seizure propagation to the contralateral (right) brain hemisphere. The more diffuse and robust hyperperfusion in the propagated areas (RIGHT frontotemporal and insular regions) is indirectly suggestive of an underlying structural abnormality in the epileptogenic left frontal cortex, with impaired (less robust) hyperemic response to seizure activities [3].

Technically, the radioactive tracer injection at 20-second ictal onset is acceptable but not desir-

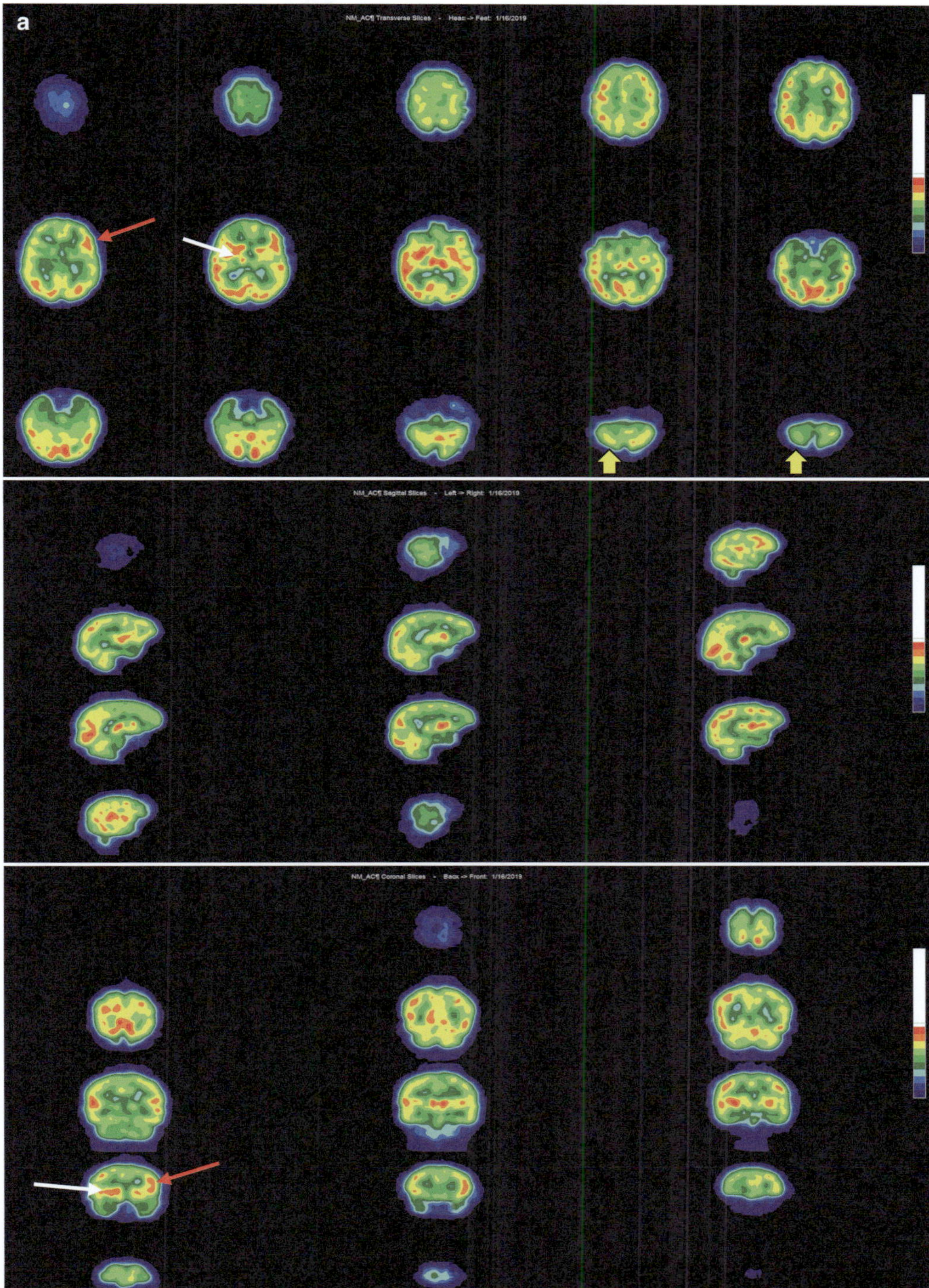

Fig. 4.7 (**a**) A 5-year-old right-handed boy with probable left frontal lobe epilepsy (FLE) – *an ictal study*. (**b**) A 5-year-old right-handed boy with probable left frontal lobe epilepsy (FLE) – *an interictal study*. (**c**) A 5-year-old right-handed boy with probable left frontal lobe epilepsy (FLE) – SISCOM analysis

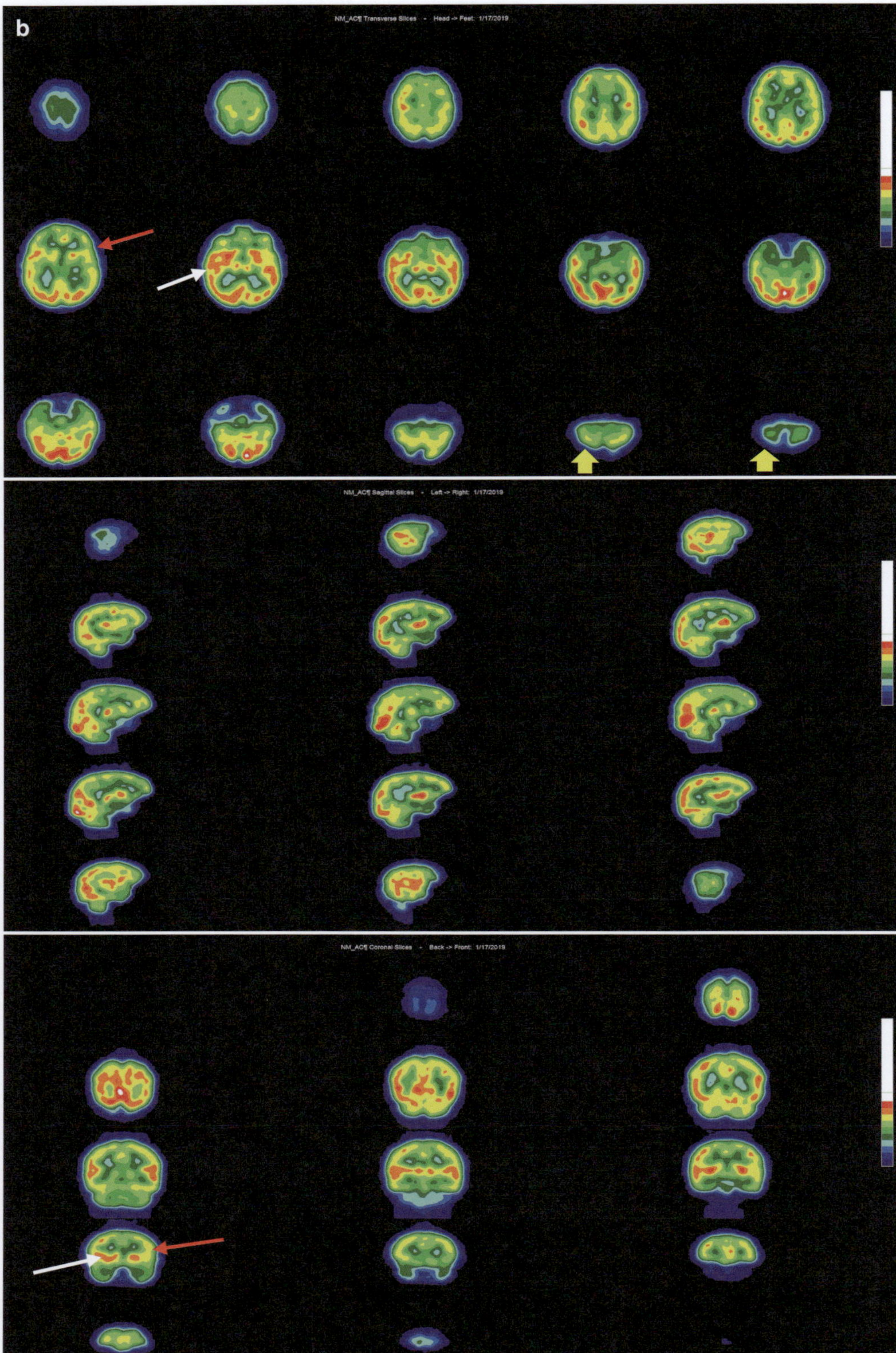

Fig. 4.7 (continued)

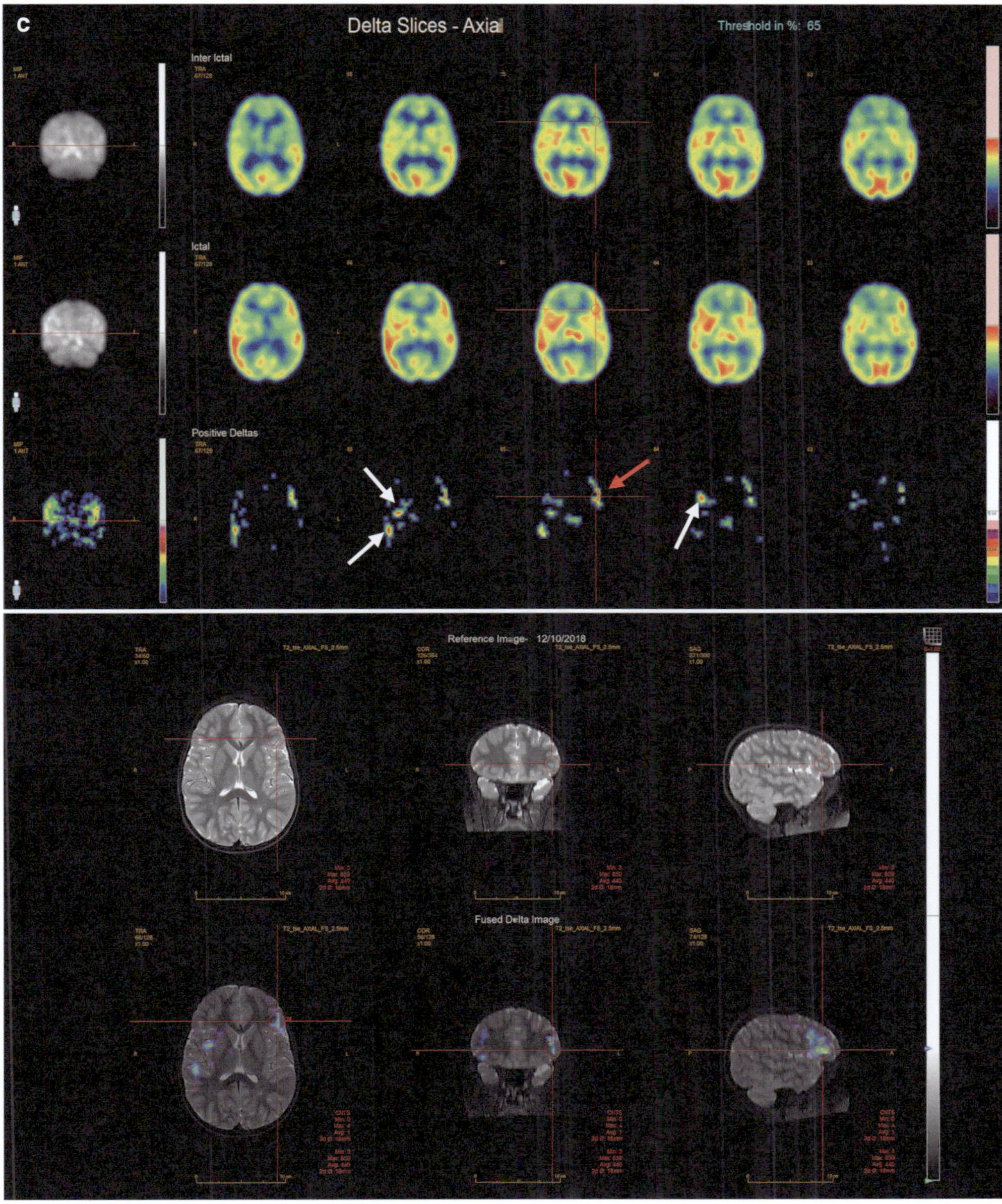

Fig. 4.7 (continued)

able. This was probably compensated by the additional 97 seconds of seizure duration following the tracer administration. The relatively late injection and subsequent long seizure duration are likely contributory to the extensive seizure propagation activities observed in the right brain as well.

Approximately 3 months after the ictal/interictal scintigraphic studies, the patient underwent stereo-EEG electrode implantation. The invasive EEG monitoring confirmed an epileptogenic focus in the lateroinferior portion of the left frontal cortex.

Six months after the ictal/interictal SPECT studies, the patient underwent stereotactically guided laser ablation of the left frontal lobe epileptogenic cortex. Two weeks after the laser ablation, the patient was brought back for follow-up, and his mother reported no seizures observed since the laser treatment. The patient is presently maintained on levetiracetam and trileptal, and he tolerates the medications well.

Case Summary

Frontal lobe epilepsies (FLEs) often manifest as focal motor seizures and usually associated with rapid seizure propagation not only within the ipsilateral but also to the contralateral brain hemisphere [1]. Prior to the scintigraphic studies, clinical semiology, brain FDG PET, and EEG studies in this case were concordantly suggestive of left frontotemporal epilepsy. The ictal/interictal SPECT findings were essentially confirmatory, but the SISCOM analysis further coregistered the potential epileptogenic focus to the lateroinferior portion of the left frontal cortex. Although extensive seizure propagation to the right brain was noted, there was no involvement of the left temporal lobe. This precise imaging localization guided stereo-EEG electrode implantation, leading to a successful laser ablation of the left frontal epileptogenic cortex.

Case 4.8 Multifocal Epilepsy Secondary to Tuberous Sclerosis (TS)

Clinical Information

Chief Complaint *Medically refractory focal seizures and known tuberous sclerosis (TS)*

The patient is a 22-month-old undifferentiated male with a reported history of tuberous sclerosis (TS) complex and infantile spasms. According to the mother, the boy also has had subtle focal seizures manifesting as staring spells while playing, with abnormal mouth movements on the right side. The episodes lasted for a few seconds and were interrupted by loud noises. There was no twitching, shaking, or stiffness noted in the past. Recently, however, his seizures have been manifested by unresponsiveness to loud stimuli with bilateral arm shaking, right hand opening, and eye deviation to the left. The patient is currently on antiepileptic medications of topiramate and sabril, with a good tolerance. However, despite maximizing the medication dose, he continues to have one or more seizures per day.

Past medical history is notable for known TS, speech delay, known cardiac rhabdomyoma, and PFO (patent foramen ovale). Birth history was unremarkable. There was no history of traumatic brain injury (TBI), meningitis/encephalitis, or family history of seizure/epilepsy.

A recent MRI of the brain revealed stable cortical/subcortical and subependymal tubers. The largest subependymal lesion in the frontal horn of the left lateral ventricle showed stable enhancement and size.

Brain FDG PET showed numerous cortical tubers involving both brain hemispheres.

Multiple EEG studies were suggestive of left frontotemporal epilepsy.

The first ictal SPECT was performed with tracer injected approximately 9 seconds into a typical burst with subtle behavioral change.

The second ictal SPECT was performed, with tracer injected 2-second ictal onset of different kind according to EEG.

Then, an interictal SPECT was performed for comparison with the two ictal studies and for SISCOM analysis.

SPECT and SISCOM Findings

The first ictal study (Fig. 4.8a) shows three areas of hyperperfusion involving the bilateral frontal lobes and the left parietal lobe (red arrows). As expected, there are numerous tubers of different sizes, with variably decreased or even absent tracer activity (white arrows). The second ictal SPECT (Fig. 4.8b) only shows two areas of hyperperfusion, scattered in the right frontal lobe and the right superolateral temporal lobe (red arrows). The previously noted left frontal hyperperfusion is less evident. The interictal SPECT (Fig. 4.8c) shows more prominent cortical tubers, all with decreased tracer activity (white arrows), while the previously noted multiple areas of hyperperfusion are not evident, as expected.

The SISCOM analysis of the first ictal SPECT versus the interictal study (Fig. 4.8d) reveals a focus (red arrow, top panel) in yellow-green color indicating the difference being about 2 SD, coregistered to the left frontal lobe on the patient's MRI (bottom panel). In addition, there are at least two similar foci in green color (indication their difference being less than 2 SD) involving the right frontal lobe (white arrow, top panel) and the left parietal lobe (data not shown), suspicious for additional epileptogenic tubers.

In contrast, the SISCOM analysis of the secondary ictal versus the interictal study (Fig. 4.8e) only shows one dominant focus in red-orange color indicating the difference being >2 SD, coregistered to the right frontal lobe, suspicious for an epileptogenic tuber.

Discussions and Follow-Up

Medically refractory seizures are one of the most common neurological features of TS. As shown in this case, this 22-month-old boy with known genetic TS has several different types of drug-resistant seizures. Although literature is suggestive of the usefulness of alpha-[C^{11}]-methyl-L-tryptophan (AMT) PET for pre-surgical identification of epileptogenic tubers [4, 6], this approach is only available in a few academic PET centers with on-site cyclotron and research laboratory for AMT synthesis. There is increasing evidence to use ictal/

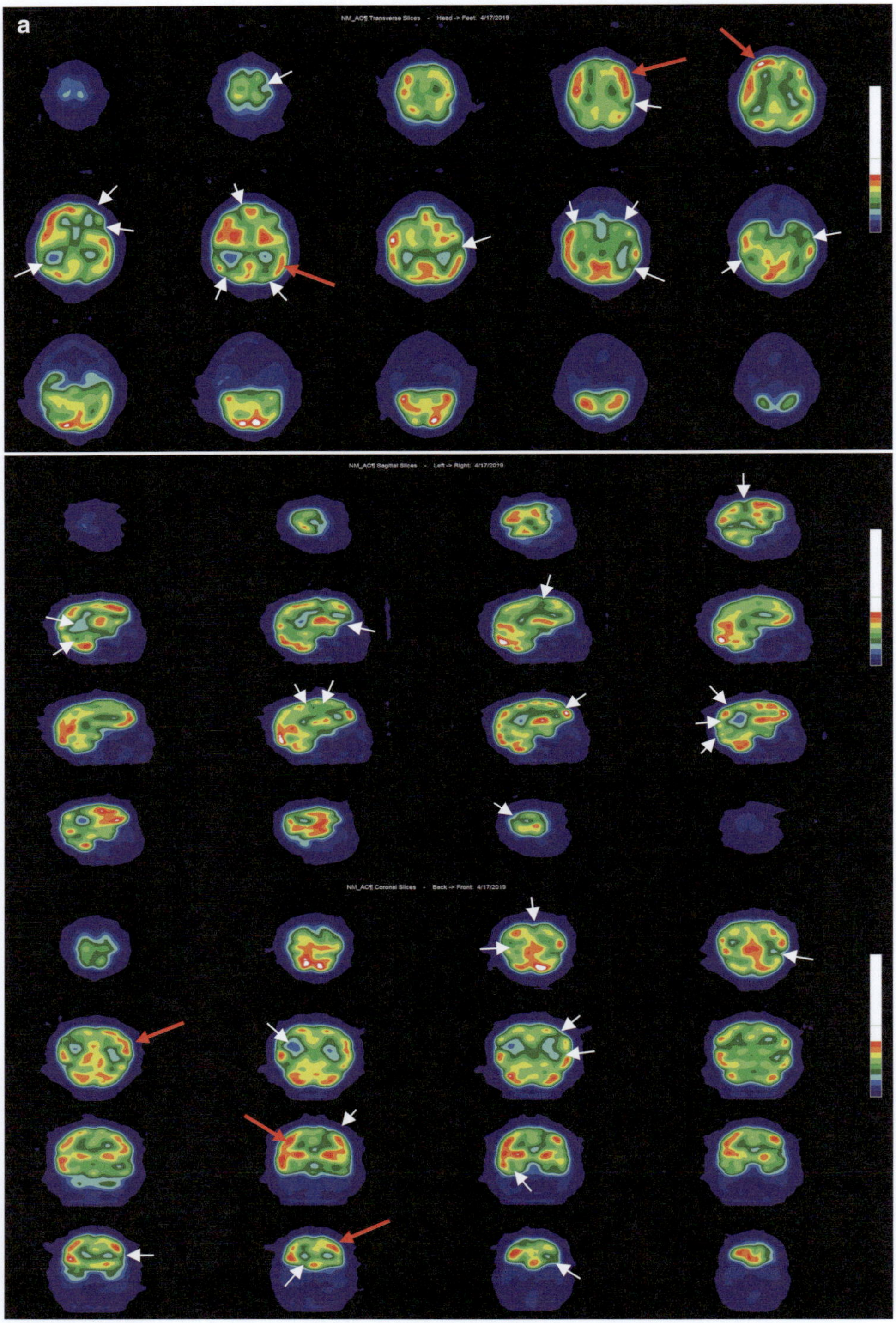

Fig. 4.8 (**a**) A 22-month-old boy with intractable seizures and known tuberous sclerosis (TS) – the first ictal study. (**b**) A 22-month-old boy with intractable seizures and known tuberous sclerosis (TS) – the second ictal study. (**c**) A 22-month-old boy with intractable seizures and known tuberous sclerosis (TS) – an interictal study. (**d**) A 22-month-old boy with intractable seizures and known tuberous sclerosis (TS) – the first SISCOM analysis. (**e**) A 22-month-old boy with intractable seizures and known tuberous sclerosis (TS) – the second SISCOM analysis

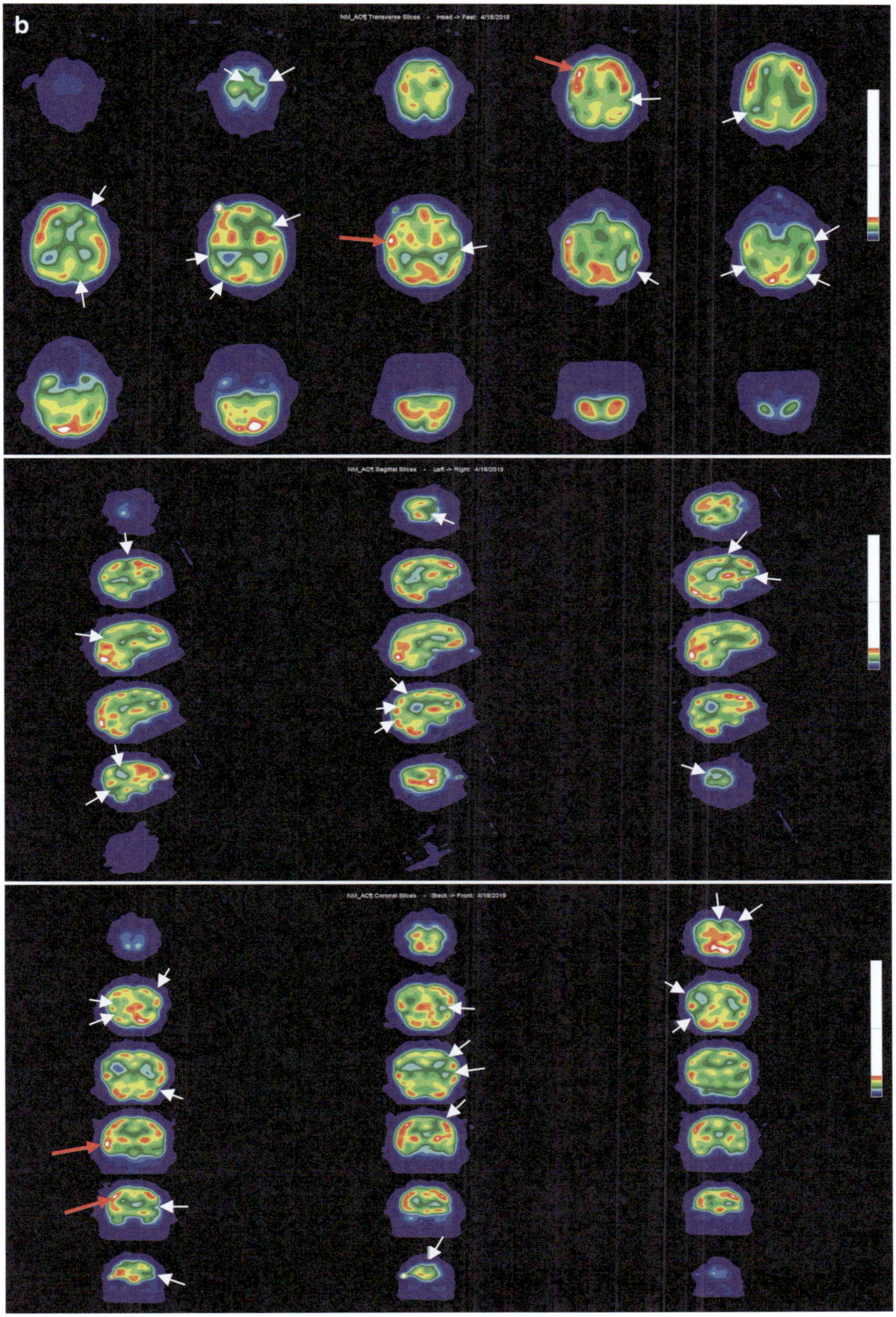

Fig. 4.8 (continued)

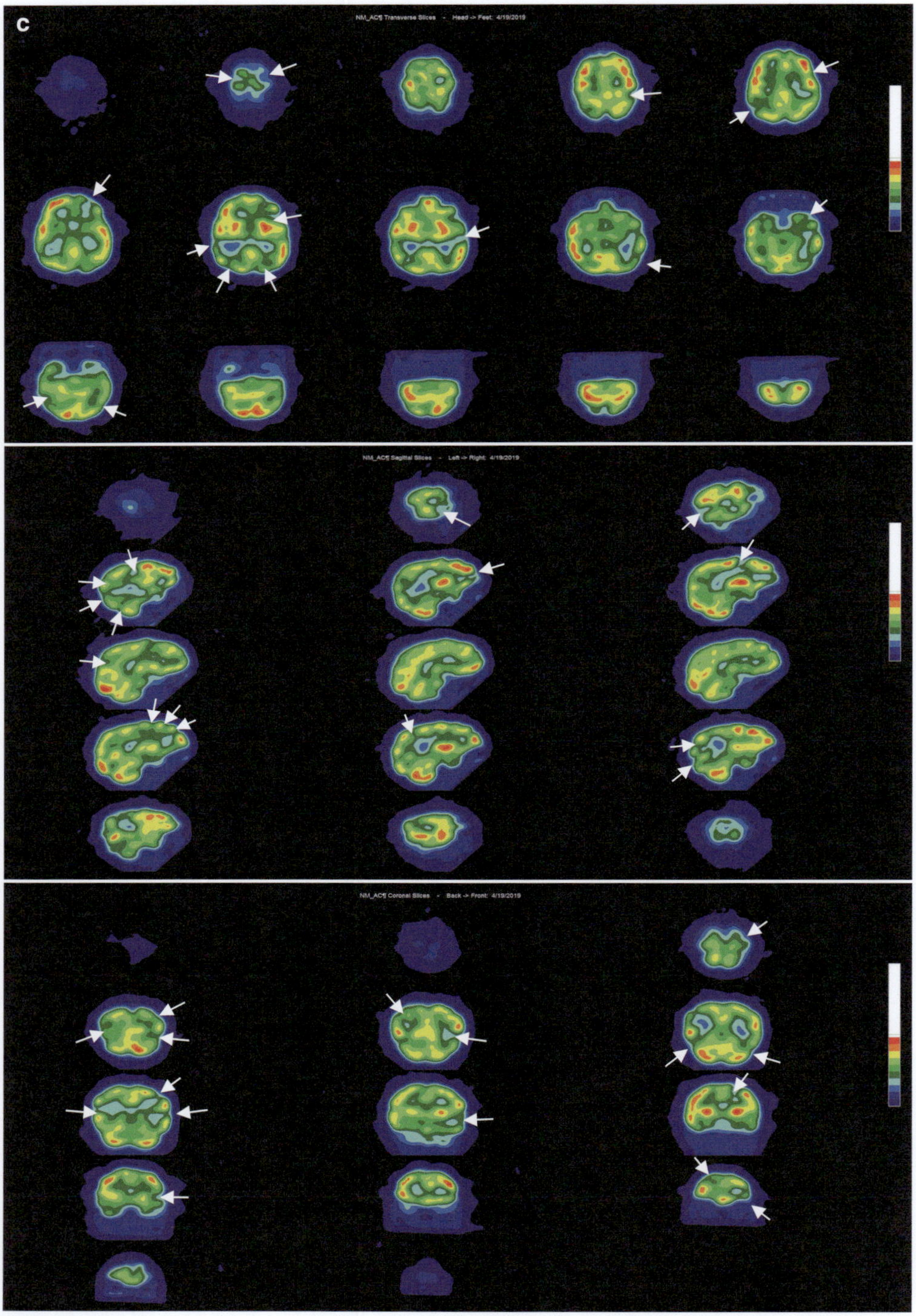

Fig. 4.8 (continued)

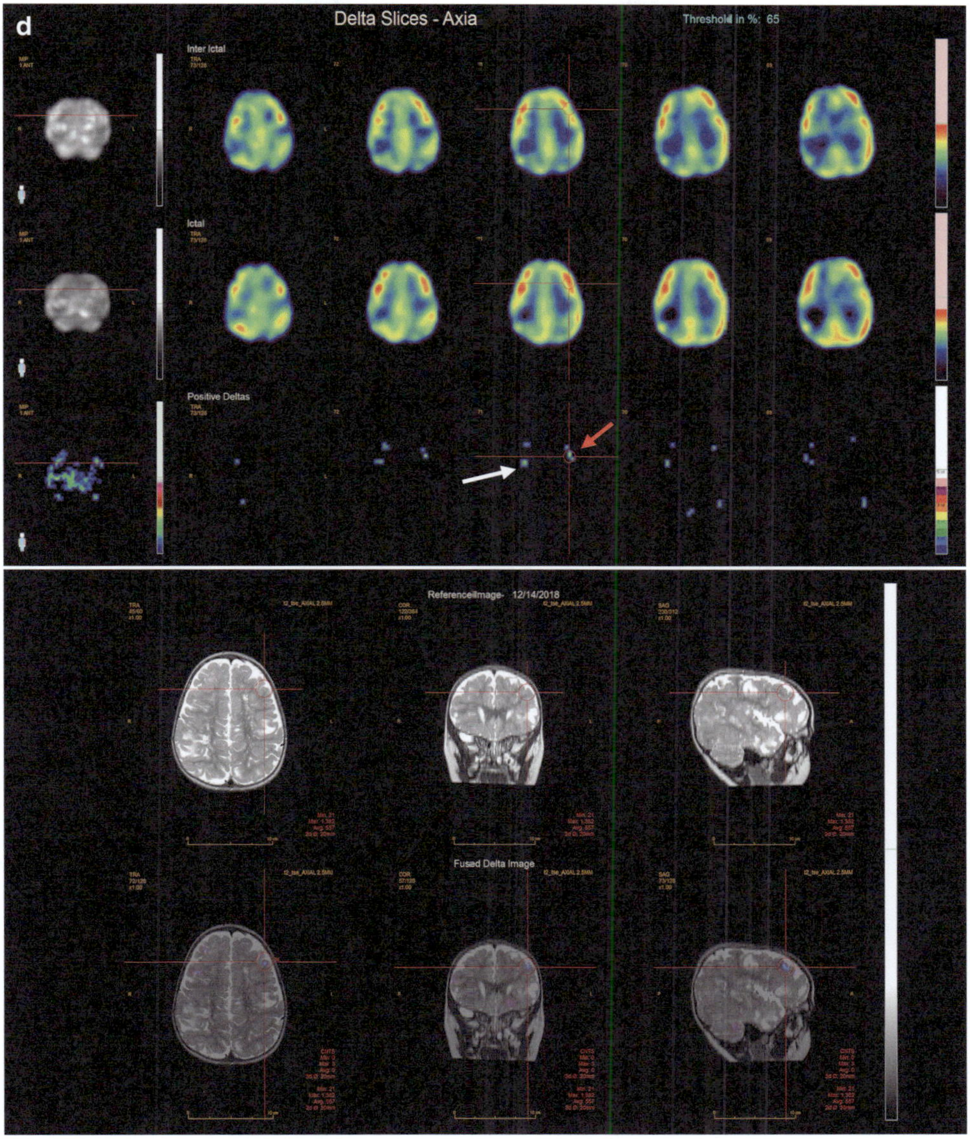

Fig. 4.8 (continued)

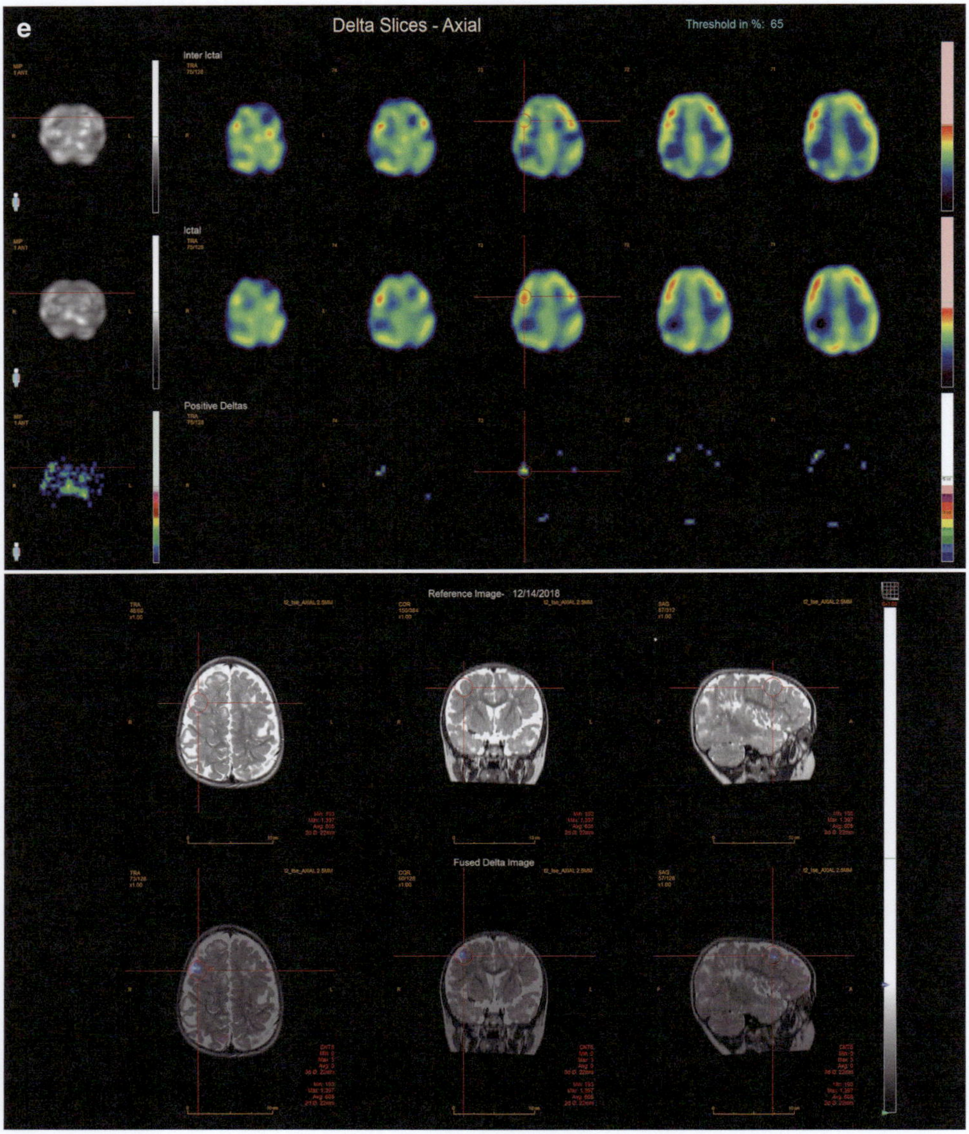

Fig. 4.8 (continued)

interictal brain perfusion studies with SISCOM analysis as an alternative approach [2, 10]. The multi-session scintigraphic studies in this case confirm the presence of numerous tubers of different size with widely variable hypoperfusion. The two ictal studies that targeted different seizure onsets revealed multiple areas of cortical hyperperfusion, overlapping with some of the tubers. As a result, the SISCOM analysis shows multiple epileptogenic tubers involving at least the bilateral frontal lobes and the left parietal lobe. After additional workup, it was concluded that the patient's left frontal tubers appeared to be the most active and causative for his current medically refractory seizures and likely contributed to his speech delay as well.

Subsequently, the patient underwent a partial left frontal brain lobectomy, with pathology confirming the presence of cortical tubers. Of note, the known left parietal epileptic tuber was not active during intraoperative monitoring. Three days after the surgery, breakthrough seizures were observed, for which fosphenytoin was added to the existing antiepileptic medications. Despite the add-on fosphenytoin maintenance, the patient was readmitted 3 weeks after the surgery due to an extended breakthrough seizure, and he was treated with levetiracetam and topiramate with increased dosage.

Case Summary

TS is a multi-system disease including the brain involvement, which often causes medically refractory seizures [1, 4, 6]. This case demonstrates the usefulness of the ictal/interictal SPECT and SISCOM analysis for pre-surgical identification of epileptogenic tubers among numerous silent/inactive tubers. After extensive workup, the patient underwent a partial left frontal lobectomy, not only for resection of the most active epileptic tuber(s) but also for alleviation of the patient's speech delay. It's not surprising to observe frequent breakthrough seizures after the surgery, given the pre-surgical scintigraphic evidence of multiple epileptogenic tubers involving at least the bilateral frontal lobes and the left parietal lobe.

References

1. Abou-Khalil BW, Gallagher MJ, Macdonald RL. Epilepsies. In: Daroff R, Jankonic J, Mazziotta J, Pemerony S, editors. Bradley's neurology in clinical practice. London: Elsevier; 2016. p. 1563–614.
2. Chen T, Guo L. The role of SISCOM in preoperative evaluation for patients with epilepsy surgery: a meta-analysis. Seizure. 2016;41:43–60.
3. Gaillard WD. Nuclear imaging (PET, SPECT). In: Wyllie E, editor. Wyllie's treatment of epilepsy: principles and practice. 5th ed. Philadelphia: Wolters Kluwer; 2011. p. 860–8.
4. Kagawa K, Chugani DC, Asano E, et al. Epilepsy surgery outcome in children with tuberous sclerosis complex evaluated with alpha-[11C]-methyl-L-tryptophan positron emission tomography (PET). J Child Neurol. 2005;20(5):429–38.
5. Krsek P, Pieper T, Karlmeier A, et al. Different presurgical characteristics and seizure outcomes in children with focal cortical dysplasia type I or II. Epilepsia. 2009;50:125–37.
6. Kumar A, Chugani HT. The role of radionuclide imaging in epilepsy, part 2: epilepsy syndromes. J Nucl Med Technol. 2017;45(1):22–9.
7. Kumar A, Chugani HT. Application of PET and SPECT in pediatric epilepsy surgery. In: Cataltepe O, Jallo GI, editors. Pediatric epilepsy surgery preoperative assessment and surgical treatment. New York: Thieme; 2010. p. 82–98.
8. O'Brien T, O'Connor M, Mullan B, et al. Subtraction ictal SPECT co-registered to MRI in partial epilepsy: description and technical validation of the method with phantom and patient studies. Nucl Med Commun. 1998;19:31–45.
9. O'Brien T, So EL, Mullan B, et al. Subtraction ictal SPECT co-registered to MRI improves postictal SPECT localization of seizure foci. Neurology. 1999;52:137–46.
10. von Oertzen TJ, Mormann F, Urbach H, et al. Prospective use of subtraction ictal SPECT coregistered to MRI (SISCOM) in presurgical evaluation of epilepsy. Epilepsia. 2011;52(12):2239–48.

5 FDG PET Imaging of Brain Tumors

Case 5.1 Primary Glioblastoma Multiforme (GBM)

Clinical Information

Chief Complaint *Sudden onset of speech difficulty and transient confusion*

The patient is a 70-year-old right-handed male presenting with sudden onset of speech difficulty and loss of consciousness for a short time. While in emergency department, neurological examination showed no dizziness, seizures, weakness, or headaches. Although CT of the head/brain showed findings suspicious for "subacute infarct involving the left middle cerebral artery (MCA) territory particularly the left temporal lobe," MRI of the brain with and without IV contrast revealed an enhancing lesion in the left temporal lobe, suspicious for "an infiltrating glioma." A lumbar puncture (spinal tap) was normal.

Past medical history is notable for peripheral neuropathy, hypertension, hyperlipidemia, and coronary artery disease (CAD).

A follow-up brain MR imaging 1 month later revealed an interval enlarged left temporal enhancing lesion (current size of 2.7 × 1.9 × 2.5 cm, relative to prior size 1.5 × 0.7 × 1.2 cm) with surrounding edema, suspicious for "a primary neoplastic process versus infection." Subsequently, the patient underwent an open brain biopsy of the known left temporal lesion, which was "without significant diagnostic abnormalities," per pathology report.

Then, whole-body FDG PET/CT was performed, with the patient's blood glucose level of 106 mg/dL prior to FDG administration.

FDG PET CT Findings (Fig. 5.1)

Due to clinical concerns of primary brain malignancy or metastasis, whole-body FDG PET CT was performed. The FDG PET images (the upper panel) show a discrete highly FDG-avid lesion in the superolateral portion of the left temporal lobe (red arrows), which corresponds to the interval enlarged and enhancing mass on the recent MRI. The abnormal FDG activity is more intense in the superoanterolateral aspects of the mass, suspicious for a malignant lesion with eccentric necrosis. Surrounding the mass is mild to moderately decreased FDG in the cortical or subcortical regions of the left temporal, frontal, parietal, and occipital lobes, as well as the left basal ganglia and thalamus, suggestive of mass effects and vasogenic edema or both. The concurrent CT without IV contrast (the middle panel) is less informative and only shows low-density changes in the medial and posterior left temporal regions (white arrow), likely sequelae of mass effects and vasogenic edema. The PET CT fused images (the lower panel) confirm the FDG-avid lesion located in the left temporal lobe.

D. Wu, *Clinical Nuclear Medicine Neuroimaging*, https://doi.org/10.1007/978-3-030-40893-0_5

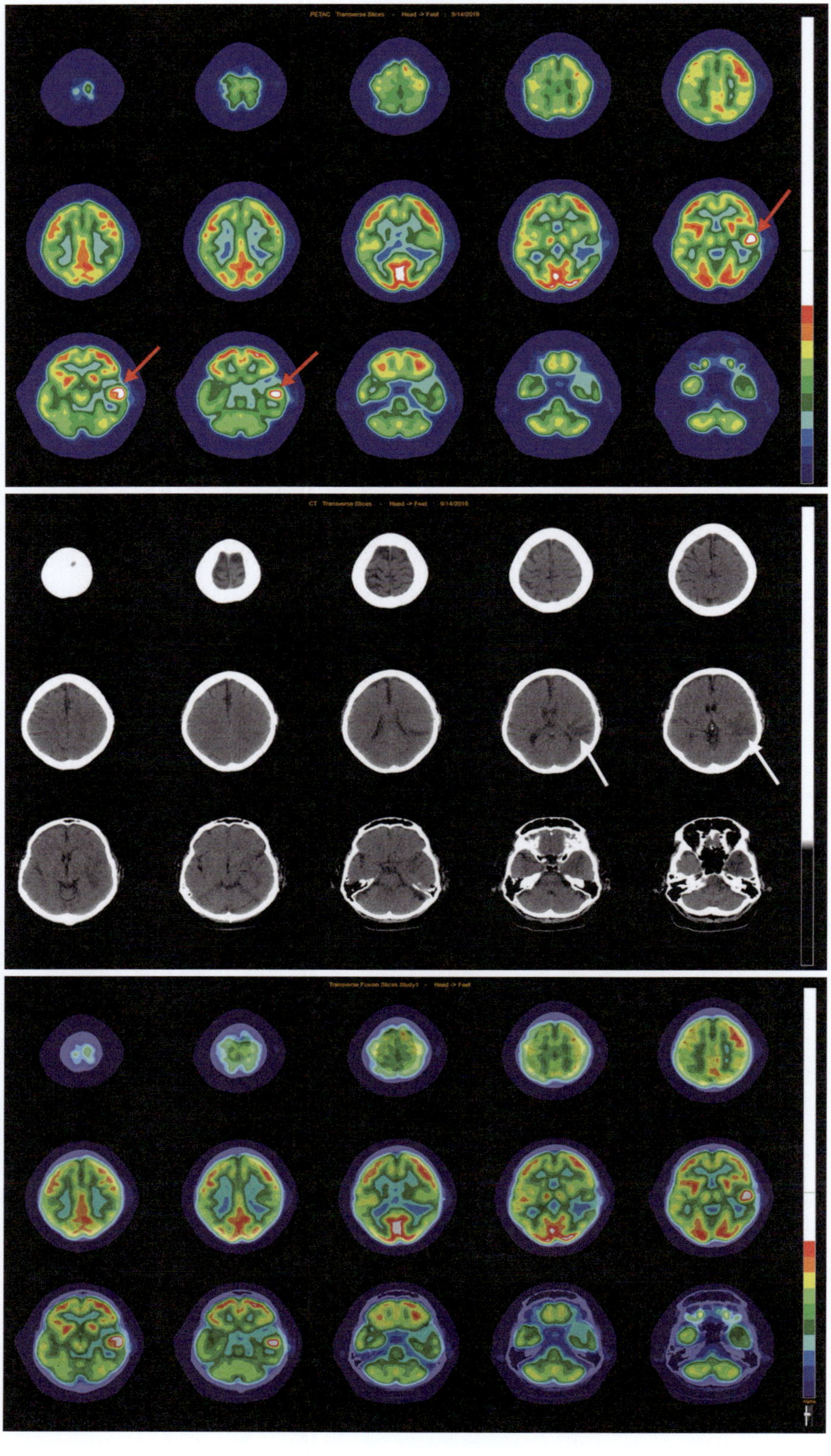

Fig. 5.1 A 70-year-old male with primary glioblastoma multiforme (GBM)

The remainder of the whole-body PET CT (images not shown) revealed no suspicious peripheral FDG-avid malignancy or metastasis, with a special reference to both lungs.

Discussion and Follow-Up

Despite clinical concerns of primary brain tumor or metastasis and a nondiagnostic brain biopsy, the abnormal FDG PET CT findings, in line with the prior MRI results, are highly suggestive of a left temporal lobe primary malignancy with eccentric necrosis, given the lack of evidence of peripheral lesions. Additionally, the PET CT images show more prominent FDG activity in the superoanterolateral aspects of the mass, which helps future biopsy planning for definite diagnosis.

Surrounding the highly metabolic tumor mass in the left temporal lobe is a large area of vasogenic edema and mass effects or both as indicated by hypometabolism. The hypometabolic involvement of the inferior left frontal lobe may explain for the sudden onset of speech difficulty (likely Broca's aphasia) in this right-handed patient.

Ten days after the abnormal FDG PET CT study, the patient underwent a neuronavigational assisted needle biopsy, which was positive for glioblastoma, WHO (World Health Organization) grade IV, IDH (isocitrate dehydrogenase) mutation wild type, and ATRX (alpha-thalassemia mental retardation syndrome, X-linked) expression retained.

Following the positive biopsy, the patient underwent surgical resection, radiation therapy, and adjuvant chemotherapy with Temodar. Follow-up has shown no clinical or imaging evidence of recurrent glioblastoma for 1 year so far.

Case Summary

Prior to FDG PET study, CT and MRI studies and open brain biopsy in this 70-year-old male patient with sudden onset of speech difficulty and loss of consciousness showed non-conclusive or falsely negative results. FDG brain PET CT, however, shows unique metabolic features as the following:

1. There is intense FDG avidity in the brain tumor mass, but no evidence of FDG-avid lesions in the peripheral, highly suggestive of primary malignant brain tumor.
2. The uneven FDG activity within the brain tumor mass not only indicates areas of necrosis but also guides future biopsy of metabolically active tumor tissues in the superoanterolateral portion of the mass.
3. There is hypometabolism in the surrounding areas, indicative of mass effects and vasogenic edema or both, which may explain the patient's symptom of speech difficulty (likely Broca's aphasia). With the guide of the FDT PET CT findings, the patient had a positive biopsy for glioblastoma, leading to successful treatments. Postsurgically, he has been disease-free for 1 year.

Case 5.2 Recurrent Glioblastoma Multiforme (GBM)

Clinical Information

Chief Complaints *History of GBM and worsening right hemiparesis*

The patient was a 56-year-old male with history of glioblastoma multiforme (GBM), status post left craniotomy with stereotactic debulking in 2005, followed by radiotherapy and chemotherapy with last treatment in 2009. He developed recurrent disease in 2012 which was treated with Avastin (Bevacizumab). Posttreatments, he developed headaches and seizures for which he was treated with levetiracetam and valproic acid, with a good seizure control. However, he reported worsening headache and weakness of right upper and lower extremities. Brain MRI revealed increasing irregular solid enhancement along posteromedial aspect of the known cystic surgical cavity in the left occipitoparietal lobe, in addition to a new 1.3 cm ring-enhancing focus in the medical left precentral gyrus. Both findings were concerning for recurrent GBM.

Due to worsening headache, increased right hemiparesis, and abnormal MR imaging findings, he was admitted to our hospital. Next day, he underwent left occipital craniotomy and excisional biopsy which showed gliotic brain tissues with features of prior irradiation and focal necrosis, no evidence of recurrent glioma. Additional pathology findings were consistent with known CLL (chronic lymphocytic leukemia).

Whole-body FDG PET CT scan was performed, with the patient's blood glucose of 88 mg/dL, prior to FDG administration.

FDG PET CT Findings (Fig. 5.2)

The PET images (the upper panel) show a focus of increased FDG activity in the medial left frontal lobe adjacent to the premotor region (red arrows). This corresponds to minimal hyperdense changes (white arrows) on the concurrent non-IV-contrasted CT (the middle panel) and also corresponds to the recent MRI finding of a ring-enhancing lesion of approximately 1.3 cm in the same region, suspicious for tumor recurrence. In contrast, moderate to severely decreased FDG activity is noted in the left occipital, parietal, and temporal lobes, in conjunction with cystic and low-density changes on the concurrent CT, consistent with posttreatment changes including at least surgical cavities, resection defect, and post-radiation necrosis. The recent MRI reported enhancing lesion in the posterior left occipital lobe shows absent FDG activity on PET (green arrows), suggestive of post-radiation necrosis. This FDG PET finding is also consistent with the recent negative excisional biopsy results, in retrospect. The PET CT fused images (the lower panel), despite slight misregistration, confirms an FDG-avid lesion in the medial left frontal lobe only.

Discussions and Follow-Up

Prior to FDG PET study, brain MRI showed two areas suspicious for recurrent disease, but excisional biopsy of the contrast-enhanced lesion in the posteromedial left occipital lobe was negative for malignancy. Consistent with the negative resection biopsy, FDG PET revealed absent or decreased FDG activity in the posteromedial left occipital region, suggestive of surgical cavity or posttreatment changes, and no evidence of FDG-avid recurrent disease. In contrast, there was a single focus of increased FDG activity in the medial left frontal lobe, corresponding to a 1.5 cm enhancing lesion on MRI, suspicious for recurrent GBM in the appropriate clinical setting.

During the follow-up for 9 months, the patient experienced progressive right hemiparesis. A new brain MRI revealed an interval enlarged left medial frontal lesion. Subsequently, the patient underwent left craniotomy and excision biopsy of the known left medial frontal lesion, which was positive for glioblastoma (WHO grade IV) along with changes of prior radiation. Postsurgically, patient's conditions continued deteriorating, and he deceased 2 weeks later.

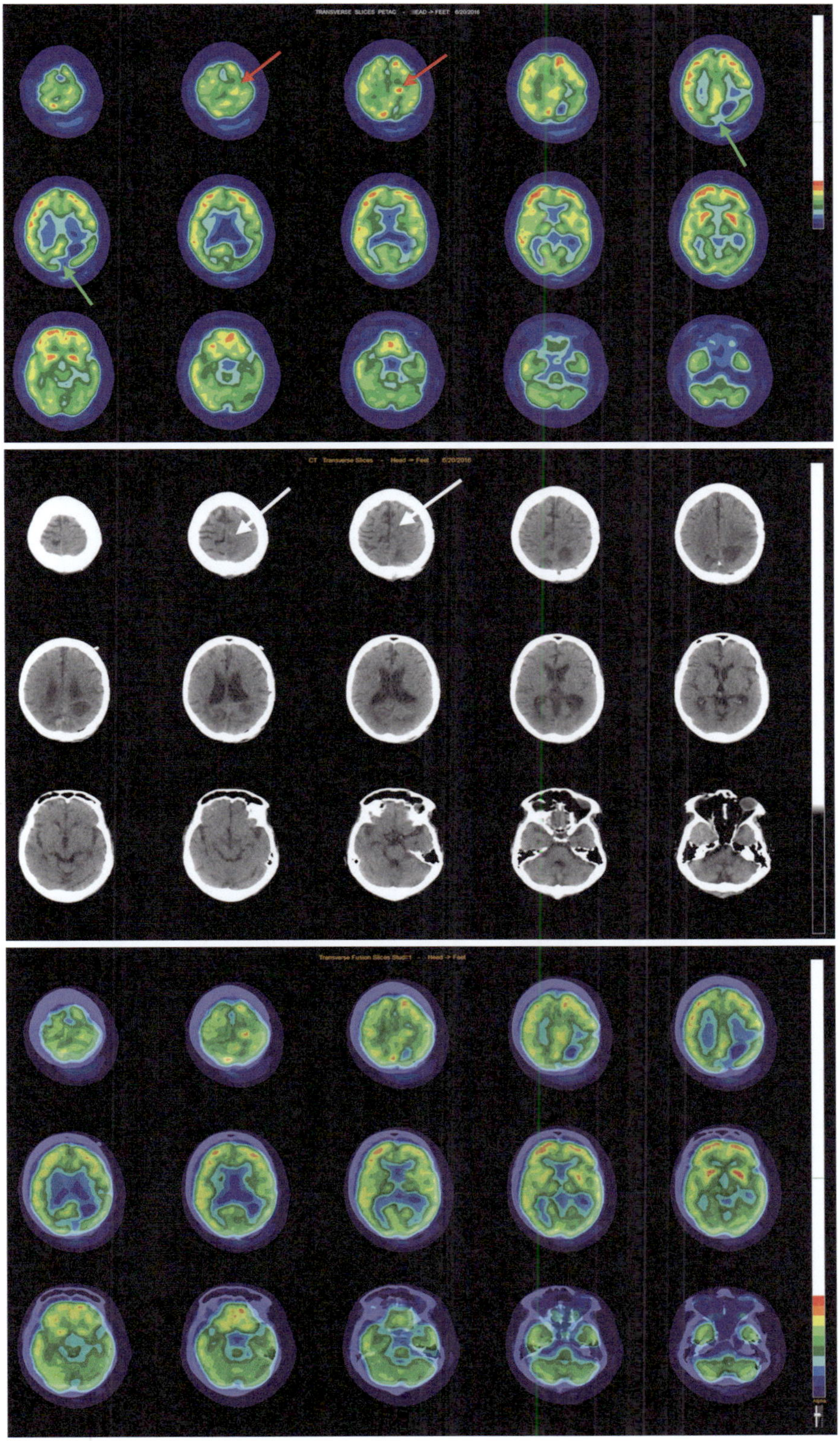

Fig. 5.2 A 56-year-old male with recurrent GBM and post-radiation necrosis

Case Summary

Since both brain tumor recurrence and post-radiation necrosis are contrast-enhancing [2, 3, 7, 9], it is often difficult to differentiate one from the other on anatomic neuroimaging (MRI and CT). This case shows that FDG PET could play an important role in this particular area. Prior to FDG PET study, brain MRI showed two enhancing lesions, both suspicious for tumor recurrence. FDG PET, however, revealed hypometabolism in the enhancing lesion in the posterior left occipital lobe, suggestive of necrosis, which, in retrospect, was in line with the recent negative excision biopsy. In contrast, focal hypermetabolism was identified, corresponding to a ring-enhancing lesion of 1.3 cm in the medial left frontal lobe, suspicious for recurrent GBM, which was biopsy proven 9 months later.

Case 5.3 Primary CNS Lymphoma (PCNSL)

Clinical Information

Chief Complaint *Recently diagnosed brain tumor and new onset of altered mental status*

The patient was a 72-year-old male with recent admission to an outside hospital due to new-onset seizure and MRI finding of a left brain tumor. Planned brain tumor biopsy was canceled due to newly developed myocardial infarction (MI). He was discharged, with levetiracetam prescribed for seizure control. However, he was brought to our hospital 1 week later, due to altered mental status after he was found by his friend lying on the ground in his apartment. While in the emergency department, CT of the head/brain showed "a hyperdense callosal mass with surrounding vasogenic edema." A new brain MRI was performed, which demonstrated "a large homogeneous enhancing mass involving the splenium of the corpus callosum with mass effect and vasogenic edema as well as a satellite enhancing lesion in the periatrial white matter on the left side," suspicious for CNS lymphoma versus GBM.

While in hospital, the patient underwent stereotactic brain lesion biopsy with pathology pending. Then, whole-body FDG PET was performed, with the patient's blood glucose level of 79 mg/dL prior to FDG administration.

FDG PET CT Findings (Fig. 5.3)

The brain PET CT images showed a large focus of intense FDG activity (red arrows), corresponding to a hyperdense mass residing in the splenium of the corpus callosum (white arrows), with maximal SUV 23.1. As a reference, max SUV of the cerebral cortices is 3.2. In addition, there is a small focus of moderately increased FDG activity in the left para-ventricular region (green arrows), maximal SUV 4.8, without CT correlate, likely due to the small size and lack of IV contrast. But this small FDG-avid lesion appears corresponding to an enhancing satellite lesion in the left para-ventricular region on the recent diagnostic brain MRI.

Global cortical hypometabolism is noted, with moderately preserved metabolism in the bilateral sensorimotor strips and the cerebella especially the vermis. Decreased FDG activity is also noted in bilateral basal ganglia and thalami.

The remainder of the whole-body FDG PET CT scan revealed no evidence of FDG-avid lymphomatous involvement in the peripheral (images not shown).

Discussions and Follow-Up

The FDG PET CT findings, in line with the brain MRI results, were highly suspicious for a malignant tumor of the splenium of the corpus callosum with a satellite lesion in the left para-ventricular region. The global cortical hypometabolism including the basal ganglia and thalami was most likely due to vasogenic edema and mass effect or both.

Two days after the FDG PET CT study, brain biopsy results came out, with flow cytometry findings consistent with diffuse large B-cell lymphoma (DLBCL). Subsequently, CSF analysis with concurrent flow cytometry also showed lymphoma involvement.

The patient had a poor response to chemotherapy including high-dose methotrexate. Moreover, he developed sepsis due to pneumonia treated with vancomycin/cefepime; then he developed fungemia with *Candida albicans* treated with IV Diflucan. Due to the complications and deteriorating metal status, the patient was transferred to inpatient hospice.

Case Summary

Primary CNS lymphoma (PCNSL) is a rare extranodal non-Hodgkin's lymphoma that mainly involves the brain, less commonly the leptomeninges, eyes, or spinal cord, without evidence of outside CNS involvement [8]. This case shows that FDG PET is an ideal and important imaging modality to help diagnose PCNSL. FDG PET features suspicious for or suggestive of PCNSL include single or multiple intracranial solid lesions, with variable hypermetabolism depending on lesion sizes, and no evidence of lymphoma involvement in the peripheral.

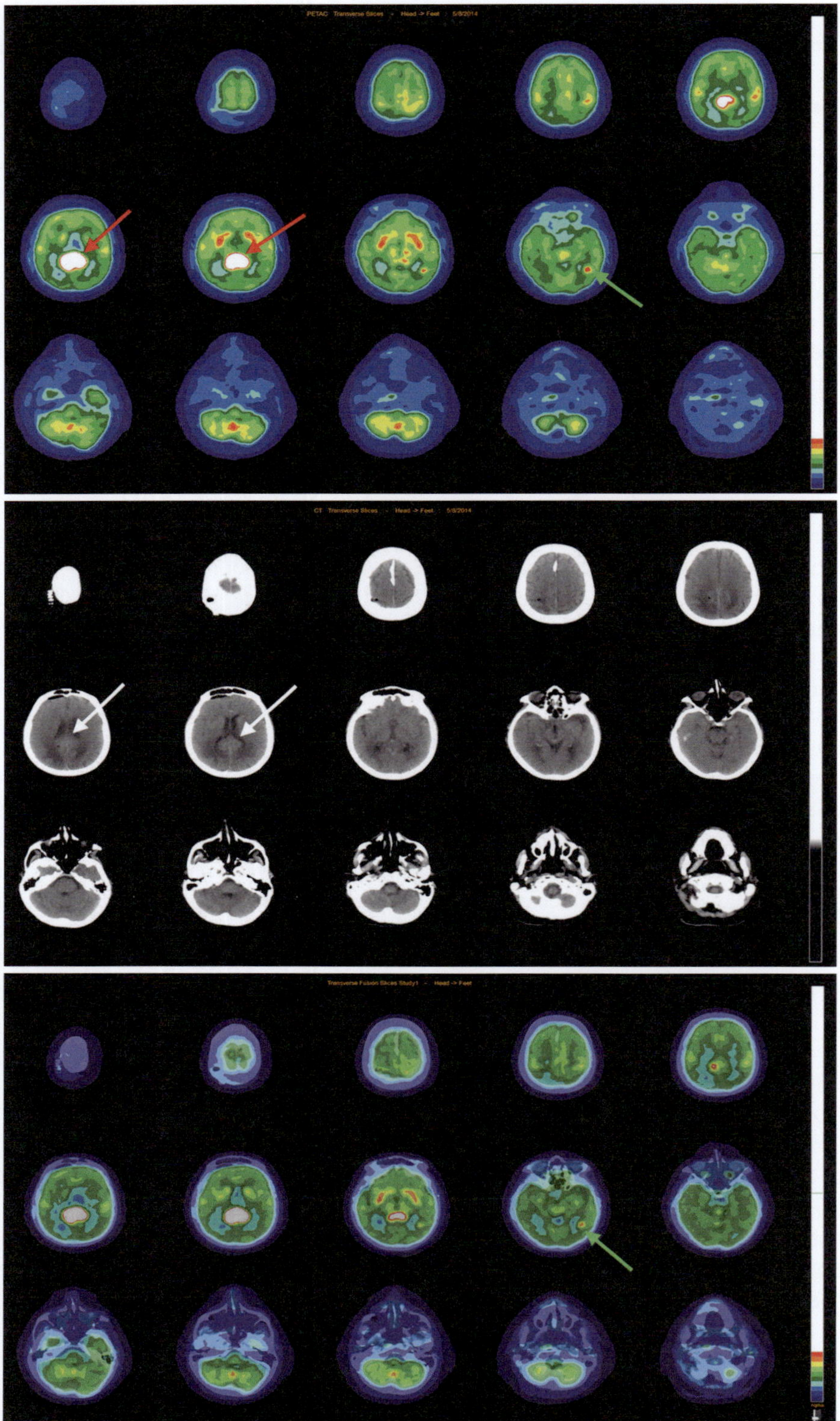

Fig. 5.3 A 72-year-old male with primary CNS lymphoma (PCNSL)

Case 5.4 Secondary CNS Lymphoma (SCNSL)

Clinical Information

Chief Complaint *History of malignant lymphoma and completed chemotherapy 1 year ago*

The patient is a 70-year-old male with longstanding history of chronic lymphocytic leukemia (CLL) which was stable until June 2017, when transformed diffuse large B-cell lymphoma (DLBCL) was diagnosed via lymph node and bone marrow biopsies at an outside institution. He received chemotherapy with RCHOP (rituximab, cyclophosphamide, doxorubicin hydrochloride, oncovin, and prednisolone) which was completed in December 2017 and currently on rituximab maintenance. The patient had achieved complete remission after six cycles of RCHOP, and there was no evidence of recurrent or residual disease on multiple FDG PET CT studies from October 2017 to August 2018. Clinical exam and laboratory tests were also negative, and the patient was asymptomatic.

A routine follow-up whole-body FDG PET CT was performed, with the patient's blood glucose level of 76 mg/dL prior to FDG administration.

FDG PET CT Findings (Fig. 5.4)

The brain PET images show a focus of intense FDG uptake (red arrows), corresponding to a low-density mass in the lateral right cerebellum on the concurrent CT (white arrows). Maximal SUV of the right cerebellar mass was 23.8, relative to max SUV 10.1 of the lateral left cerebellar cortex, suspicious for a malignant mass. Surrounding the mass is moderate hypometabolism noted in the remainder of the right cerebellum, suggestive of mass effect and vasogenic edema or both.

FDG activity in the remainder of the brain is within normal limits.

The remainder of the whole-body PET CT study was also negative for FDG-avid recurrent lymphoma in the peripheral (images not shown).

Discussion and Follow-Up

This 70-year-old male patient had a history of CLL and transformed DLBCL. After he received six cycles of standardized chemotherapy, he had achieved a complete remission for more than 1 year. This routine follow-up whole body FDG PET CT study, however, is suspicious for a newly developed right cerebellar malignant mass with mass effect and vasogenic edema in the surrounding right cerebellar parenchyma. The remainder of the whole-body FDG PET CT study shows no evidence of FDG-avid recurrent lymphoma in the peripheral. Brain MRI was performed at our recommendation, which confirmed "an approximately 2.3 × 1.9 cm right lateral cerebellar mass with mild adjacent edema," suspicious for malignancy.

Subsequently, biopsy of the right cerebellar mass was positive for extensive diffuse large B-cell lymphoma (DLBCL).

Given the history of treated DLBCL in the peripheral, this case is consistent with secondary CNS lymphoma (SCNSL), which is a rare and aggressive non-Hodgkin's lymphoma that mainly involves the leptomeninges and less commonly the brain parenchyma, the spinal cord, or eyes [5]. After the pathological diagnosis of SCNSL, the patient was treated with two cycles of IV methotrexate and rituximab in addition to intrathecal methotrexate. Additional chemotherapy could not proceed due to the patient's worsening chronic kidney disease. Nevertheless, a new FDG PET CT and MRI were negative for residual or recurrent disease in the brain. Again, there was no evidence of recurrent lymphoma in the peripheral on the follow-up FDG PET CT study.

Case Summary

This case shows an incidental finding of an FDG-avid right cerebellar lesion on a routine follow-up

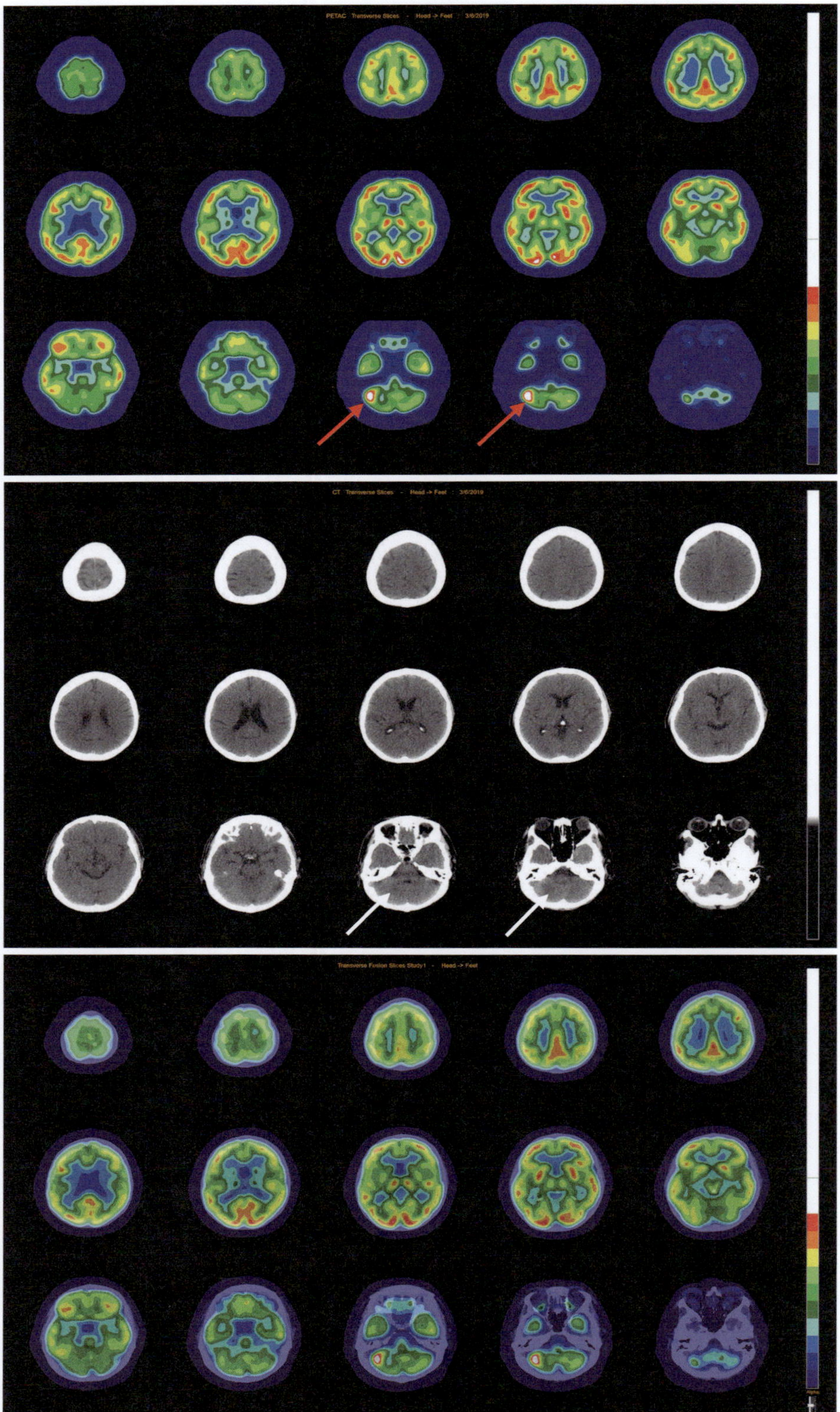

Fig. 5.4 A 70-year-old male with secondary CNS lymphoma (SCNSL)

whole body FDG PET CT for this 70-year-old male patient with history of DLBCL treated with standardized chemotherapy and achieved complete remission. Max SUV of the right cerebellar mass was 23.8, relative to max SUV 10.1 on the contralateral cerebellar cortex, suspicious for malignancy. Subsequently, the patient underwent a brain MRI and biopsy which was positive for DLBLC. Given the history of treated DLBCL in the peripheral, this case is consistent with secondary CNS lymphoma (SCNSL), a rare and aggressive non-Hodgkin's lymphoma that often involves the leptomeninges and less commonly the brain parenchyma, the spinal cord, or eyes [5]. Due to worsening chronic kidney disease, the patient only completed two cycles of IV and intrathecal chemotherapy but with a favorable response, based on the limited follow-up data.

Case 5.5 Left Temporal Ganglioglioma

Clinical Information

Chief Complaint *New-onset seizures with increasing frequencies*

The patient is a 1.5-year-old right-handed otherwise healthy male presenting with episodes of seizures, which were described by his father as staring look in his eyes, with lips turned blue and breath holding lasted for a few seconds. The seizure occurred even in his primary care pediatrician's office yesterday. On the day of his hospital admission, the patient has had several seizures already. Between seizures, he returned to normal activities.

Birth history is unremarkable. However, the patient has developmental delay in speech.

There is no history of traumatic brain injury, meningitis, or encephalitis.

Family history is significant for seizures and Down syndrome in the patient's uncles.

Brain MRI showed an approximately 1.7 × 1.8 × 4.1 cm circumscribed lesion involving the medial inferior left temporal lobe with avid enhancement.

EEG revealed seizure activity in the left temporal region.

Brain FDG PET CT was performed, with the patient's blood glucose of 72 mg/dL prior to FDG administration.

FDG PET Findings (Fig. 5.5)

The PET images show diffusely decreased FDG activity in the entire left temporal lobe, more prominent in the medial inferior portion (red arrows), corresponding to a circumscribed lesion on the prior brain MR T2 imaging (white arrows), suspicious for a left medial temporal tumor. Moderately decreased FDG activity is also noted in the adjacent left occipital, parietal, and frontal lobes, as well as the left basal ganglia and thalamus, likely due to mass effect or vasogenic edema or both.

FDG activity in the remainder of cerebral cortices is within normal limits.

Discussions and Follow-Up

It's well-known that low-grade gliomas could exhibit hypometabolism relative to the surrounding normal gray matter or contralateral cerebral cortex [2–4, 7]. The diffuse hypometabolism in the left temporal lobe, more prominent in the medial portion, is well corresponding to a circumscribed mass in the same location on the prior MRI. Constellation of the metabolic and anatomic neuroimaging features is highly suggestive of a left temporal tumor with a low metabolic rate, likely a low-grade primary brain tumor. The moderate hypometabolism in the surrounding is likely due to mass effects or vasogenic edema or both. FDG activity in the remainder of the cerebral cortices is within normal limits, indicating no surgical contraindications.

Subsequently, the patient underwent left temporal craniotomy and left temporal tumor resection. Pathological examination was consistent with a low-grade ganglioglioma, WHO grade I. After the surgery, the patient has been maintained on anti-seizure medication of levetiracetam. During the follow-up, the patient tolerated the medication well and has been seizure-free for nearly 3 years, with improved mood and general health.

Case Summary

Gangliogliomas are rare and low-grade primary brain tumors that often occur in the temporal lobes leading to medically refractory seizures, as presented in this case. Although brain MRI showed a well-circumscribed lesion, hypometabolism is identified not only in the lesion but also in the surrounding areas suggesting mass effects or vasogenic edema or both. The preserved metabolism in the remainder of the cerebral cortices indicates no surgical contraindications.

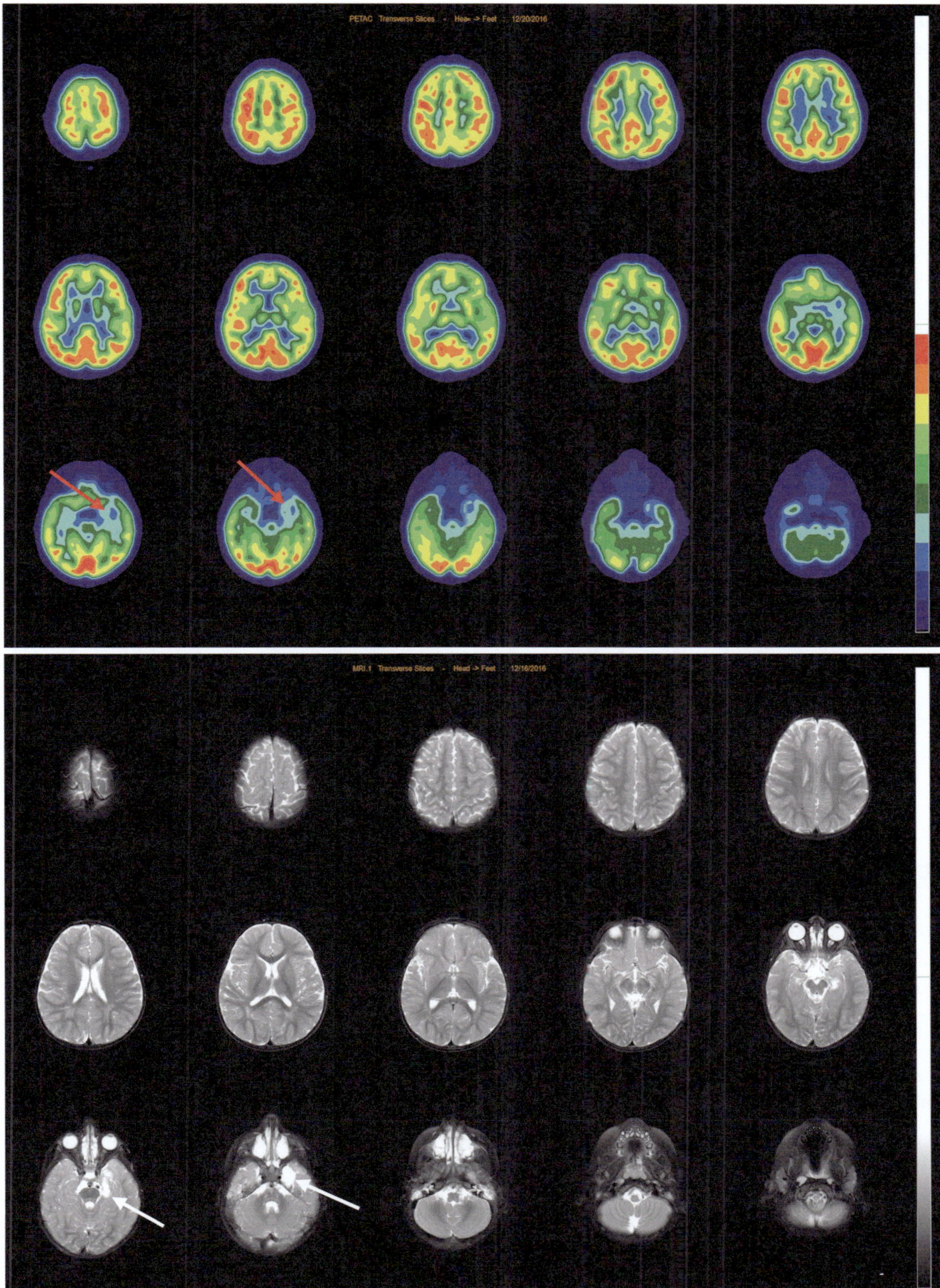

Fig. 5.5 A 1.5-year-old boy with left temporal ganglioglioma

Case 5.6 Leptomeningeal Melanoma

Clinical Information

Chief Complaint *Recently diagnosed brain melanoma with incomplete resection*

The patient is a 52-year-old male with recently diagnosed left cerebellopontine angle melanoma, status post incomplete surgical resection twice at an outside institution. According to the outside pathology report, the melanoma was moderate to severe nuclear pleomorphism, with focal necrosis, increased mitotic activity (9 mitoses per hpf), immunostains positive for S100, HMB-45, and melan-A. Postsurgical MRI showed a persistent mass with interval enlargement. In addition to known complete left ear deafness, the patient reports constant headache. Also, he reports waxing and waning left facial weakness, gait instability, and mild nausea, which were treated with dexamethasone. He's referred to our hospital for adjuvant radiotherapy.

Past medical history is notable for type I diabetes mellitus on insulin pump and hypertension.

Whole-body FDG PET CT was performed for restaging, with the patient's blood glucose level of 183 mg/dL prior to FDG administration.

FDG PET CT Findings (Fig. 5.6)

This is a technically limited study owing to the patient's hyperglycemia, indicating a poor blood glucose control. Therefore, maximal SUV measurements in this study are underestimated.

Nevertheless, the PET images show an irregular FDG-avid lesion in the left cerebellopontine angle (red arrows), corresponding to a hyperdense mass on the concurrent CT (white arrows), in line with the recent MRI findings, highly suggestive of residual leptomeningeal melanoma. In contrast, FDG activity in the majority of the left cerebellum is mild to moderately decreased, suggesting mass effects and vasogenic edema or both. Maximal SUV of the mass is 11.8, while the max SUV of the cerebral cortices is 6.8. Both values are likely markedly underestimated, due to the patient's hyperglycemia. However, there is no discrete focal abnormality in the remainder of the brain to suggestive additional involvement. On the concurrent CT, post-resection changes are noted in the left mastoid/ear channel region.

The remainder of the whole-body FDG PET CT study was unremarkable, without evidence of FDG-avid malignancy or metastasis in the peripheral (images not shown).

Discussion and Follow-Up

Despite the technical limitation due to hyperglycemia, the FDG PET CT findings, in line with prior MRI results, are highly suggestive of residual leptomeningeal melanoma located in the left cerebellopontine angle. The max SUV of the mass is nearly twice as high as that of the cerebral cortices, and this high metabolic rate is consistent with known aggressive features of the melanoma on immunostains and the recent interval enlargement on MRI. The hypometabolism in the surrounding left cerebellar parenchyma is likely due to mass effects or vasogenic edema or both. There is no evidence of FDG-avid malignancy or metastasis in the remainder of the CNS nor the peripheral. However, MRI of the lumbar spine showed a punctate intradural/extramedullary lesion posterior to the conus medullaris at the L1–L2 level, suspicious for a leptomeningeal seeding tumor, although MRI of the cervical and thoracic spine was unremarkable. The patient is currently under further evaluation for adjuvant radiation of the left cerebellopontine angle residual melanoma, which will be followed by systemic therapy, given the presence of leptomeningeal seeding in the lumbar spine region.

Case Summary

FDG PET CT study in this diabetic patient is technically limited, due to hyperglycemia (183 mg/dL), which is a common clinical issue. Nevertheless, the value of FDG PET CT in this particular case is at least threefold: (1) Although

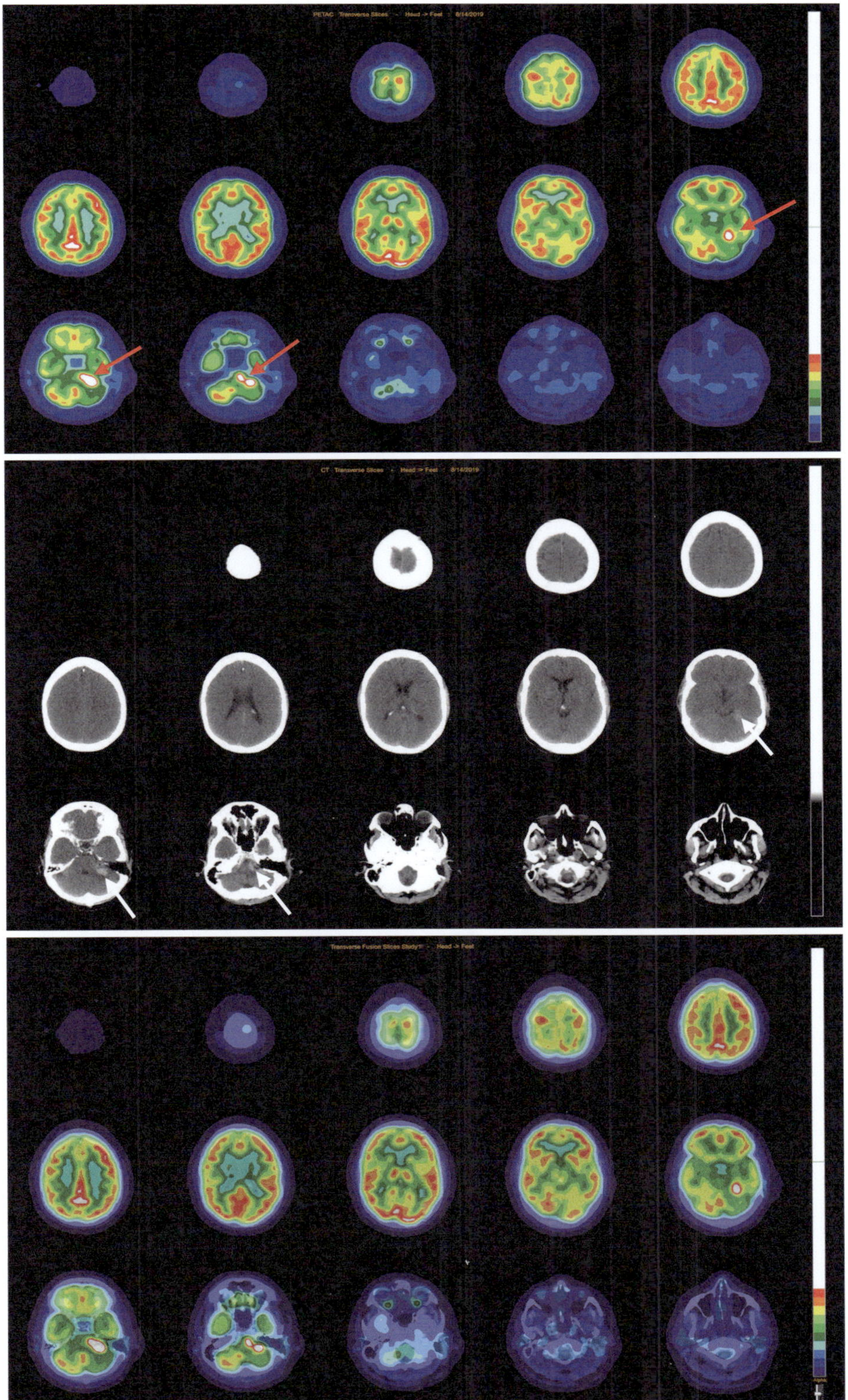

Fig. 5.6 A 52-year-old male with residual leptomeningeal melanoma

the max SUV is underestimated due to hyperglycemia, the nearly twice high max SUV of the left cerebellopontine angle tumor mass, relative to that of the normal cerebral cortex, is consistent with the known aggressive features of the malignant melanoma. (2) The hypometabolism in the adjacent left cerebellum is suggestive of mass effects and vasogenic edema or both, indirect evidence of a malignant tumor. And (3) there is no evidence of FDG-avid additional sites of malignancy or metastasis in the remainder of CNS or the peripheral. Subsequent MRI, however, shows subtle findings suspicious for a tiny leptomeningeal seeding in the lumbar region that deems undetectable on FDG PET CT. MRI and FDG PET CT play a complementary rule in this patient's leptomeningeal melanoma restaging and radiation therapy planning.

Case 5.7 Multifocal Brain Metastases of Lung Origin

Clinical Information

Chief Complaint *Recently diagnosed lung cancer and new-onset seizure*

The patient was a 76-year-old female with recently diagnosed right lung poorly differentiated adenocarcinoma. Mediastinoscopy with lymph node sampling (one level 7 node and two level R4 nodes) was negative for metastasis. She deemed not a good candidate for surgery due to her poor pulmonary function status and other comorbidities. While waiting for radiation therapy, she developed one episode of myoclonic jerking at home that lasted for a few minutes, without recollection of the event and no reported loss of consciousness or fall. Since then, she reported left lower extremity weakness and intermittent mixing up of words for about 10 days.

Medical oncology history was notable for remote left breast cancer, status post left mastectomy 15 years ago, without chemotherapy or radiation.

Past medical history was notable for extensive smoking for more than 50 years, COPD, anemia, hypertension, dyslipidemia, depression, and chronic kidney disease (stage IV).

FDG PET CT including a dedicated brain imaging was performed, with the patient's blood glucose of 94 mg/dL prior to FDG administration. Due to markedly abnormal findings in the brain as described below, MRI of the brain was performed subsequently at our request.

Imaging Findings (Fig. 5.7)

The dedicated brain PET imaging revealed three discrete small foci of increased FDG activity, two in the right frontal lobe and one in the left frontal lobe (red arrows), corresponding to ring-enhancing lesions on the MRI (white arrows), highly suspicious for brain metastases. In addition, multiple areas of cortical hypometabolism are noted, involving at least the bilateral frontal lobes, the superomedial right parietal lobe, and the right cerebellum (hatched yellow arrows), suggestive of vasogenic edema and/or diaschisis. However, there is no discrete focally increased FDG activity to correspond to at least four other enhancing lesions on the MRI, scattered in the lateral right frontal lobe, left lateral inferior parietal lobe, and the right cerebellum (green arrows), which are also suspicious for brain metastases, despite the lack of FDG PET correlation. In retrospect, focal normometabolism is noted in the lateral right frontal lobe and the lateral right cerebellum, where three enhancing lesions are appreciated on the MRI.

The FDG PET CT scan of the chest demonstrated a right upper lung mass, consistent with known right lung primary malignancy, with several satellite nodules in the adjacent right lung parenchyma, and multiple FDG-avid lymph nodes scattered in the right hilum and bilateral mediastinum, suspicious for metastases (images not shown).

Discussion and Follow-Up

Brain metastasis of lung origin is the most commonly diagnosed metastatic brain tumors and accounts for 40–50% of the total cases [1]. It's estimated that approximately 10% of newly diagnosed patients with advanced non-small cell lung cancers (NSCLC) would develop brain metastasis [1, 6]. Initial clinical workup in this patient, however, was suggestive of early stage of right lung cancer, given the negative mediastinal lymph node biopsies. A dedicate brain PET scan was requested as part of the initial staging with FDG PET CT, mainly because of newly developed seizure and other neurological symptoms (left lower extremity weakness and difficulty in wording). Although the FDG PET findings were highly abnormal, and suggestive of at least three discrete FDG-avid metastatic lesions, there were multiple areas of cortical hypometabolism likely due to vasogenic edema and concerning for more metastatic involvement. Brain MRI was subsequently performed at our request, which indeed revealed a total of seven discrete enhancing lesions, three with FDG PET correlate and the

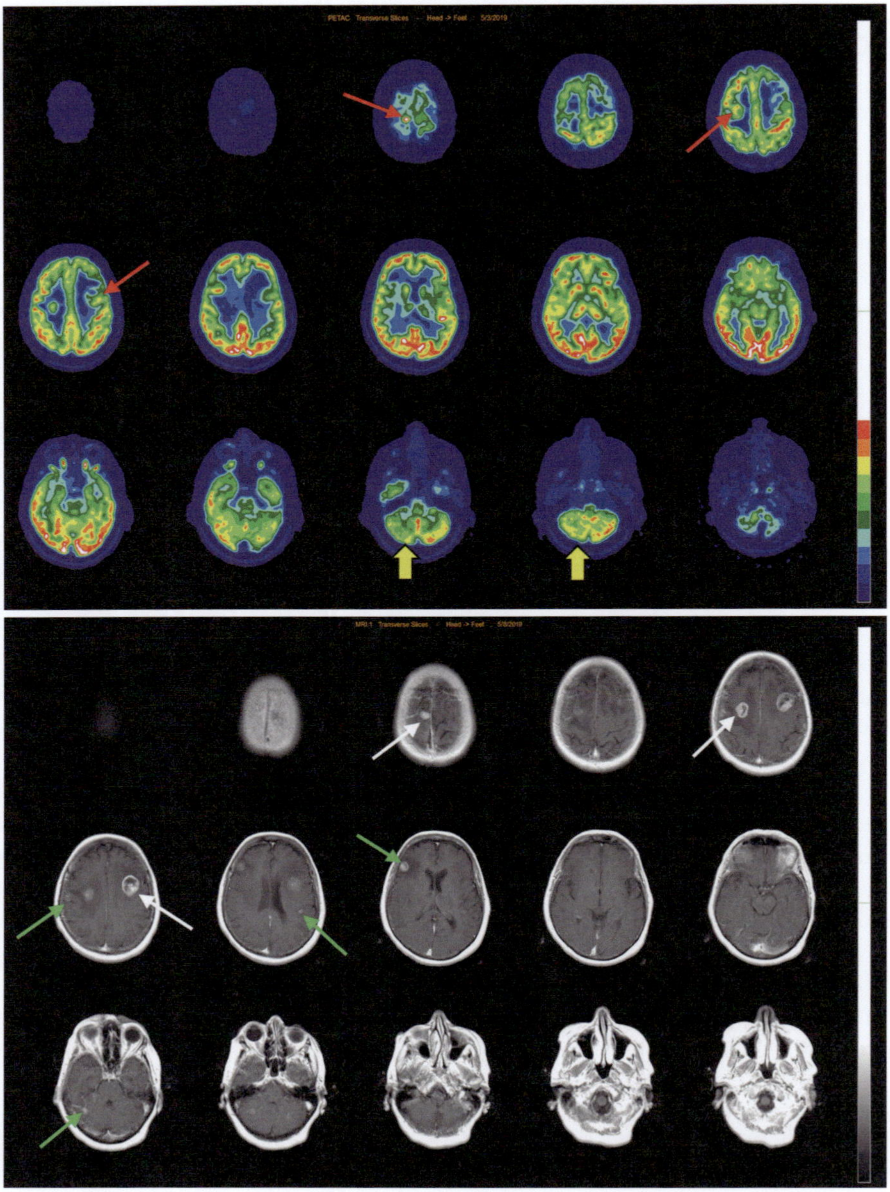

Fig. 5.7 A 76-year-old female with multifocal metastatic lung cancer to the brain

other four without, in retrospect, all suspicious for brain metastasis. The suboptimal detection sensitivity of FDG PET CT, relative to that of MRI, appears independent of lesion size, contrast enhancement or location.

On the same day of the brain MRI study, the patient was admitted to our hospital due to altered mental status. She was treated with Decadron and levetiracetam, with a good seizure control. Then, per multidisciplinary discussion, the patient started whole brain radiation, which was stopped 2 weeks later due to lack of improvement. Systemic chemotherapy was planned but could not proceed due to acute blood loss anemia from Mediport placement. The patient deceased several days later, due to a poor response to therapy, deteriorating anemia and hypoxia, and multiple organ failure.

Case Summary

Metastatic lung cancer to brain is the most commonly diagnosed brain metastatic tumor [1]. This case highlights the importance of a dedicated brain FDG PET as part of the initial staging of patients with newly diagnosed lung cancer, especially for patients with new onset of neurological symptoms. Brain metastatic lesions of lung origin could manifest on FDG PET as hypermetabolic foci (positive findings), or normometabolism or even hypometabolism (falsely negative findings), independent of lesion size, contrast-enhancing, or location. Therefore, correlation with brain MRI is always recommended, which is a first-line neuroimaging modality with the highest sensitivity for detection of brain metastasis.

Case 5.8 Recurrent Brain Metastasis of Breast Origin

Clinical Information

Chief Complaint *History of metastatic breast cancer involving the brain, lung, and bone*

The patient is a 63-year-old female with history of right breast cancer diagnosed in 2014, treated with multiple lobectomies eventual mastectomy followed by radiation. Four years ago, she developed left frontal brain metastasis of breast origin (biopsy proven) in addition to a small metastatic lesion to the right occipital lobe, status post right frontal craniotomy/tumor resection, and Gamma Knife stereotactic radiosurgery (GK SRS) of the small right occipital lesion. Also, the patient developed metastases to the right mid lung and several sites of the bone, for which she received palliative radiation.

Current symptoms include progressive back pain, weakness, and gait instability. A new brain MRI showed an enhancing lesion at the prior left frontal surgical site, measuring approximately 2.1 × 1.7 × 2.4 cm. However, MR spectroscopy analysis was in favor of posttreatment inflammatory changes.

Whole-body FDG PET CT scan was performed, with the patient's blood glucose of 97 mg/dL prior to FDG administration.

FDG PET CT Findings (Fig. 5.8)

The PET images (the upper panel) show a moderate-sized focus of increased FDG uptake in the lateral left forefrontal lobe (red arrow), surrounded by a large area of moderate to severe hypometabolism, even involving the left basal ganglia and thalamus, in line with the prior MRI findings, highly suggestive of recurrent brain metastasis with extensive mass effects and vasogenic edema.

In the right orbitofrontal region, there is an area of absent FDG activity (green arrow), consistent with the history of right frontal lobe metastasectomy. Diffuse, mild hypometabolism is noted in the right cerebellum (hatched yellow arrows), relative to the left, consistent with diaschisis. There is diffusely increased FDG activity in the remainder of the right frontal lobe and bilateral parietal and occipital lobes of unknown etiology.

On the concurrent CT (the middle panel), low-density changes are noted in the left frontal lobe and the right orbitofrontal area (white arrows), consistent with mass effects/vasogenic edema and postsurgical changes.

The PET CT fused images (the lower panel) confirm an FDG-avid lesion located in the lateral left frontal lobe.

The remainder of the whole-body FDG PET CT shows interval improvement in multiple bone lesions involving at least the left T7, the T11, and the left proximal tibia, indicating a partial response to ongoing chemotherapy (images not shown).

Discussion and Follow-Up

Prior to FDG PET CT study, MRI and MR spectroscopy showed suspicious but non-conclusive findings in the left frontal lobe. In contrast, FDG PET CT findings as described are highly suggestive of recurrent metastasis in the left forefrontal lobe, surrounded by mass effects and vasogenic edema. Follow-up brain MRIs consistently showed interval enlargement of the left frontal lesion. Subsequently, the patient underwent surgical resection of approximately 3 cm left frontal tumor mass, which was consistent with metastatic carcinoma of breast primary, per pathology.

Case Summary

Breast cancers are one of the common causes of brain metastasis [6], which, as demonstrated in this case, is characterized by hypermetabolism in metastatic tumors surrounded by hypometabolism due to mass effect and vasogenic edema. FDG PET played a significant role in the diagnosis of current metastasis in this patient with prior non-conclusive/conflicting MRI and MR spectroscopy results. The positive FDG PET finding of a left frontal recurrent metastasis was further supported by follow-up MRIs and finally confirmed by surgical resection and definite pathological diagnosis.

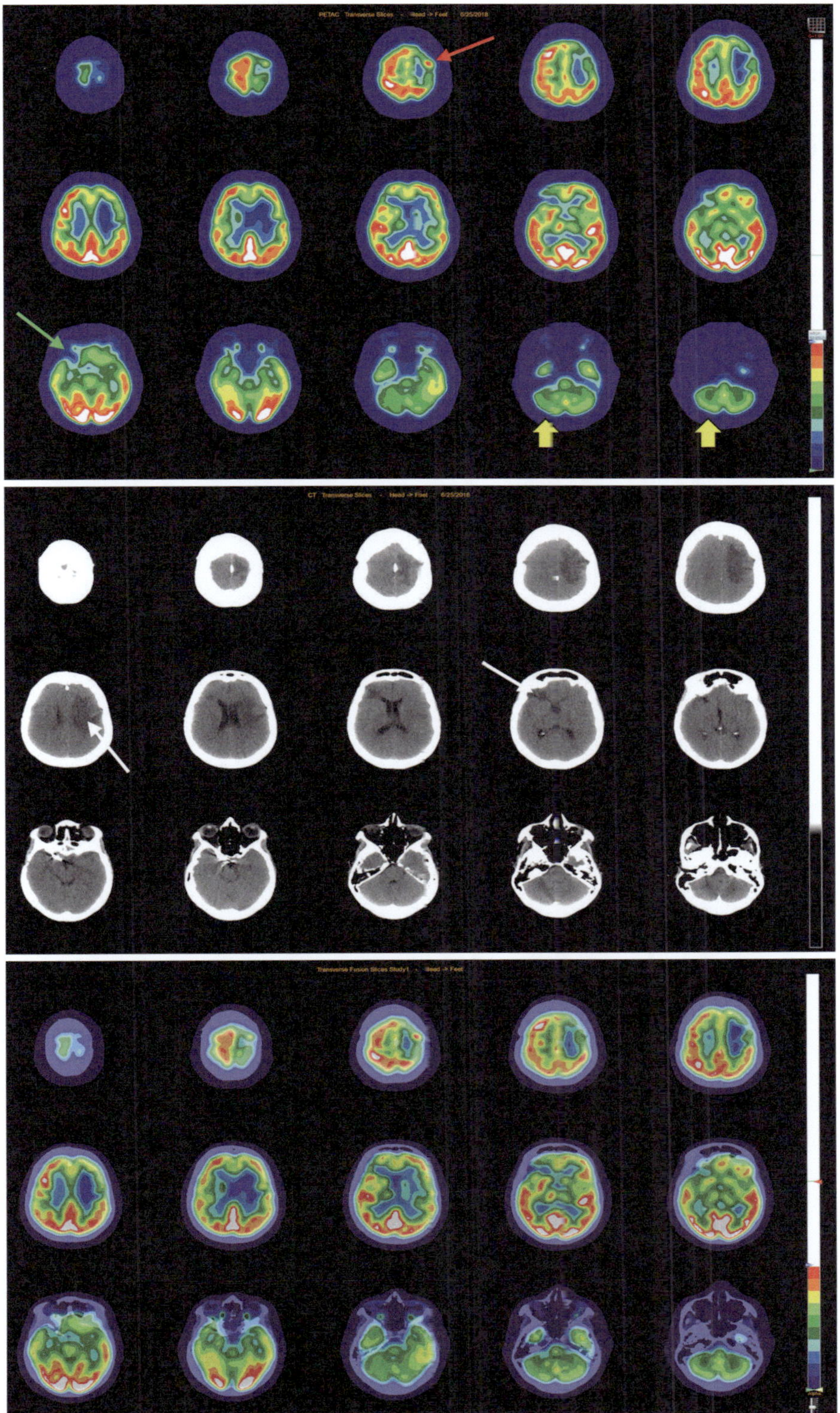

Fig. 5.8 A 63-year-old female with recurrent metastatic breast cancer to the brain

References

1. Barnholtz-Sloan JS, Sloan AE, Davis FG, et al. Incidence proportions of brain metastases in patients diagnosed (1973-2001) in the Metropolitan Detroit Cancers Surveillance System. J Clin Oncol. 2004;22:2865–72.
2. Chen W. Clinical applications of PET in brain tumors. J Nucl Med. 2007;48(9):1468–81.
3. Demetriades AK, Almeida AC, Bhangoo RS, et al. Application of positron emission tomography in neuro-oncology: a clinical approach. Surgeon. 2014;12(3):148–57.
4. Hustinx R, Fosse P. PET in brain tumors. PET Clin. 2010;5(2):185–97.
5. Malikova H, Burghardtova M, Koubska E, et al. Secondary central nervous system lymphoma: spectrum of morphological MRI appearances. Neuropsychiatr Dis Treat. 2018;14:733–40.
6. Schouten LJ, Rutten J, Huveneers HA, et al. Incidence of brain metastases in a cohort of patients with carcinoma of the breast, colon, kidney, and lung and melanoma. Cancer. 2002;94:2698–705.
7. Seqtnan EA, Hess S, Grupe P, et al. ^{18}F-fluorodeoxyglucose PET/computed tomography for primary brain tumors. PET Clin. 2015;10(1):59–73.
8. Tang YZ, Booth TC, Bhogal P, et al. Imaging of primary central nervous system lymphoma. Clin Radiol. 2011;66(8):768–077.
9. Wang X, Hu X, Xie P, et al. Comparison of magnetic resonance spectroscopy and positron emission tomography in detection of tumor recurrence in posttreatment of glioma: a diagnostic meta-analysis. Asia Pac J Clin Oncol. 2015;11(2):97–105.

6 Dopamine Transporter Scan (DaTscan)

Case 6.1 Probable Normal DaTscan Consistent with Essential Tremor (ET)

Clitnical Information

Chief Complaint *Right hand and head tremor for 3 years*

The patient is a 54-year-old right-handed male who has noted right hand tremor for approximately 3 years. This followed shortly by head tremor that bothers him, and sometimes he wakes up with head tremor. His hand writing is sloppy. Past medical history is notable for ankylosing spondylitis and right hemifacial spasm. The patient is a never smoker and denies alcohol or drug abuse. Family history is significant for essential tremor in his father who also has restless legs syndrome in his paternal aunt and a paternal grandmother. The patient was evaluated at an outside institution, but several tests including brain MRI, electromyography (EMG), and DaTscan were reported unremarkable. Since November 2016, he has been on propranolol (Inderal), 20 mg by mouth, twice a day, with a good tremor control.

DaTscan Findings

Review of DaTscan starts with color normalization. Since the highest tracer activity is normally seen in caudate nuclei, the color of caudate nuclei shall be adjusted in red on the 10-step color spectrum. Then, I recommend to centralize the striatal imaging transaxial slides on a panel of 15 in order to appreciate any asymmetry and/or patient's head tilting.

After color normalization and appropriate image display, the DaTscan of this case (Fig. 6.1) shows striatal tracer activity in a crescent shape, with highest activity in caudate nuclei (red arrow) as expected and tapering into putamen body and tail (white arrow), on both sides, in a continuum and essentially symmetric pattern. The striatal tracer activity is distinct and is at least threefold higher, when compared to that of the surrounding brain parenchyma (green arrow), which is in blue to sky-blue color, indicating approximately 20–30% of the striatal tracer activity.

Discussion and Follow-Up

This patient has a strong family history of essential tremor (ET). He has had right hand and head tremors for several years; however, neurological tests/studies at an outside institution including brain MRI, EMG, and DaTscan were unremarkable. Furthermore, the patient has been treated with a beta-blocker (propranolol) that shows a good response. This current DaTscan at our hospital is again normal, consistent with ET rather than PD [1].

D. Wu, *Clinical Nuclear Medicine Neuroimaging*, https://doi.org/10.1007/978-3-030-40893-0_6

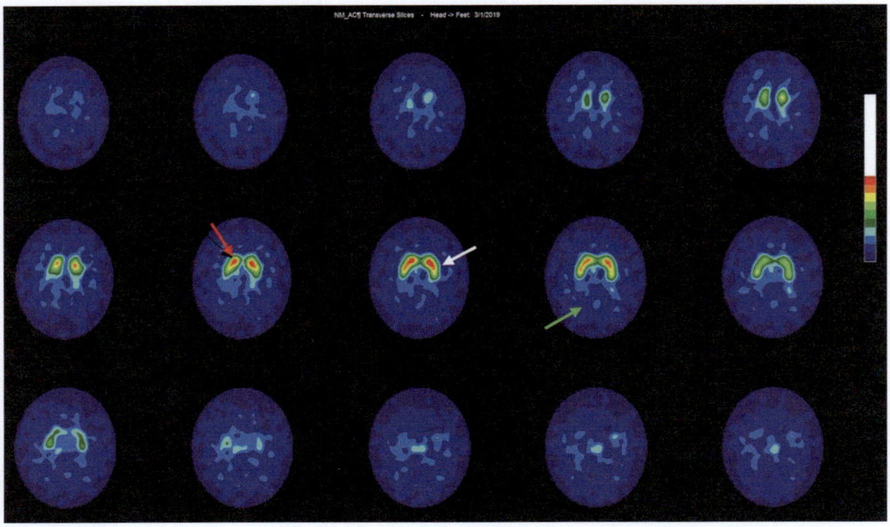

Fig. 6.1 A 54-year-old right-handed male with probable normal DaTscan consistent with essential tremor (ET)

Of note, although the patient is on multiple medications, none of them has significant interfering effects on DaTscan.

During the follow-up, the patient's tremor is well controlled on Inderal (propranolol) 20 mg daily.

Case Summary

A normal DaTscan is characterized by essentially symmetric, crescent-shaped tracer activity in bilateral basal ganglia, which is distinct, relative to that of the surrounding brain tissue. Normal DaTscan findings are consistent with ET rather than neurodegenerative disorders [8]. The sustained good response to a beta-blocker (Inderal) in this patient further supports for the scintigraphic diagnosis of ET.

Case 6.2 Abnormal DaTscan Likely due to PD and Coexisting AVM

Clinical Information

Chief Complaint *Right hand tremor for 1 year and history of AVM*

The patient is a 65-year-old female presenting with right hand tremor for 1 year, for which she even cannot hold a glass. Past medical history is notable for right brain arteriovenous malformation (AVM) status post embolization and surgical treatments, seizure disorder, right cerebrovascular accident (CVA) due to thrombosis, and left hemiplegia.

Current medications include citalopram, divalproex, filgrastim, gabapentin, imipramine, phenobarbital, and nitrofurantoin.

DaTscan Findings (Fig. 6.2)

The images show absent tracer activity in the entire right striatum, with overall decreased brain parenchyma background activity (magenta arrow) in nearly entire right hemisphere, consistent with known AVM, CVA, and posttreatment changes. Interpretation of the left striatum is a challenge, due to lack of comparison to the right, but there is moderately decreased tracer activity in the left putamen (white arrow). Although tracer activity in the left caudate nuclei appears preserved, the mildly elevated background activity in the left brain parenchyma (green arrow) is suggesting globally decreased left striatal activity, probably including the left caudate nuclei.

Discussion and Follow-Up

Interpretation of this patient's DaTscan is difficult, due to known right brain large AVM, CVA, and extensive posttreatment changes. Also, the patient is currently on multiple medications, although they appear to have no significant interference. Despite the lack of comparison to the right, the DaTscan shows moderately decreased tracer activity in the left putamen, corresponding to the patient's recent onset of right hand tremor, in conjunction with likely globally decreased left striatal tracer activity, suspicious for left-sided PD.

Shortly after the abnormal DaTscan, the patient has started pharmacotherapy with Sinemet, 25/100 mg, one tablet by mouth, twice a day, at an outside institution. She tolerated the medication well, with a good tremor control.

Case Summary

This case emphasizes the importance of clinical history and current presentation, especially lateralized symptoms, in the interpretation of DaTscan results. This 65-year-old female patient has an extensive history of right brain AVM and CVA, treated with embolization and surgeries, which explains the absent tracer activity in the entire right striatum and even decreased background activity in the right brain parenchyma on DaTscan. Imaging of the left striatum, however, shows moderately decreased tracer activity in the left putamen and likely mild global decreased left striatal activity. The finding is well corresponding to the patient's recent onset of right hand tremor, therefore, suspicious for left-sided PD, which was supported by a good response to L-dopa pharmacotherapy during the follow-up.

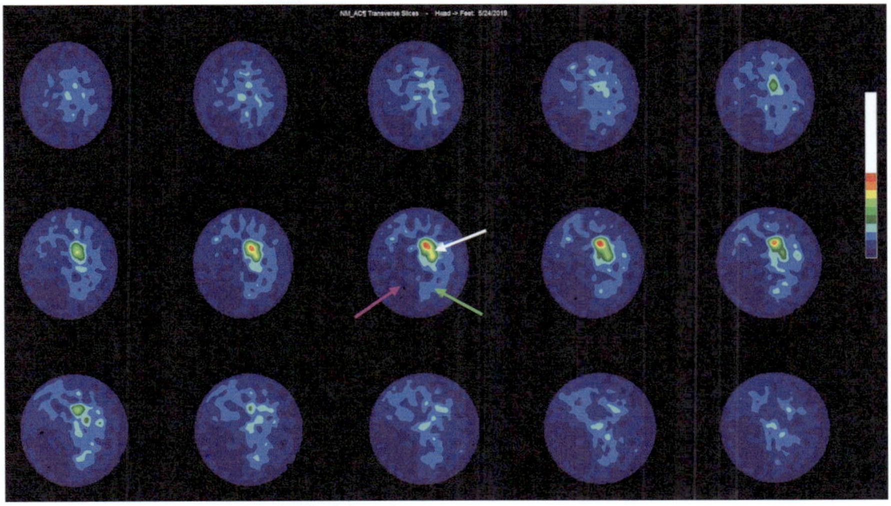

Fig. 6.2 A 65-year-old female with abnormal DaTscan likely due to PD and AVM

Case 6.3 Abnormal DaTscan due to Left-sided Stroke

Clinical Information

Chief Complaint *Occasional tremor in both hands for 3 years*

The patient is a 72-year-old female presenting with occasional tremor of both hands for 3 years. Neurological examination has been unremarkable, although there is a clinical concern for conversion disorder. Past medical history is notable for hypertension, non-insulin-dependent diabetes, peripheral vascular disease, paroxysmal atrial fibrillation, mitral valve disorder, uterine cancer, and stroke in 2011.

The patient is a current smoker, but denies alcohol or drug abuse.

Current medications include atorvastatin, digoxin, lisinopril, and metoprolol.

DaTscan Findings (Fig. 6.3)

The images show normal, crescent-shaped tracer activity in the entire right striatum. In contrast, the left caudate nuclei (red arrow) and putamen are shrunk (white arrow) and both with severely decreased tracer activity.

Discussion and Follow-Up

Interpretation of this DaTscan is challenging due to lack of anatomic neuroimaging for correlation. Nevertheless, the DaTscan shows normal tracer intensity in the right caudate nuclei and putamen. The severely decreased tracer activity in the left caudate nuclei and putamen is abnormal, but is atypical for PD that often affects putamen more than caudate nuclei. Given the history, the left-sided abnormal findings are most likely secondary to prior left-sided stroke, probably in the middle cerebral artery territory.

Clinically, the patient has occasional tremor of both hands, which is atypical for Parkinson's disease. During the follow-up for 5 years, the patient developed symptoms, in conjunction with the abnormal DaTscan finding, leading to clinical diagnosis of vascular Parkinsonism.

Case Summary

This is an extraordinary case showing abnormal DaTscan due to prior left-sided stroke. The prior ischemic insult causes shrunk left striatum, with severely decreased tracer activity, equally affecting the caudate nuclei and putamen, a pattern atypical for idiopathic PD. This case highlights that unilateral involvement of one entire striatum with spared contralateral striatum, especially contralateral putamen on DaTscan, is an imaging "red flag" suspicious for neurological conditions other than PD.

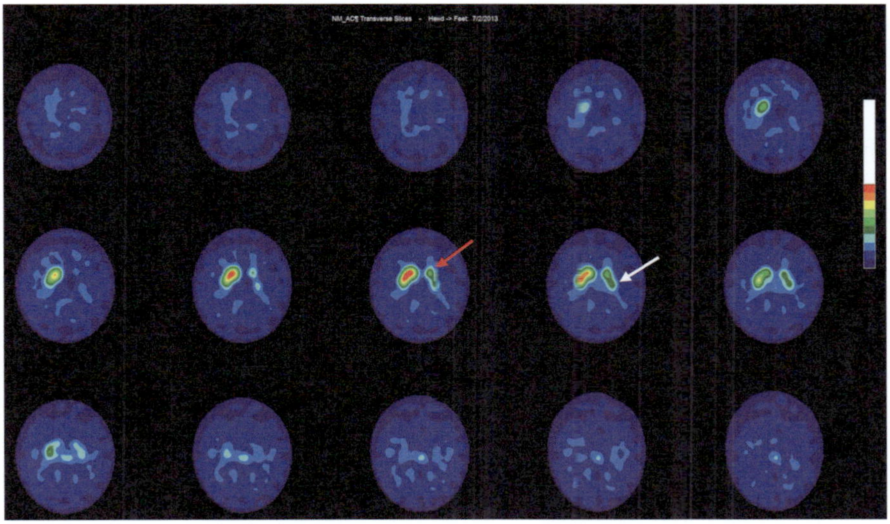

Fig. 6.3 A 72-year-old female with abnormal DaTscan due to left stroke

Case 6.4 Abnormal DaTscan with Right Striatum Being More Affected Than the Left

Clinical Information

Chief Complaint *Right arm and hand tremor for 5 months*

The patient is a 62-year-old male presenting with right arm and hand tremors for 5 months. He has been on Sinemet for 2 months, with a good response, and now only has occasional tremor. Past medical history is notable for hypertension, hyperlipidemia, spinal stenosis, chronic neck pain, asthma, thoracic outlet syndrome, gastroesophageal reflux disease (GERD), and obstructive sleep apnea (OSA).

Current medications include Sinemet (25/100 mg, twice a day), atorvastatin, gabapentin, hydrocodone-acetaminophen, and omeprazole.

DaTscan Findings (Fig. 6.4)

The images show nearly absent tracer activity in the putamen of both hemispheres (white arrow). Decreased tracer activity is also noted in the right caudate nuclei (red arrow) when compared to the left. There is mildly elevated tracer activity in the surrounding brain parenchyma (green arrow) relative to the striata, which is indirect evidence of global decreased striatal activity including that of the left caudate nuclei.

Discussion and Follow-Up

At the time of the DaTscan, the patient has been treated with Sinemet that shows a good response. This DaTscan shows global and regional abnormalities, in a classic imaging pattern highly suggestive of PD, right striatum being more affected than the left. This laterality is disconcordant to the patient's right-sided tremor. According to the recent literature [5], approximately 76% patients have contralateral clinical symptoms corresponding to lateralized striatal dopamine transporter depletion on DaTscan. However, disconcordant DaTscan findings relative to lateralized tremor symptom do occur in at least 15% patients.

During the follow-up, the Sinemet dose was increased from 25/100 mg, one tablet by mouth, twice a day, to 25/250 mg, two tablets by mouth, three times a day, with further improved tremor control.

Case Summary

The neuropathology of idiopathic PD is characterized by vulnerability-dependent loss of striatal dopamine neurons, e.g., putamen being more vulnerable than caudate nuclei [2, 10]. This DaTscan shows nearly absent dopamine transporter activity in bilateral putamens and, to a lesser degree, decreased activity in both caudate nuclei, the right being more affected than the left, in a classic imaging pattern, highly suggestive of PD rather than ET. This scintigraphic diagnosis has been further supported by an improved tremor control with increased dosage of Sinemet.

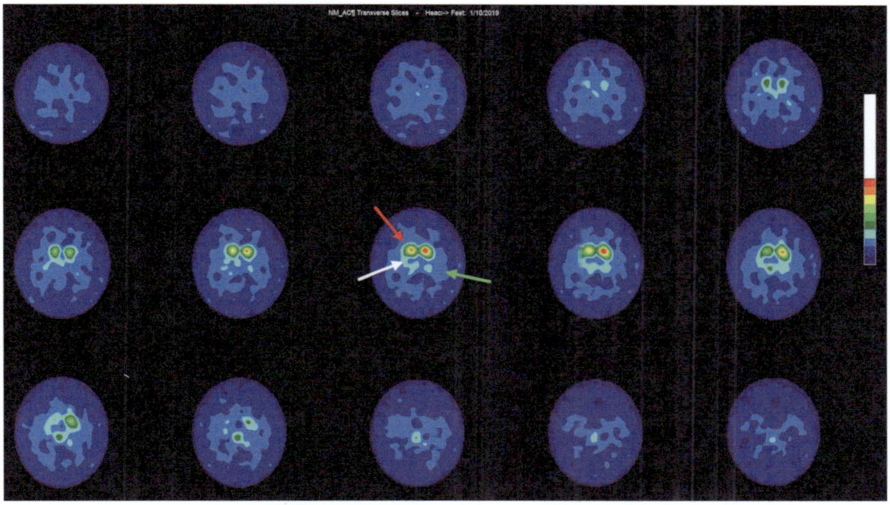

Fig. 6.4 A 62-year-old male with abnormal DaTscan consistent with PD

Case 6.5 Probable Normal DaTscan Consistent with Neuroleptic-Induced Parkinsonism

Clinical Information

Chief Complaint *Tremor in left arm/hand and history of bipolar disorder*

The patient is a 63-year-old male presenting with left arm and hand tremor for 8 weeks. Past medical history is notable for essential hypertension, hyperlipidemia, cervical spinal stenosis, and bipolar disorder with depression. Current medications include Risperdal Consta (risperidone) IM injection every 2 weeks for long-term treatment of his bipolar disorder. At the request of the referring physician, DaTscan was performed without stopping Risperdal Consta IM injection.

DaTscan Findings (Fig. 6.5)

The images show crescent-shaped, normal tracer activity in caudate nuclei (red arrow) and putamen (white arrow) of both hemispheres. The striatal activity relative to the surrounding brain parenchyma is distinct and is at least three times higher, based on the 10-step color scale. Of note, the appearance of minimal decreased tracer activity in the left striatum relative to the right is likely due to head-tilting to the right.

Discussion

The patient has a history of bipolar disorder treated with Risperdal Consta IM injection every other week. According to the manufacturer's instruction and literature [3–5], risperidone needs to be discontinued, but DaTscan proceeded without stopping the injection at request of the referring neurologist. It turned out that that DaTscan is essentially normal, without evidence of a neurodegenerative process. Therefore, the scintigraphic findings are supportive of neuroleptic-induced Parkinsonism.

Case Summary

Risperidone is a medication with highest property to cause Parkinsonism. This case shows that DaTscan can be performed without stopping risperidone injections if clinically needed. Moreover, the normal DaTscan finding is highly suggestive of drug-induced Parkinsonism rather than a dopamine neurodegenerative disorder.

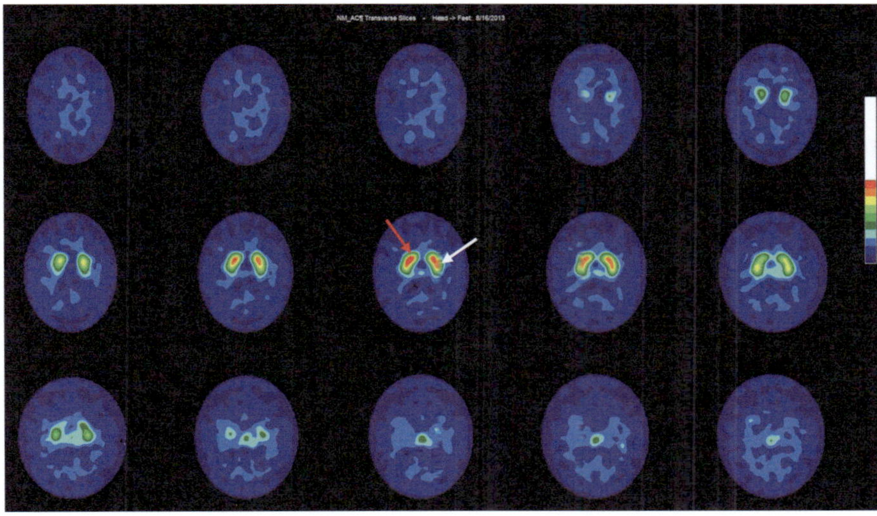

Fig. 6.5 A 63-year-old male with probable normal DaTscan consistent with neuroleptic-induced Parkinsonism

Case 6.6 Abnormal DaTscan with Left Striatum Being More Affected Than the Right

Clinical Information

Chief Complaint *Right hand rest tremor for 4 months*

The patient is a 72-year-old male presenting with right hand tremor for 4 months. The tremor is more prominent when he is sitting still. When he stands up, the tremor seems improved. His writing is shaky, but balance is fine. He denies a family history of tremor. Past medical history is notable for hypercholesterolemia, GERD, and anxiety disorder treated with neuroleptics in the past.

Current medications include Mucinex D, Prevacid, Vicodin ES, vitamin D3, and Xanax.

DaTscan Findings (Fig. 6.6)

The images show decreased tracer activity in the left caudate nuclei (red arrow) and more severely decreased/nearly absent tracer activity in the left putamen (white arrow). To a lesser degree, decreased tracer activity is also noted in the right putamen. Tracer activity in the right caudate nuclei is relatively preserved. However, the mildly elevated background tracer activity in the surrounding brain parenchyma (green arrow) is suggestive of globally decreased striatal activity including the right caudate nuclei.

Discussion and Follow-Up

The patient has a history of anxiety disorder treated with neuroleptics in the past and recently developed right hand rest tremor. DaTscan was requested to evaluate PD versus neuroleptic-induced Parkinsonism. The abnormal DaTscan findings as described are consistent with a dopamine neurodegenerative process rather than drug-induced Parkinsonism. Furthermore, the scintigraphic finding of dominant loss of left striatal dopamine transporters corresponds to the patient's right-sided hand tremor.

Following the abnormal DaTscan, the patient has been on Sinemet 25/100 mg, with initial dosage of one table by mouth, twice a day, and adjusted in 3 months to two tablets by mouth, three times a day. He tolerated the medication well and has achieved a good and sustained tremor control over the last five and a half years.

Case Summary

Progression of Parkinson's neuropathology follows a pattern characterized by first involvement of putamen on one or both sides and then spreading into one or two caudate nuclei. DaTscan in this case reveals profound loss of dopamine transporters in putamens, to a lesser degree in caudate nuclei. The predominant loss of dopamine transporters in left striatum is concordant with the patient's right hand rest tremor. During the follow-up, the patient has had a good and sustained response to Sinemet for more than 5 years, further supporting the scintigraphic diagnosis of PD, rather than drug-induced Parkinsonism.

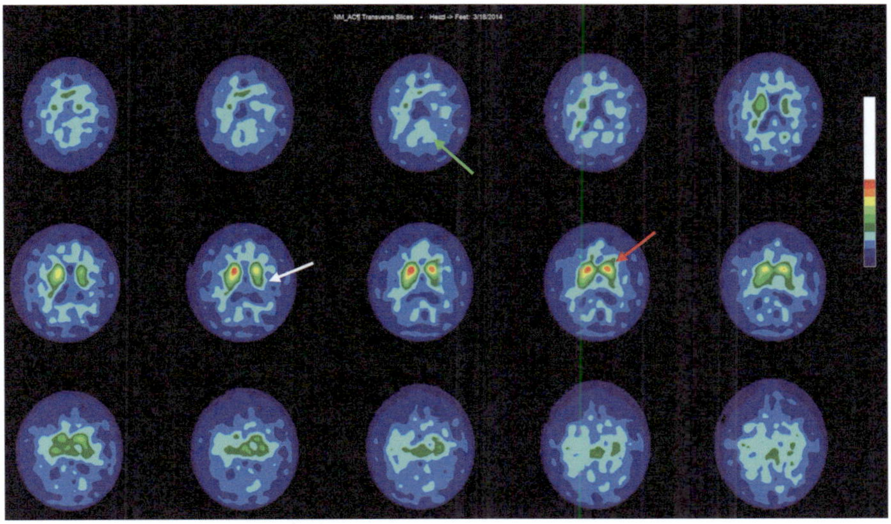

Fig. 6.6 A 72-year-old male with abnormal DaTscan consistent with PD

Case 6.7 Probable Abnormal DaTscan Suspicious for Early-Stage PD

Clinical Information

Chief Complaint *Slight and occasional right hand tremor*

The patient is a 76-year-old female with self-reported slight and occasional right hand tremor of uncertain duration. Past medical history is notable for hyperlipidemia, headache, neck pain, and breast cancer status post right mastectomy and chemotherapy.

Current medications include aspirin, biotin, vitamin D, coenzyme Q-10, and simvastatin. Brain MRI was read unremarkable.

DaTscan Findings (Fig. 6.7)

The images show moderately reduced tracer activity in the left putamen (white arrow), while tracer activity in the left caudate nuclei is well preserved (red arrow), despite slight head-tilting. Tracer activity in the entire right striatum (both caudate nuclei and putamen) is crescent-shaped, which is distinct, relative to the surrounding brain tissue.

Discussion and Follow-Up

The DaTscan images show moderately decreased tracer activity confined to the left putamen, corresponding to the contralateral symptom, therefore suspicious for early stage of PD. However, given the presence of head-tilting and atypical clinical features, a normal variant cannot be excluded.

Following the DaTscan, the patient has been observed, without evidence of worsening tremor for one and a half years.

Case Summary

Abnormal DaTscans have several categories, mainly depending on stages of PD. One of the common features, however, is asymmetry. It is well-known that dopamine neurons in putamen are more vulnerable to neurodegenerative insults compared to those in caudate nuclei. This case shows moderately decreased tracer activity confined to the left putamen, corresponding to patient's mild and occasional right hand tremor, therefore, suspicious for early stage of Parkinson's disease. Due to head-tilting during imaging acquisition, however, a normal variant needs to be considered as well.

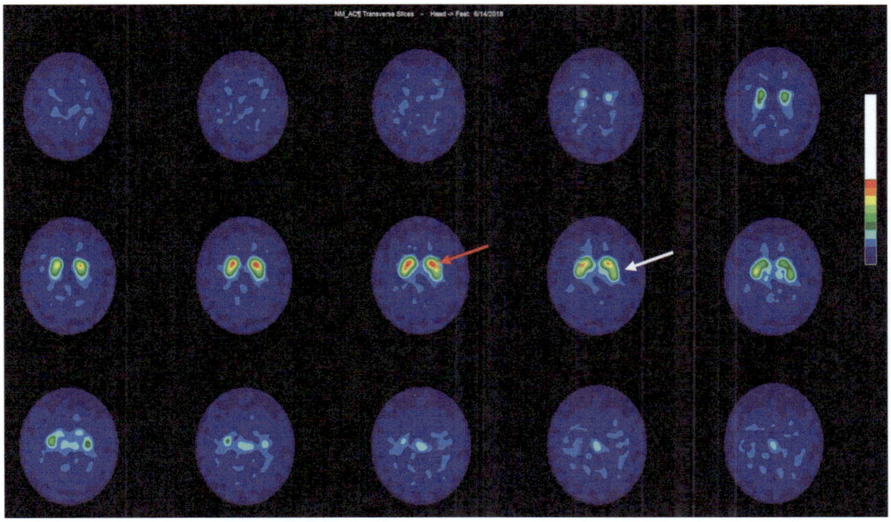

Fig. 6.7 A 76-year-old female with abnormal DaTscan suspicious for early stage of PD

Case 6.8 Abnormal DaTscan due to CVA and Likely Early Stage of PD

Clinical Information

Chief Complaint *Mild hand tremor, right greater than left*

The patient is an 86-year-old male presenting with some imbalance, fatigue, and mild tremor especially with writing and eating, the right more prominent than the left. Past medical history is notable for a cerebral vascular accident in 2016, vascular dementia without behavioral disturbance, type 2 diabetes, gout, hyperlipidemia, carotid artery disease treated with bilateral carotid endarterectomy (CEA), and coronary artery disease (CAD) status post bypass graft ×3.

Several CTs of the head/brain showed brain atrophy and bilateral lacunar infarcts, left being more affected than the right.

DaTscan Findings (Fig. 6.8)

The images show diffusely reduced tracer activity in the left caudate nuclei (red arrow) and putamen (white arrow), in a typical pattern suggestive of sequelae of prior left lacunar infarcts. While tracer in the right caudate nuclei is preserved, there is mild to moderately decreased tracer activity in the right putamen (green arrow).

Discussion and Follow-Up

This patient has a medical history of prior cerebral vascular accidents (CVA) and known vascular dementia (VD). Several CTs of the head/brain consistently showed brain atrophy and bilateral lacunar infarcts, left more affected than the right. This DaTscan shows greatly reduced tracer activity, equally involving the left caudate nuclei and putamen, a pattern inconsistent with neurodegenerative changes of PD type, instead, compatible with known prominent left lacunar infarcts. However, there is mild to moderately reduced tracer activity in the right putamen, concerning for early stage of PD [1, 8].

Despite the atypical clinical symptoms and complicated medical history, this abnormal DaTscan helps clinical diagnosis and management of this 86-year-old patient. One month after the DaTscan, the patient was put on a trial of Sinemet 25–100 mg, one tablet PO, three times a day, with a good response. Half a year later, however, he developed sepsis of unknown organism and passed away.

Case Summary

Parkinson's disease (PD) often coexists with other neurological conditions, especially in elder patients, which complicates the interpretation of DaTscan images. This case shows diffusely decreased tracer activity in the entire left striatum (equally involving the left caudate nuclei and putamen), in line with the prior CT findings of left lacunar infarcts, highly suggestive of sequela of prior CVA, rather than PD. In contrast, there is mild to moderately decreased tracer activity confined to the right putamen, raising concerns of early stage of Parkinson's disease, although superimposed or coexisting vascular parkinsonism cannot be excluded. The good response to Sinemet further supports the imaging diagnosis of early stage of PD during the limited follow-up.

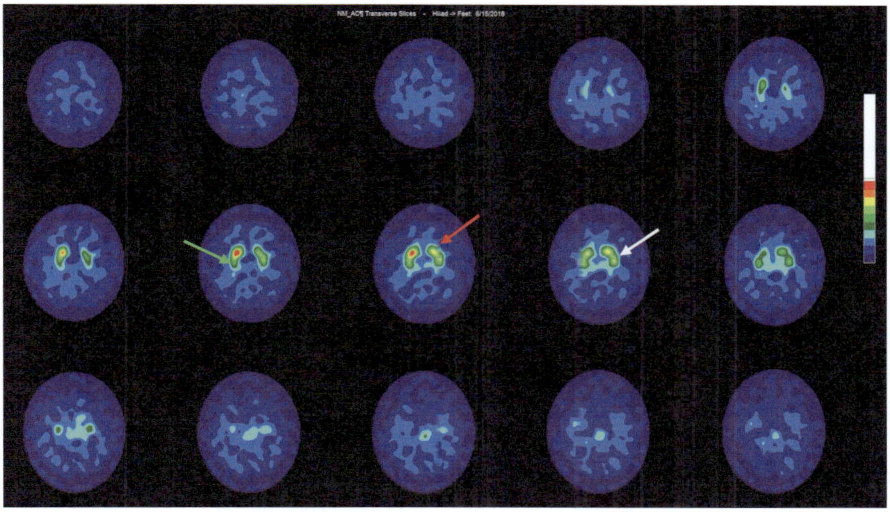

Fig. 6.8 An 86-year-old male with abnormal DaTscan due to CVA and early stage of PD

Case 6.9 Abnormal DaTscan Likely due to Corticobasal Degeneration (CBD)

Clinical Information

Chief Complaint *Memory loss and right-sided limb weakness leading to a recent fall*

The patient is a 64-year-old right-handed female with mild cognitive difficulty, slowly deteriorating executive functions (*e.g.*, stopping driving and unable taking care of family financials), and self-reported weakness of the right hand and right leg. There is no mood or behavior change. She denies any tremor or muscle rigidity or shuffling.

Past medical history is notable for asthma, depression, and osteoporosis. Family history is significant for dementia affecting her mother, her maternal uncle, and her sister.

Brain MRI performed half a year ago was unremarkable except for mild senescent changes, likely representing white matter chronic ischemic changes.

An EEG test was negative for seizure activity.

Laboratory tests showed TSH, B_{12}, and homocysteine in normal ranges.

A recent brain FDG PET showed hypometabolism involving left frontal lobe, left basal ganglion, and thalamus, with crossed diaschisis in the right cerebellum. Constellation of the FDG PET findings was suspicious for cortical basal degeneration (CBD, images not shown).

DaTscan Findings

The initial DaTscan images (Fig. 6.9a) showed normal tracer activity in a crescent shape in the right striatum. In contrast, tracer activity is diffusely reduced in the left caudate nuclei (red arrow) and putamen (white arrow). Given the mildly elevated background activity in the surrounding brain parenchyma (green arrow), mild global decreased striatal activity cannot be excluded.

Approximately 14 months later, the follow-up DaTscan (Fig. 6.9b) revealed the same abnormalities, but further decreased tracer activity in the left caudate nuclei (red arrow) and putamen (white arrow), when compared to the prior study. Mildly elevated background activity in the brain parenchyma is still noted, but overall stable (green arrow). Tracer activity in the right striatum remains unchanged and in a normal pattern.

Discussion and Follow-Up

The clinical presentation in this case was concerning for neurodegenerative dementias rather than PD. DaTscan was requested for further evaluation of abnormal FDG PET findings suspicious for cortical basal degeneration (CBD). Consistently, the DaTscan confirmed diffuse involvement of the entire left striatum, while the right striatum, especially the right putamen, is preserved. This is in support of the diagnosis of left sided CBD, rather than PD [1].

Approximately 2 weeks after the first DaTscan, the patient underwent a brain Vizamyl (amyloid) PET, which was negative, with special reference to the left frontal cortex. This adds more imaging evidence to support the diagnosis of CBD, rather than AD.

During the ensuring 1-year follow-up, patient has been treated with low doses of Aricept and Namenda, and she also undergoes physical therapy. Despite the treatments, she reports multiple recent falls. Neurological exam reveals progressive dementia with severe apraxia.

Case Summary

This DaTscan revealed diffusely decreased tracer in the entire left striatum, while tracer activity in the right striatum especially the right putamen is preserved. This imaging pattern shall be considered as a “red flag” suggestive of neurological disorders/diseases other than PD. In this case, both clinical presentation and prior brain FDG PET study results are suggestive of left-sided CBD. This imaging diagnosis has been further supported by a negative brain amyloid PET, a follow-up DaTscan showing progression of left striatal dopamine transporter depletion, and the clinical follow-up data.

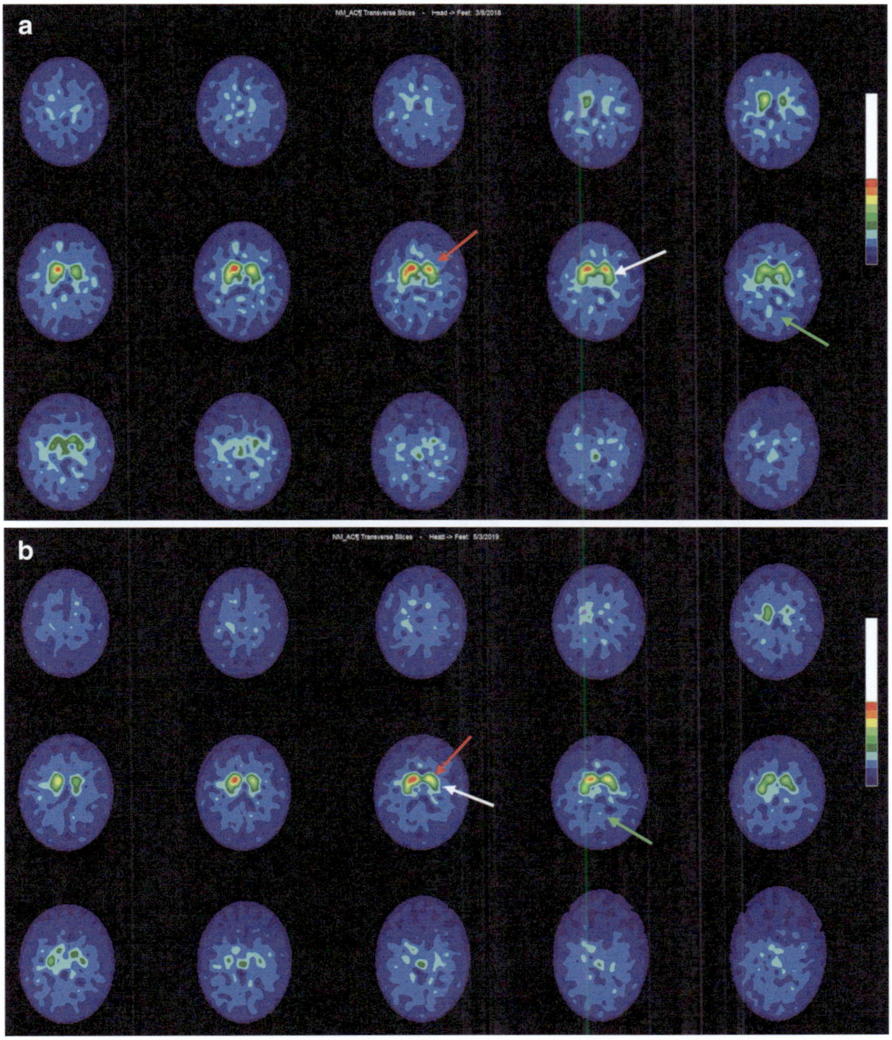

Fig. 6.9 (**a**) A 64-year-old female with abnormal DaTscans likely secondary to cerebrobasal degeneration (CBD). (**b**) A follow-up DaTscan study 14 months later showed worsening loss of left striatal dopamine transporters, indicating progression of CBD

Case 6.10 Abnormal DaTscan Consistent with Advanced PD

Clinical Information

Chief Complaint *Left hand rest tremor and slow movement for 1 year*

The patient is a 68-year-old ambidextrous male with a history of essential tremor for a few years. Since 2015, however, he has developed bilateral hand tremor, left > right, slow movement, increasing fatigue, and shuffling gait. He denies history of head injury, seizure, or stroke. There is no family history of movement disorder. Past medical history is notable for depression, prostate cancer status post prostatectomy, and essential tremor.

A recent brain MRI showed numerous foci of T2/FLAIR signal abnormality in the bilateral subcortical and deep white matter, likely relating to chronic small vessel ischemic changes.

Current medications include escitalopram, aspirin, ibuprofen, and multiple vitamins.

DaTscan Findings (Fig. 6.10)

This is a technically limited study due to patient's motion during imaging acquisition.

Nevertheless, the images show absent tracer activity in the right putamen (white arrow) and severely decreased tracer activity in the right caudate nuclei (red arrow). Tracer activity in the left putamen is also reduced, but to a lesser degree when compared to the right putamen. Tracer activity in the left caudate nuclei appears preserved relative to the contralateral; however, there is markedly elevated background activity in the surrounding brain parenchyma (magenta arrow) in green to yellow-green color, indicating 50–60% of the striatal activity (normal 20–30% or less), suggesting marked globally decreased striatal activity including the left caudate nuclei.

Discussion and Follow-Up

Patients' motion is a common problem while performing DaTscan. Another limitation in the imaging review is the high brain background tracer activity, likely due to marked globally reduced striatal activity.

Nevertheless, the DaTscan study is abnormal, with findings classic for a dopamine neurodegenerative process, right striatum being more affected than the left, corresponding to the patient's left-sided dominant symptoms, in conjunction with global reduced striatal tracer activity, suspicious for advanced PD [1, 8].

Nearly 1 year after the DaTscan, the patient started Sinemet 25/100 mg, initially one tablet by mouth three times a day, gradually increased to three tablets, PO, three times a day, with general improvement of mobility, facial expression, and rest tremor as well as essential tremor.

Case Summary

Patient's motion is a common problem or a limitation factor in the interpretation of neuroimaging studies including DaTscans. Despite the technical limitation, this patient's abnormal DaTscan is characterized by involvement of striata on both sides, but more diffuse and severe on the right. This laterality corresponds to the patient's contralateral symptoms (left-sided dominant hand rest tremor and slow movement), suggestive of advanced PD. The scintigraphic diagnosis of PD has been further supported by a good response to L-dopa therapy (Sinemet).

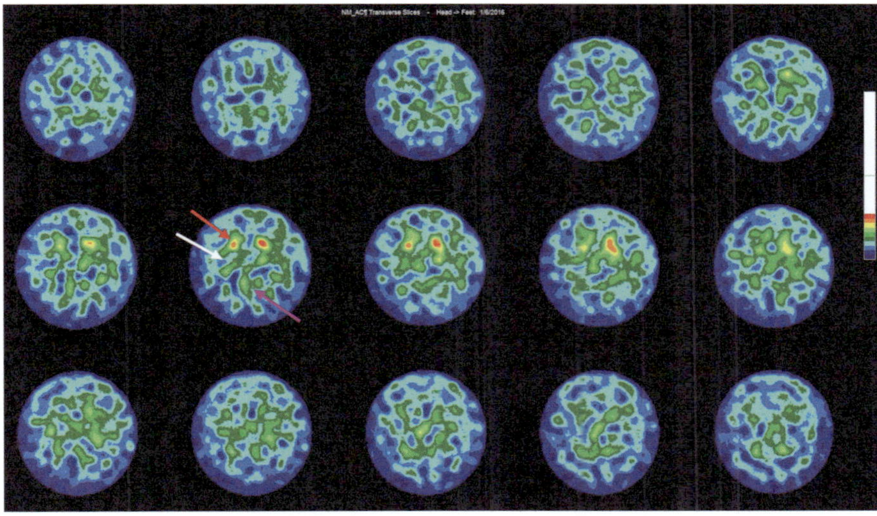

Fig. 6.10 A 68-year-old male with abnormal DaTscan suggestive of advanced PD

Case 6.11 Abnormal DaTscan due to Progressive Supranuclear Palsy (PSP)

Clinical Information

Chief Complaint *Rapid decline in balance and frequent falls*

The patient is a 77-year-old female presenting with rapid decline in balance and multiple falls last year and one recent fall this year. In addition, she has impaired memory and tremor of both hands. She denies dizziness and has no seizures. Past medical history is notable for hypertension, dyslipidemia, diabetes mellitus, and obesity.

Brain MRI showed findings suspicious for progressive supranuclear palsy (PSP).

EEG revealed no focal or epileptiform features.

Laboratory tests showed TSH, vitamin B_{12}, and folate in normal ranges.

Imaging Findings

The DaTscan images (Fig. 6.11, the upper panel) show decreased tracer activity in the right caudate nuclei (red arrow) and, to a greater extent, in the right putamen (white arrow). In contrast, tracer activity in the left caudate nuclei is preserved, while there is questionable decreased tracer activity in the left putamen.

As shown in the lower panel of Fig. 6.11, a sagittal view of the prior MRI exhibits a "hummingbird sign" (hatched white arrow) due to midbrain atrophy, which is an imaging hallmark for diagnosis of PSP.

Discussion and Follow-Up

The chief complaint of frequent falls in this patient, in conjunction with impaired memory, and rapid decline in balance, is suggestive of atypical Parkinsonian syndromes. Consistently, prior MRI showed midbrain atrophy with a "hummingbird sign," which is an imaging hallmark for diagnosis of PSP (also called "Richardson-Olszewski syndrome"), a rare neurodegenerative disorder linked with four-repeat tauopathy [6, 7]. However, the patient also presents with tremor of both hands; DaTscan was requested to rule out underlying PD. As expected, the DaTscan is abnormal, but the involvement of both right putamen and caudate nuclei, but essentially normal left striatum, is in line with the recent literature report by Ogawa and associates [9], further in support of the diagnosis of PSP rather than PD.

Case Summary

This 77-year-old female patient has clinical features suggesting PSP, which was supported by MRI finding of midbrain atrophy, *e.g.,* a hummingbird sign. However, she also presents with tremor of both hands, concerning for underlying PD. DaTscan shows dopamine transporter depletion involving the entire right striatum, but essentially normal left striatum. The pattern is inconsistent with a classic neurodegenerative process of idiopathic PD, instead, further supporting an atypical Parkinsonian syndrome and consistent with the established diagnosis of PSP.

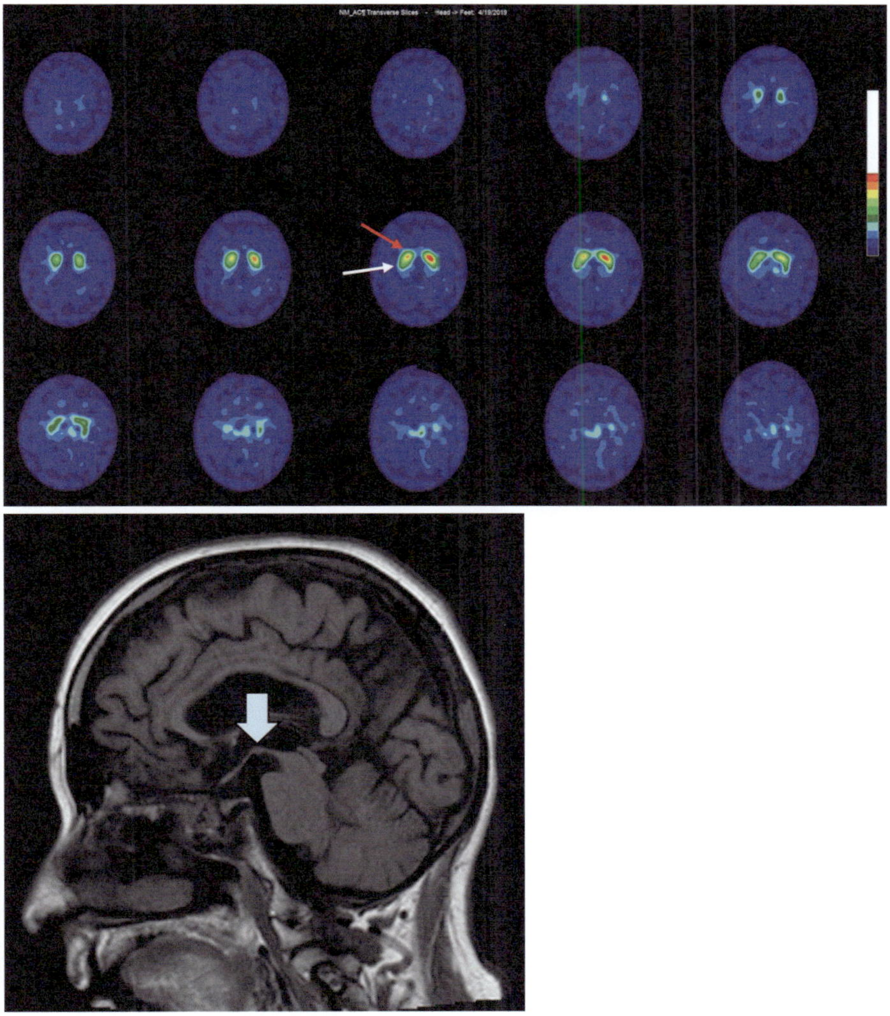

Fig. 6.11 A 77-year-old female with abnormal DaTscan secondary to PSP

Case 6.12 Abnormal DaTscan due to Multiple System Atrophy (MSA)

Clinical Information

Chief Complaint *Progressive weakness and ataxia*

The patient is a 76-year-old male presenting with progressive weakness and ataxia. In addition, he has dysarthria (difficulty speaking) and swallowing impairment for more than 10 years. There is no tremor. The patient denies history of head injuries, and there is no history of being exposed to significant chemicals or toxins or endemic infections.

Past medical history is notable for known cerebellar/pontine degeneration, hypothyroidism, dysphonia, anemia, urinary retention, coronary artery disease, bradycardia, blood pressure short turn frequently, erectile dysfunction, and dyspnea.

Family history is negative for neurodegenerative disorders.

He is a non-smoker, and denies the use of illicit drugs.

Brain MRI showed "cerebellar and pontine atrophy," suspicious for multiple system atrophy (MSA).

Imaging Findings

The DaTscan is a technically limited study due to head-tilting. Nevertheless, the images (Fig. 6.12, the upper panel) show an essentially crescent-shaped tracer activity in the RIGHT striatum. In contrast, moderately decreased tracer activity is noted in the left putamen (white arrow), while tracer activity in the left caudate nuclei is preserved.

As shown in the lower panel of Fig. 6.12 (hatched white arrow), brain MRI shows marked cerebellar atrophy, worsening when compared to the prior MRIs (images not shown).

Discussion and Follow-Up

Multiple system atrophy (MSA, originally referred to as *Shy-Drager syndrome*, also sometimes referred to as olivopontine cerebellar degeneration) is a rare neurodegenerative disorder, with clinical features falling into two major categories: MSA Parkinsonian variant and MSA cerebellar variant [7]. Prior to DaTscan, this patient has been diagnosed with MSA, which was established with neuroimaging findings and clinical presentation including nonmotor features including cardiovascular autonomic failure and urogenital dysfunction. The DaTscan is abnormal and shows asymmetric, focally decreased tracer activity confined to the left putamen. This is essentially in line with the literature [7, 9], further supporting MSA rather than PD. The left striatal involvement may explain the patient's extensive history of speech difficulty, indicating neurodegenerative changes involving motor speech cortex (Broca's area), usually in the LEFT frontal lobe.

The preserved dopamine neuron activity in the entire RIGHT striatum and the LEFT caudate nuclei effectively rules out MSA Parkinsonian variant or advanced PD, although the finding is indistinguishable from early stage of PD. Therefore, this patient is unlikely to benefit from L-dopa therapy. Indeed, the patient was treated briefly with chlorzoxazone (a muscle-relaxing agent) and Flomax (an alpha-blocker for the treatment of benign prostate hyperplasia). Both medications were stopped due to their side effects leading to significantly decline in functional status and causing confusion. During the follow-up for 4.5 years, the patient is overall stable.

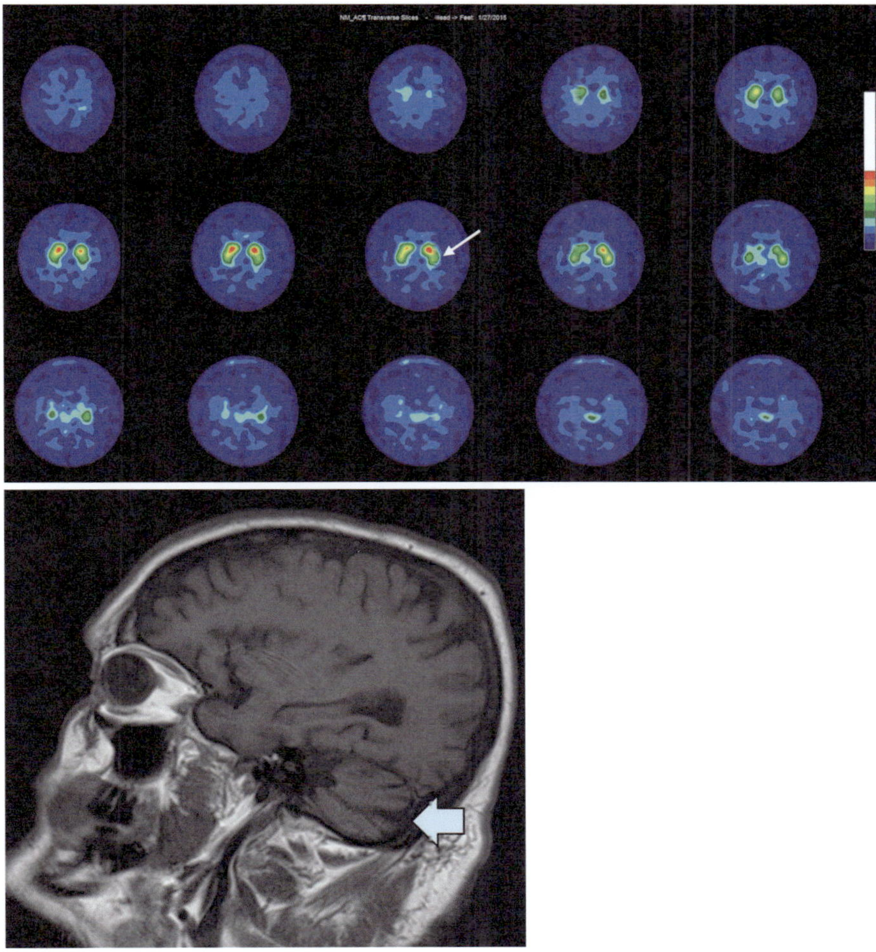

Fig. 6.12 A 76-year-old male with abnormal DaTscan due to MSA

Case Summary

Differential diagnosis of an abnormal DaTscan includes at least PD, PSP, MSA, and CBD [4, 5, 10]. This 76-year-old male patient has an outstanding history of MSA, likely cerebellar variant. The DaTscan finding of moderate involvement of only left putamen is indistinguishable from early stage of PD, but effectively rules out MSA Parkinsonian variant or underlying advanced PD. This helps choose pharmacotherapy other than L-dopa and improves the patient's care. The scintigraphic diagnosis of abnormal DaTscan likely secondary to MSA has been supported by clinical follow-up data.

References

1. Booij J, Teune LK, Verberne HJ. The role of molecular imaging in the differential diagnosis of parkinsonism. Q J Nucl Med Mol Imaging. 2012;56:17–26.
2. Brooks DJ. Parkinson's disease: diagnosis. Parkinsonism Relat Disord. 2012;18S1:S31–3.
3. Davidsson A, Georgiopoulos C, Dizdar N, et al. Comparison between visual assessment of dopaminergic degeneration pattern and semi-quantitative ratio calculations in patients with Parkinson's disease and atypical Parkinsonian syndromes using DaTSCAN SPECT. Ann Nucl Med. 2014;28(9):851–9.
4. Gayed I, Joseph U, Fanous M, et al. The impact of DaTSCAN in the diagnosis of Parkinson disease. Clin Nucl Med. 2015;40(5):390–3.
5. Kuo PH, Lei HH, Avery R, et al. Evaluation of an objective striatal analysis program for determining laterality in uptake of I-123-ioflupane SPECT images: comparison to clinical symptoms and to visual reads. J Nucl Med Technol. 2014;42(2):105–8.
6. Ling H. Clinical approach to progressive supranuclear palsy. J Mov Disord. 2016;9(1):3–13.
7. La M, Micallef C, Paviour DC, et al. Conventional magnetic resonance imaging in confirmed progressive supranuclear palsy and multiple system atrophy. Mov Disord. 2012;27:1754–62.
8. Meles SK, Tenue LK, de Jong BM, et al. Metabolic imaging in Parkinson disease. J Nucl Med. 2017;58:23–8.
9. Ogawa T, Fujii S, Kuya K, et al. Role of neuroimaging on differentiation of Parkinson's disease and its related disease. Yonago Acta Medica. 2018;61:145–55.
10. Pagano G, Niccolini F, Politis M. Imaging in Parkinson's disease. Clin Med (Lond). 2016;16(4):371–5.

Cerebrospinal Fluid (CSF) Scintigraphy

7

CSF Imaging in Normal Pressure Hydrocephalus (NPH)

Case 7.1 Normal CSF Scintigraphy

Clinical Information

Chief Complaint *Headache and abnormal brain MR imaging*

The patient is a 45-year-old female presenting with headache, vertigo, short-term memory loss, and abnormal brain MR imaging suggestive of mild to moderate ventriculomegaly. In addition, she complains of visual disturbance and some unsteadiness of gait.

Past medical history is notable for migraine, spastic bladder, Langerhans cell histiocytosis, COPD, immunocompromised state, hypotension, endometriosis, rheumatoid arthritis, chronic pain, and chronic narcotic use.

The patient denies history of stroke, seizure, or head trauma.

Laboratory tests showed TSH, folate, and vitamin B_{12} in normal ranges.

CT of the head/brain was read normal. However, brain MR imaging revealed mild to moderate ventriculomegaly of the lateral and third ventricles with a normal fourth ventricle. Concurrent MRA of the intracranial circulation was normal.

Imaging Findings (Fig. 7.1)

The top panel of the images was obtained 4 hours after intrathecal tracer injection at lumbar spine, which shows CSF tracer activity ascending to the basal cisterns (red arrows), the superior cisterns (blue arrows), reaching the bilateral Sylvian fissures (green arrows). Imaging of the spine shows CSF ascending within the spinal canal and no appreciable tracer activity in the kidney regions.

The middle panel of the images that were obtained 24 hours after tracer administration reveals CSF tracer diffusely spreading into the subarachnoid spaces in both hemispheres and over the top cerebral convexities (hatched yellow arrows). Clearance of tracer activity is noted in the basal and superior cisterns. Clearance of tracer activity from soft tissues of the head/neck and the visualized portion of the chest is also noted. There is no appreciable tracer activity in the lateral ventricles.

The imaging 48 hours after tracer administration as shown in the lower panel reveals further clearance of CSF tracer activity from the entire brain including the convexities. There is no appreciable tracer activity at the basal cisterns by this time (red arrows). Again, there is no appreciable tracer activity in the lateral ventricles.

Discussion and Follow-Up

Since normal CSF turnover time in adult human subjects is about 4–6 hours, the visualization of basal and superior cisterns on the 4-hour imaging indicates normal CSF flow along the spinal canal [1]. At 24 hours, CSF tracer activity is not only significantly cleared from the cisterns but also

D. Wu, *Clinical Nuclear Medicine Neuroimaging*, https://doi.org/10.1007/978-3-030-40893-0_7

ascending into the convexities/arachnoid villi where CSF absorption occurs into blood circulation, without evidence of ventricular reflux, consistent with a normal CSF dynamic. The imaging obtained at 48 hours confirms that there is normal clearance of CSF in the entire brain. Therefore, this cisternographic study is normal, without evidence of normal pressure hydrocephalus (NPH).

During the follow-up for nearly 3 years, the patient was diagnosed with low-grade trigeminal neuralgia. The symptoms of headache and memory loss have improved without treatment. However, she has had frequent doctor office visits and hospital admissions due to acute-on-chronic pain, recurrent viral infection, and recent infection with *C. difficile*, likely secondary to her known immunocompromised state.

Case Summary

The findings on a normal CSF scintigraphy reflect the normal CSF dynamics: tracer injected at the lumbar spine arachnoid space, following the CSF flow, will ascend to the basal cisterns and Sylvian fissures at 2–4 hours and normally will reach the cerebral convexities by 24 hours, without ventricular reflux. Further imaging is optional in clinic; if performed, it will confirm near-complete clearance of tracer activity at the cisterns by 48 hours, with minimal residual tracer activity only at cerebral convexities where CSF absorption takes place into blood circulation. A normal CSF scintigraphy effectively rules out NPH, despite CT or MRI finding of ventriculomegaly, thereby avoiding unnecessary neurosurgical ventricular-peritoneal (VP) shunt placement.

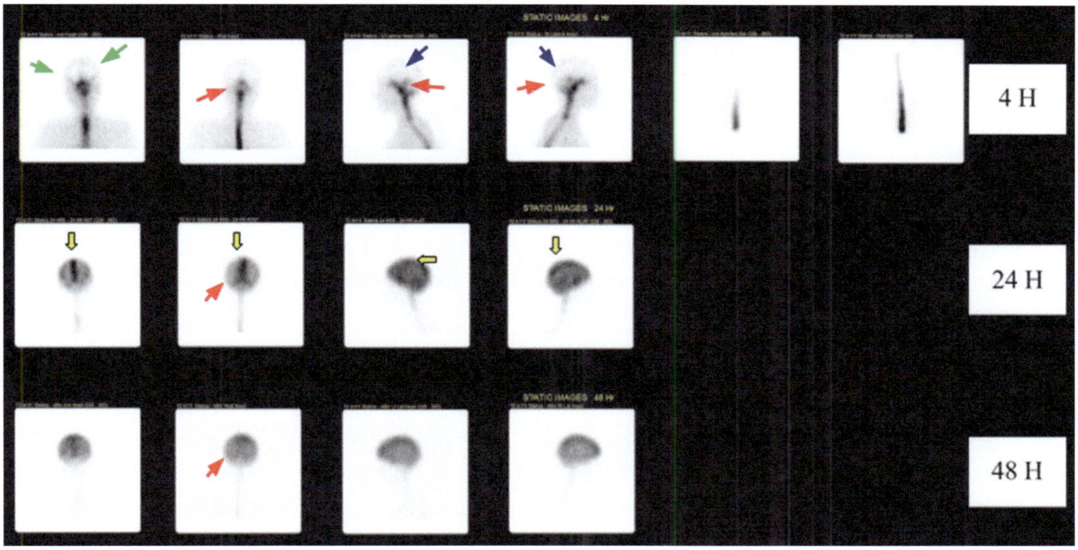

Fig. 7.1 A 45-year-old female with normal CSF scintigraphy

Case 7.2 Slow CSF Flow and Transient Ventricular Reflux Likely Secondary to Brain Atrophy

Clinical Information

Chief Complaint *Progressive memory loss and abnormal brain MR imaging*

The patient is a 73-year-old female who has had a 5-year history of progressive short-term memory loss. She was previously treated with donepezil and memantine, without improvement in her symptoms. She was then started on citalopram for the treatment of presumed depression, again without improvement. She has no delusions or hallucination. She denies history of TIA (transient ischemic attack), stroke, or closed head injury.

Past medical history is notable for hypertension, hypercholesterolemia, diabetes mellitus type II, CLL (chronic lymphocytic leukemia), fibromyalgia, neuropathy, restless leg syndrome, dizziness, sexual dysfunction, anxiety/depression, obstructive sleep apnea, and morbid obesity.

Family history is negative for stroke, seizures, or hydrocephalus.

EEG performed in May 2016 was normal, per neurologist's note.

Laboratory tests showed TSH, folate, and vitamin B_{12} in normal ranges.

Brain MRI revealed mild, age-appropriate cortical atrophy. In addition, there was prominence of the lateral ventricles out of proportion of the degree of cortical atrophy concerning for normal pressure hydrocephalus (NPH). Prior brain MRA in 2015 showed unremarkable cerebral vasculature including the basilar artery and the upper vertebral arteries; there was no evidence of proximal branch occlusion or high-grade stenosis.

Imaging Findings (Fig. 7.2)

The planar imaging at 24 hours (top panel, upper row) shows persistent tracer activity at the basal cisterns (red arrows), indicating slow CSF flow. However, this improves at 48 hours and resolves at 72 hours (top panel, middle and bottom rows). Tracer ascends bilaterally, but does not reach the top cerebral convexities until 48 hours or later (hatched yellow arrows). Meanwhile, there is continuous tracer clearance from the entire brain from 24 to 72 hours. Moderate tracer activity is noted in the lateral ventricles (blue arrows) only at 24 hours (blue arrows), and resolves by 48 hours, indicating transient ventricular reflux.

The SPECT imaging at 24 hours (middle panel) shows mild tracer activity in the lateral ventricles (blue arrows); again, this is resolved by 48 hours (bottom panel) on the SPECT imaging, consistent with transient ventricular reflux.

Discussion and Follow-Up

The findings indicate slow CSF flow and transient ventricular reflux. Despite the delay, CSF flow is seen over the top cerebral convexities at 48 and 72 hours in addition to steady clearance of the entire brain subarachnoid space activity. There is no focal abnormality in the CSF tracer distribution. Therefore, the slow CSF flow and transient ventricular reflux are likely due to moderately enlarged ventricles and expanded subarachnoid spaces secondary to known brain atrophy as shown on MRI. This study is abnormal, but there is no definite scintigraphic evidence of NPH, and there is no typical abnormal CSF pattern suggestive of benefits from VP shunting [3].

During the follow-up for 3 years, neurological evaluations showed stable memory loss. Her symptoms were likely due to pseudodementia secondary to depression, anxiety and OSA (obstructive sleep apnea).

Case Summary

This case shows abnormal CSF scintigraphic findings of delayed CSF flow and transient ventricular reflux. However, combination of steady clearance from the basal cisterns without persistent ventricular activity and improved CSF flow over the top cerebral convexities effectively rules out NPH despite suspicious MRI findings. Without evidence of focal abnormality, the delayed CSF flow and transient ventricular reflux are likely secondary to moderately enlarged ventricles and expanded subarachnoid spaces due to known brain atrophy. The scintigraphic impression has been supported by clinical follow-up data.

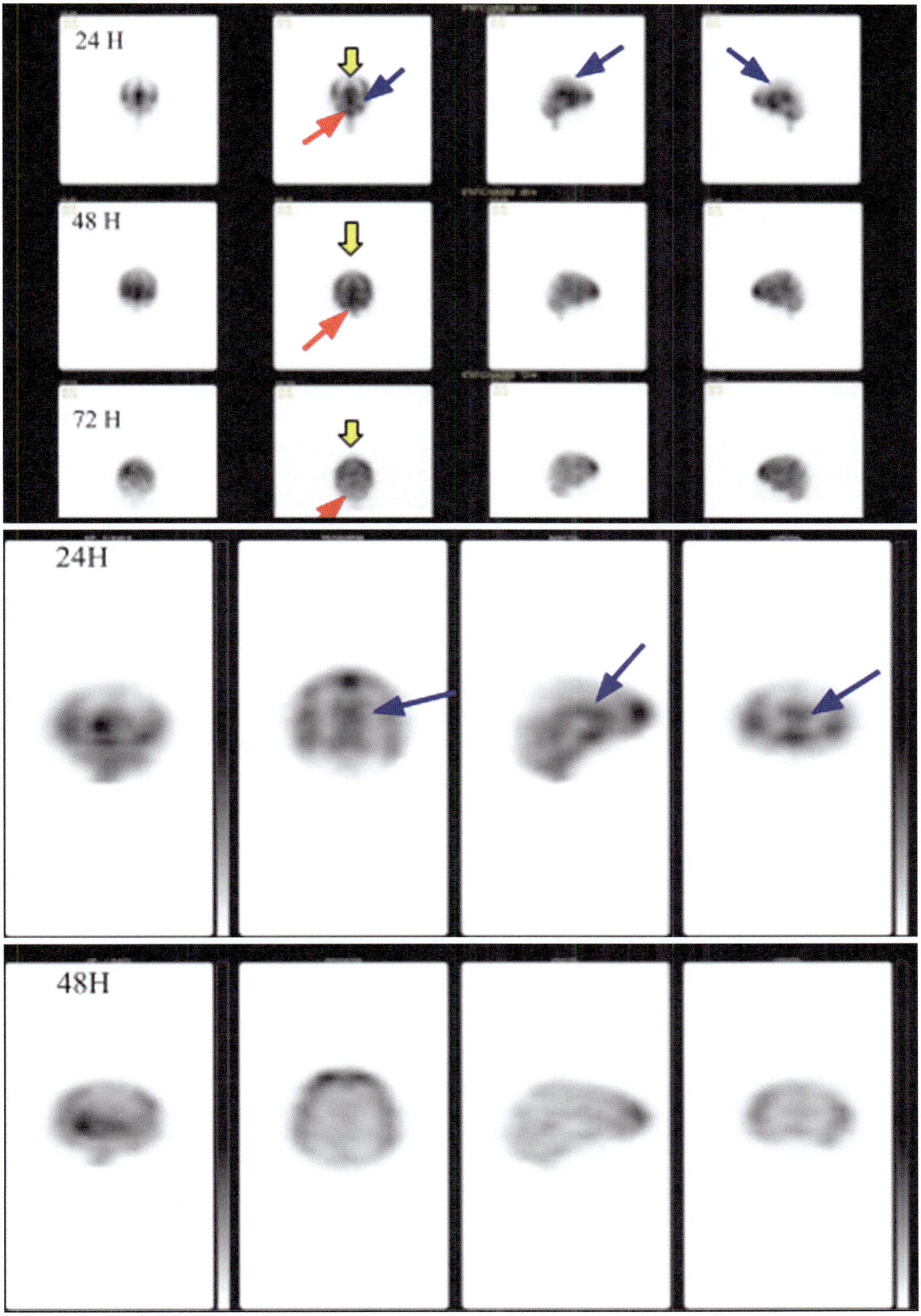

Fig. 7.2 A 73-year-old female with slow CSF flow and transient ventricular reflux likely due to brain aging/atrophy

Case 7.3 Abnormal CSF Scintigraphy Likely due to Hydrocephalus *Ex Vacuo*

Clinical Information

Chief Complaint *Memory loss, confusion, unstable gait, and urinary incontinence*

The patient is a 79-year-old male presenting with short-term memory loss, confusion, unstable gait, and urinary incontinence. CT of the head/brain showed lateral ventriculomegaly, right greater than left, suspicious for normal pressure hydrocephalus (NPH), for which he underwent a high-volume CSF removal at an outside institution. However, his symptoms did not improve.

The patient denies headache, nausea, vomiting, dizziness, visual changes, or extremity numbness. On exam he has no speech difficulties. He is a former smoker who quit over a decade ago, and he denies drug abuse.

Past medical history is notable for TIA (transient ischemic attack), GERD (gastroesophageal reflux disease), IBM (inclusion body myositis), UTI (urinary tract infection), peripheral neuropathy, and penile skin cancer.

Laboratory tests show borderline normal TSH and normal folate and vitamin B_{12}.

Brain MRI showed lateral ventriculomegaly, right > left. Similarly, CT of the head/brain, as mentioned earlier, also revealed right >left ventriculomegaly.

Imaging Findings (Fig. 7.3)

As shown on the prior MR imaging (bottom panel), this patient has marked lateral ventriculomegaly, RIGHT > LEFT, and posterior > anterior. The CSF imaging at 24 hours (top panel, upper row) shows persistent, intense tracer activity at the base cisterns (red arrow), indicating slow CSF flow; however, this is cleared steadily at 48 and 72 hours (top panel, middle and lower rows).

There is asymmetric, severely decreased tracer activity in nearly the entire right hemispheric subarachnoid spaces (blue arrows), and more prominent in the right parietal region.

Despite the abnormalities, CSF flow is present over the top cerebral convexities at 24 hours (hatched yellow arrows). There is no evidence of ventricular reflux throughout the study. Imaging at 48 hours and 72 hours shows steady clearance not only from the basal cisterns but also the entire brain including the right brain hemispheric subarachnoid spaces.

Discussion and Follow-Up

This 79-year-old patient has a classic clinical triad of ataxia, dementia and urinary incontinence for NPH. Prior MRI demonstrates marked ventriculomegaly, also supporting the clinical diagnosis of NPH. The CSF imaging shows slow CSF flow and asymmetric, severely decreased CSF distribution into the right hemispheric subarachnoid spaces. However, there is no evidence of ventricular reflux throughout the study. Furthermore, CSF flow ascending over the top cerebral convexities is seen as early as 24 hours, with further clearance over 48–72 hours.

The etiology of the diffusely decreased tracer activity in the right brain is unknown, but it is likely secondary to the more severe right-sided ventriculomegaly and the potential enlarged subarachnoid spaces of the right brain hemisphere. Despite the delayed CSF flow and the asymmetry between the right and left hemispheric CSF distribution, there is no definite scintigraphic evidence of NPH. Instead, the findings, in conjunction with marked ventriculomegaly on MRI, are suggestive of hydrocephalus *ex vacuo* [1].

A few months after the CSF imaging study, the patient was admitted to our hospital due to progressive left extremity weakness, which spontaneously resolved.

Due to worsening symptoms and progressive head/brain CT findings, the patient underwent a repeat high-volume CSF removal 1 year later, again without significant symptom relief.

During the ensuing follow-up, the patient underwent physical therapy for neck pain for a while, and then he gave it up due to transportation issues.

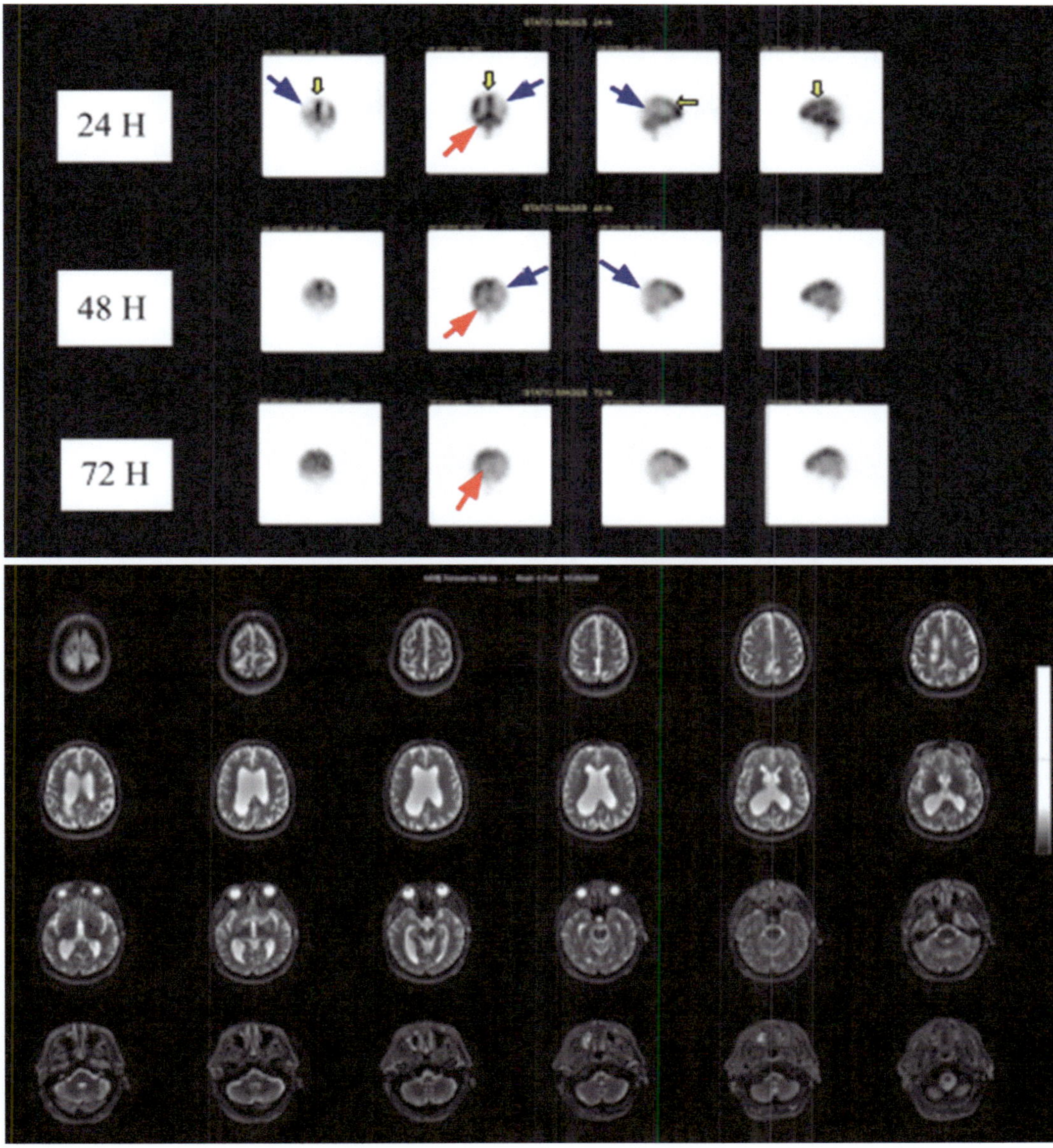

Fig. 7.3 A 79-year-old male with hydrocephalus *ex vacuo*

Case Summary

This case illustrates the value of CSF scintigraphy to show evidence of hydrocephalus *ex vacuo* in a patient with classic clinical symptoms and typical anatomic neuroimaging findings collectively suggestive of NPH. The lack of ventricular reflux, despite delayed and slow CSF clearance, does not entertain the diagnosis of NPH. Instead, the constellation of CSF imaging and anatomic neuroimaging findings, in conjunction with the clinical presentation, is suggestive of hydrocephalus *ex vacuo*. This differential diagnosis is important, as VP shunt placement may not be beneficial for symptom relief.

Case 7.4 Abnormal CSF Scintigraphy Consistent with NPH

Clinical Information

Chief Complaint *Memory loss, urinary incontinence, gait problems, and frequent falls*

The patient is a 79-year-old male brought in by family members due to progressive short-term memory difficulty. He has also had falls several times recently due to loss of balance. He has a very slow shuffling gait which has progressively worsened for the last 2–3 years. In addition, the patient sometimes has urinary incontinence. He denies any history of head injury, seizures, focal extremity weakness/numbness, neck pain, or back pain.

Past medical history is notable for high cholesterol, hypertension, and hepatitis C.

CT of the head/brain showed disproportional cerebral ventriculomegaly.

Laboratory tests showed TSH and vitamin B_{12} in normal ranges.

Imaging Findings (Fig. 7.4)

The planar imaging at 24 hours (upper panel, top row) shows mild to moderate tracer activity at the basal cisterns, with slow but steady clearance over time at 48 and 72 hours (upper panel, middle and bottom rows, red arrows). There is persistent abnormal tracer activity in the lateral ventricles throughout the study up to 72 hours (blue arrows), indicating persistent ventricular reflux. The planar imaging at 48 hours (middle panel) and 72 hours (bottom panel) confirms persistent tracer activity within the lateral ventricles consistent with ventricular reflux (blue arrows). In addition, delayed CSF flow is noted, without reaching the top (parasagittal) cerebral convexities at 24 and 48 hours, although there is improvement at 72 hours (hatched yellow arrows). Even on the imaging at 72 hours, intracerebral tracer activity is observed, indicating tracer transependymal diffusion/uptake into paraventricular brain parenchyma, which is further evidence of persistent ventricular reflux.

The SPECT imaging at 24 hours (middle panel) and 48 hours (lower panel) confirms persistent ventricular reflux, without interval improvement (blue arrows).

Discussion and Follow-Up

There is abnormal tracer activity within lateral ventricles at 24, 48, and even 72 hours, indicating persistent ventricular reflux. In addition, there is very slow and delayed CSF flow over the top (parasagittal) cerebral convexities, suggestive of poor CSF absorption at the subarachnoid villi, or severe blockage of CSF flow, or both [2, 3]. This abnormal CSF pattern is not only classical for NPH but also indicates potential benefit from a shunting procedure.

Three months after the positive cisternogram, the patient underwent VP shunt placement. However, the patient only achieved a short-term symptom relief for approximately 1.5 years. Then, the patient was admitted to our hospital due to falls and mental status change. VP shunt survey and subsequent CT showed RUQ abdominal subcutaneous fluid collection indicating a CSF pseudocyst, for which a surgical distal shunt exploration was performed with improvement in symptoms. Two months later, however, the patient was admitted again due to abdominal pain, fever, nausea, and vomiting. CT imaging showed coiling of the VP shunt within the right mid-abdomen, with adjacent soft tissue thickening within the abdominal wall, suspicious for an infection or abscess formation. The patient underwent VP shunt removal the second day after admission due to infection.

During the follow-up for 1 year, the patient's condition further worsened due to obstructive uropathy, CHF, and advanced Alzheimer's dementia.

Case Summary

This patient presented with a classic clinical triad of NPH, *e.g.*, gait disturbance, dementia, and urinary incontinence. Consistent with the symptoms, CSF imaging showed persistent ventricular reflux and severely delayed CSF flow, highly suggestive of NPH. The scintigraphic diagnosis was further supported by symptom relief after VP shunt placement.

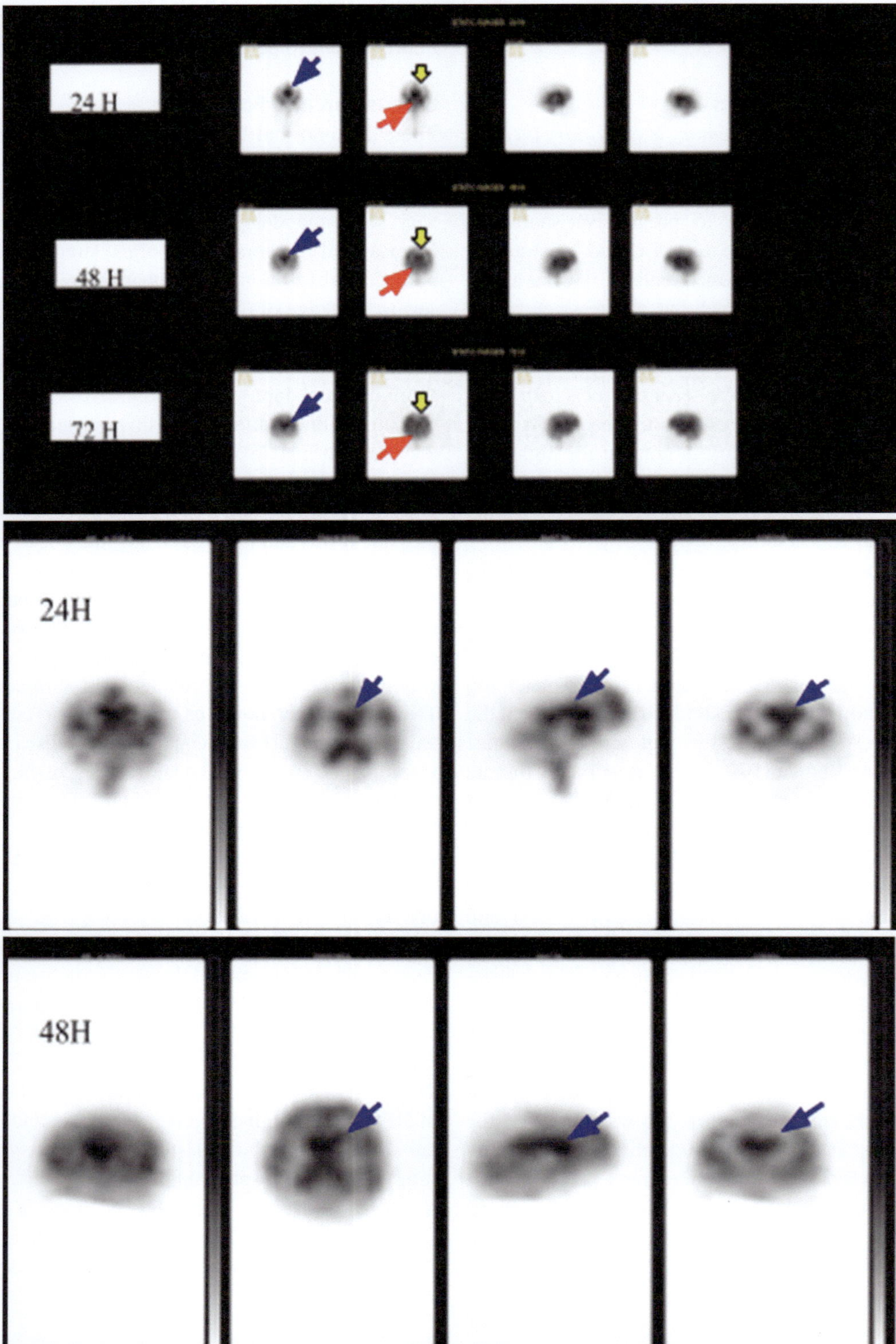

Fig. 7.4 A 79-year-old male with NPH

Case 7.5 NPH with a Favorable and Sustained Response to VP Shunting

Clinical Information

Chief Complaint *Progressive memory loss and worsening gait difficulty*

The patient is a 79-year-old right-handed female presenting with memory impairment for 5 years, which has been worsening over the last 1–2 years. She tried donepezil and Exelon patch, both without benefit. Additionally, her family members have noticed that she had gait difficulties over the last 2 years. She tends to shuffle and needed to use a walker for the past several years.

In addition, she has developed behavior changes with agitation, intermittent hallucinations, delusions, and confabulation. She denies prior head injuries, loss of consciousness, seizure, or stroke.

Past medical history is notable for hypertension, hyperlipidemia, hypoglycemia, TIA (transient ischemic attack), and tremor of arms and legs.

Brain MRI showed moderate brain atrophy, ventriculomegaly, and chronic ischemic changes of the white matter.

Laboratory tests showed TSH, free T4, and vitamin B_{12} in normal ranges.

Imaging Findings (Fig. 7.5)

The planar imaging at 24 hours (upper panel, top row) shows moderate tracer activity at the basal cisterns (red arrow), with minimal clearance at 48 and 72 hours (upper panel, middle and lower rows). There is abnormal ventricular tracer activity bilaterally, which is persistent from 24 to 72 hours (blue arrows) . This finding is confirmed on the SPECT imaging at 24 hours and 48 hours (middle and bottom panels, blue arrows). CSF ascends extremely slowly, and there is no complete ascending over the top cerebral convexities even at 72 hours (hatched yellow arrows).

Discussion and Follow-Up

The clinical presentation in this patient does not have the classic triad for NPH. However, brain MRI showed ventriculomegaly suspicious for NPH. This cisternogram clearly demonstrates persistent ventricular reflux throughout the study up to 72 hours, and extremely slow CSF flow without reaching the top cerebral convexities even at 72 hours, highly suggestive of NPH with potential benefit from VP shunting [1].

In addition, a high volume of CSF removal during the lumbar puncture for the cisternogram study resulted in some improvement in her gait, further evidence in favor of VP shunting. Subsequently, the patient underwent VP shunt placement. After the procedure, her gait significantly improved. She finished outpatient physical therapy and no longer needed a walker. Her family members also noticed that there was mild improvement of her memory, and she was more alert.

Four years later, she developed recurrent memory loss and gait difficulty. She recently underwent VP shunt reset, again with reported improvement of memory and gait during the follow-up.

Case Summary

This case shows concordant MRI (ventriculomegaly) and cisternographic findings (persistent ventricular reflux and extremely slow CSF flow/ascent), both suggestive of NPH with potential benefits of VP shunting. In addition, high-volume CSF removal during lumbar puncture resulted in some gait improvement, further evidence in favor of shunting. After VP shunt placement, the patient achieved a favorable response, *e.g.,* significant gait improvement and some improvement of memory for 4 years, and sustained benefits after recent VP shunt reset.

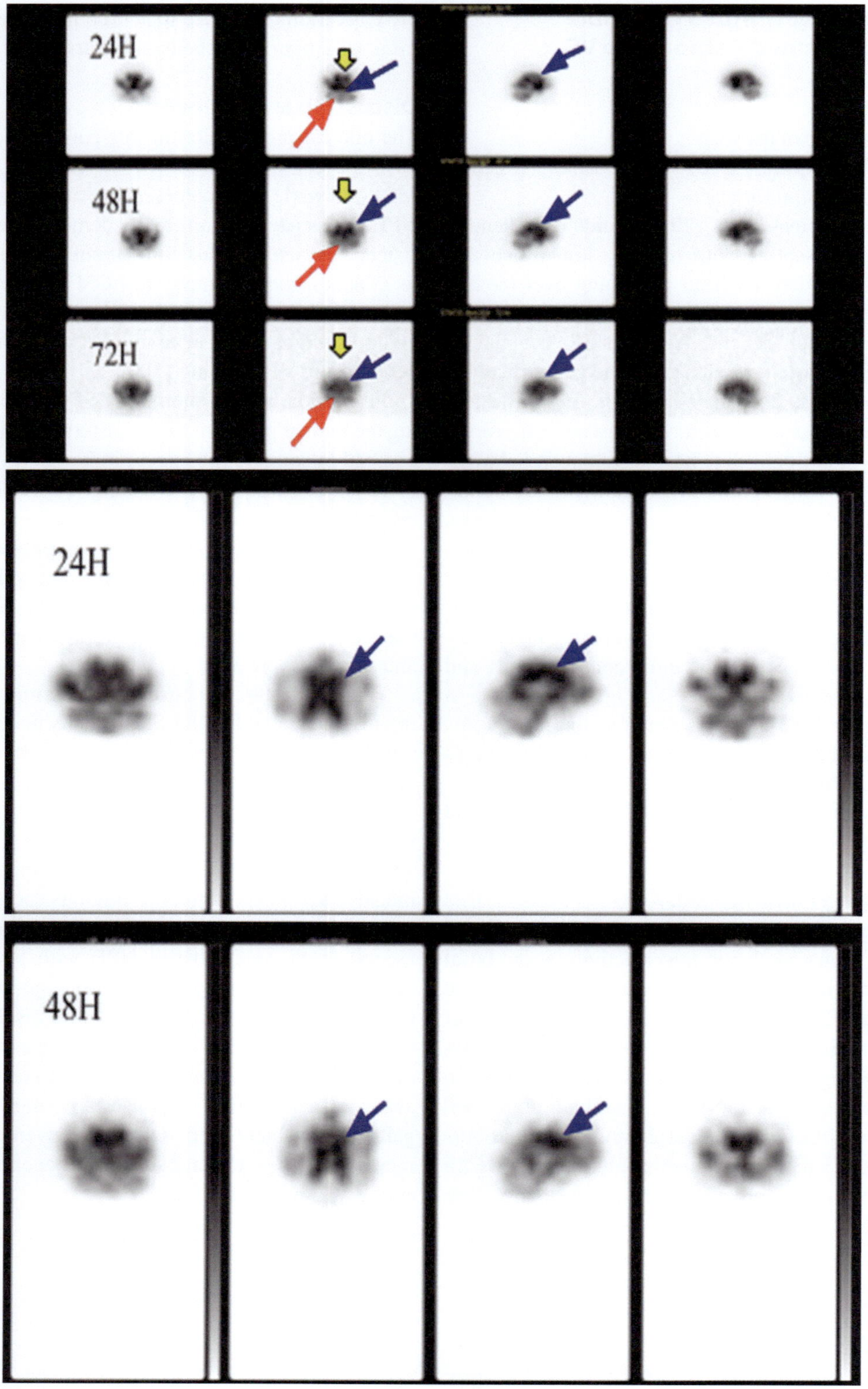

Fig. 7.5 A 79-year-female with NPH

CSF Leak Imaging

Case 7.6 Normal Study Without Scintigraphic Evidence of CSF Leak

Clinical Information

Chief Complaint *Recent LP shunt removal and persistent positional tension headache*

The patient is a 46-year-old female with a complex history including idiopathic intracranial hypertension/pseudotumor cerebri since age 8, status post lumbar-peritoneal shunt placed at age of 16, in addition to hypertension, pituitary adenoma, glaucoma, and intermittent headaches over the last 2 years. Her headaches were tension type and worsened with position changes. Therefore, CSF leak was suspected, for which she underwent LP shunt removal 2 months ago. After the procedure, her headache improved, but she still complained of a residual positional tension headache that worsened with bending over or prolonged standing.

She denies any blurred vision, double vision, speech changes, lateralized weakness, or numbness/tingling. There is no history of head trauma or stroke.

She has never smoked and denies alcohol or drug abuse.

Imaging Findings (Fig. 7.6)

Imaging 0.5 hours after radioactive tracer injection (upper row) at the lumbar spine shows normal CSF distribution and ascent within the spinal canal. Further imaging at 3 hours and 5 hours (second and third rows) shows normal CSF ascent to the basal cisterns (blue arrows), and minimal radioactive tracer activity in the urinary bladder (black arrow), likely due to free In-111 in the preparation. However, there is no appreciable tracer activity in the kidneys. Imaging at 24 hours (the bottom row) shows faint activity in both kidneys (green arrows) likely due to normal distribution of In-111 DTPA as complete CSF ascent is seen over the top cerebral convexities (hatched yellow arrows), while there is steady tracer clearance from the basal cisterns (blue arrow).

Tracer activity is noted in multiple bilateral thoracolumbar spinal nerve root sleeves, which are essentially symmetric and unchanged from 0.5 to 24 hours, indicating a normal variant.

Discussion and Follow-Up

Despite the complex neurological medical history in this patient, the CSF imaging shows normal flow and no direct or indirect imaging evidence of CSF leak. This negative finding indicates that the conventional therapy for CSF leak, *e.g.,* epidural blood patching, is not indicated.

During the follow-up for 1 year, her headache improved slightly without treatment. The orthostatic symptoms appear associated with hypotension, likely secondary to the medication of acetazolamide.

Case Summary

Normal CSF imaging is characterized by a normal CSF flow and lack of extra-CNS abnormal tracer distribution [4]. Additionally, normal renal tracer activity is seen only after 24 hours when a complete CSF ascent over cerebral convexities is reached. Visualization of kidneys on early imaging is an indirect evidence of CSF leak into general blood circulation system. Also, radioactive tracer activity at the spinal nerve roots could be a normal variant, which is indicated by a symmetric pattern and no interval changes over time.

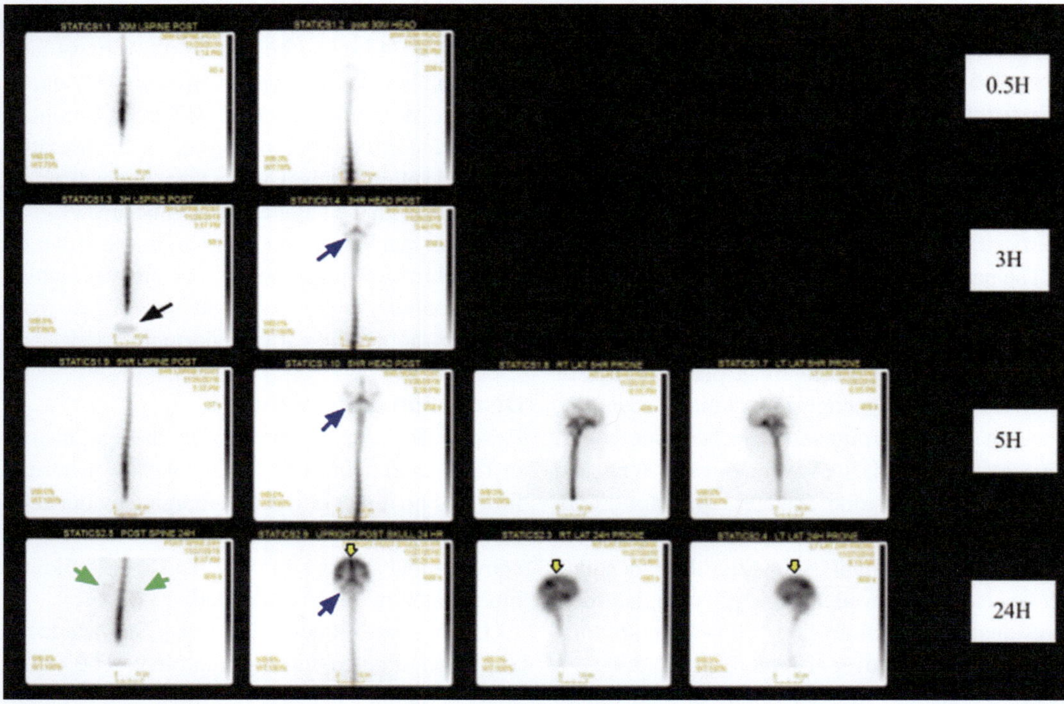

Fig. 7.6 A 46-year-old female with normal study and no scintigraphic evidence of CSF leak

Case 7.7 Normal Study Including SPECT CT of the Head/Neck Without Evidence of CSF Leak

Clinical Information

Chief Complaint *Chronic headache, prior CSF leak, and skull base surgery*

The patient is a 36-year-old male presenting with chronic headache. Past medical history is notable for right ocular sinus surgery, prior CSF leak status post skull fissure repair, chronic sinusitis, fibrous dysplasia, and recent pneumococcal meningitis diagnosed 2 months ago, likely from acute sinusitis but concerning for recurrent CSF leak.

Brain MRI showed postsurgical changes of the anterior cranial fossa and cribriform plate.

Imaging Findings (Fig. 7.7)

Imaging at 3 and 6 hours post tracer intrathecal administration (top panel, the 1st and 2nd rows) show normal CSF ascent along the spinal canal up to the basal cisterns (blue arrows), which decreases steadily over time. Minimal tracer activity is seen in the urinary bladder (black arrows); in the absence of renal activity, this is suggestive of free In-111 in the radiopharmaceutical preparation.

Imaging at 24 hours reveals normal CSF clearance from the basal cisterns (blue arrows) and complete ascent over the top cerebral convexities (hatched yellow arrows).

Due to prior history of CSF leak/skull fissure repair and clinically suspected CSF rhinorrhea, SPECT CT imaging of the head/brain was performed at 24 hours (bottom panel), which confirmed complete CSF ascent over the convexities and no evidence of CSF leak at the skull base.

Discussion and Follow-Up

Although this patient has a complex medical history, the planar imaging show normal CSF flow. There is no direct or indirect imaging evidence of a CSF leak. SPECT CT imaging confirms normal CSF ascent over the cerebral convexities and no evidence of CSF leak at the skull base.

During the follow-up for 1 year, the patient's headache resolved without treatment.

Case Summary

This patient has chief complaint of chronic headache and clinically suspected recurrent CSF leak. However, the CSF imaging shows a normal CSF flow, without direct or indirect evidence of CSF leak. SPECT/CT imaging confirms a complete CSF ascent over the cerebral convexities and no CSF leak at the skull base.

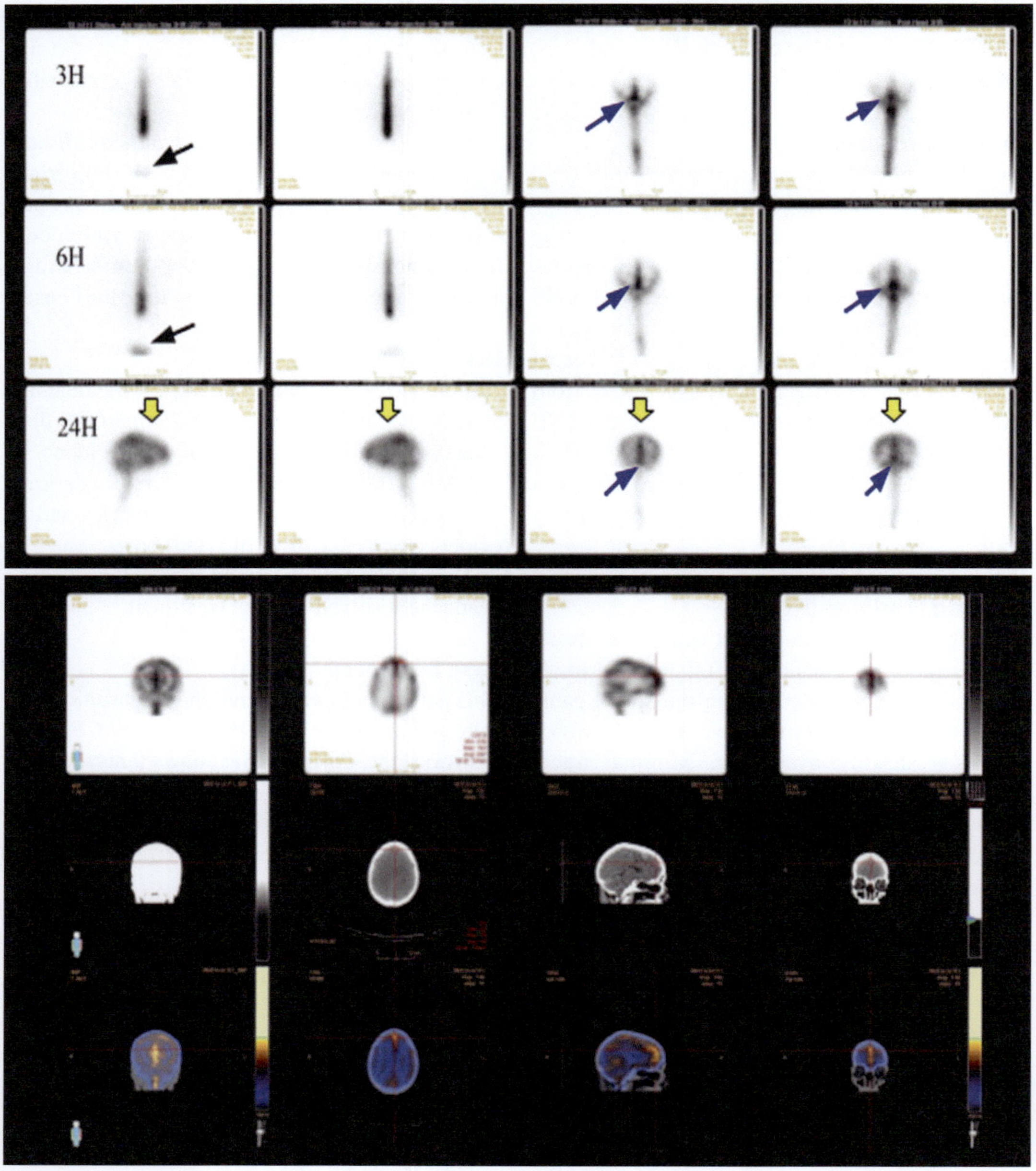

Fig. 7.7 A 36-year-old male with normal planar and SPECT CT CSF imaging

Case 7.8 CSF Leaks from T6 to L3

Clinical Information

Chief Complaint *Positional headache for months*

The patient is a 23-year-old female presenting with positional headache for 6–7 months. CSF leak and spontaneous intracranial hypotension were suspected, for which the patient had two empiric high-volume blood patches at an outside institution 2 months prior, but without significant symptom relief. The patient states that her headache began several years ago and worsens when standing but improves upon lying supine. She denies any brain/spinal procedures or prior trauma.

Past medical history is otherwise unremarkable.

A recent MR imaging of the spine at an outside institution showed findings suggestive of intracranial hypotension.

Imaging Findings (Fig. 7.8)

Imaging at 0.5 hours shows asymmetric, abnormal tracer at right T8 through L3 (red arrow). Imaging at 3 hours confirms the abnormal findings on the right, more prominent at right L1. Additionally, new abnormal tracer activity is demonstrated at left T6–T8, and more prominently at left T6 [red arrows]. The abnormalities are persistent with fluctuating intensities at 5 hours and 24 hours (red arrows).

In addition to multiple sites of CSF leak, the CSF flow is delayed, as there is persistent tracer activity at the basal cistern from 3 hours to 24 hours (blue arrows), but with complete ascent over the convexities. Imaging at 48 hours (data not shown) confirms the delayed CSF flow.

Bilateral renal tracer activity (green arrows) is seen on the 24-hour imaging, which is abnormal in the presence of delayed CSF flow (without complete ascent over convexities at 24 and even 48 hours). This finding is indirect evidence of CSF leak.

Discussion and Follow-Up

This patient's clinical features are very typical for spontaneous intracranial hypotension [5], which was supported by spine MRI findings at an outside institution. Prior to CSF imaging, the patient has had two high-volume epidural blood patches at an out institution without significant symptom relief. The CSF imaging clearly shows persistent, multiple sites of CSF leak involving the bilateral thoracolumbar spine, more prominent at left T6 and right L1. Additional findings indicate delayed CSF flow and abnormal renal activity, which is indirect evidence of CSF leak. The constellation of the abnormal findings is highly suggestive of severe CSF leak leading to intracranial hypotension.

Twenty days later, the patient underwent epidural patching, with injection of 32 ml of autologous blood at the level of T12–L1. The final outcome of this patient is unknown, as she did not return for any follow-up.

Case Summary

This is an extraordinary case showing classical clinical presentation and anatomic imaging features in a young female patient highly suspicious for CSF leak leading to spontaneous intracranial hypotension [5]. Her abnormal CSF imaging not only demonstrates direct evidence of multiple levels and bilateral CSF leak in the thoracolumbar spine but also indicates delayed CSF flow and abnormal renal activity that is indirect evidence of CSF leak. The abnormal CSF imaging findings help guide the treatment of high-volume epidural blood patching, which was performed 20 days later.

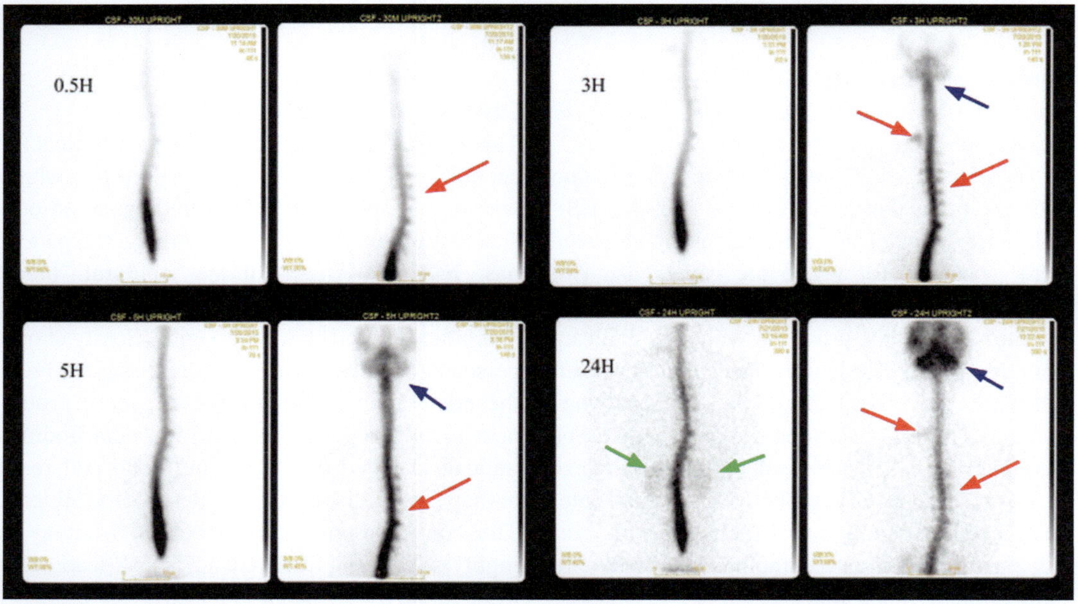

Fig. 7.8 A 23-year-old female with CSF leaks

Case 7.9 CSF Leak into Right Posterior Nasal Cavity

Clinical Information

Chief Complaint *Intractable headache and recurrent meningitis*

The patient is a 78-year-old male who was admitted to our hospital due to headache and fever similar to when he had bacterial meningitis 1 year ago. Past medical history is notable for chronic lymphocytic leukemia (CLL), hypertension, dyslipidemia, pneumonia, two brain surgeries for resection of right acoustic neuroma (2003) with bilateral hearing loss, and prior bacterial meningitis in 2013 and 2014. In-hospital workup confirms recurrent meningitis, concerning for CSF leak as the underlying cause.

Brain MRI showed diffusion restriction in the occipital horn of the right lateral ventricle, concerning for ventriculitis.

Imaging Findings (Fig. 7.9)

The planar imaging at 3, 6, and 24 hours (top panel, upper, middle, and bottom rows) shows persistent ventricular tracer activity (red arrows), slow clearance of tracer activity at the basal cisterns (blue arrows), and slow CSF ascent over the cerebral convexities at 24 hours (hatched yellow arrow). However, there is no evidence of CSF leak in the head and neck region on the planar images.

SPECT CT imaging at 24 hours (lower panel), however, demonstrates a focus of tracer activity located in the posterior right nasal cavity (cross-hairs), indicating CSF leak. Additionally, the SPECT CT imaging confirms persistent abnormal tracer activity in lateral ventricle (red arrow) and slow tracer clearance at the basal cisterns.

Radioactive count ratios (pledgets to serum ratio) were calculated as the following:

Left anterior cribriform plate	0.2
Left posterior cribriform plate	0.2
Left posterior pharynx	37.7
Right anterior cribriform plate	5.8
Right posterior cribriform plate	4.0
Right posterior pharynx	102.0

Discussion and Follow-Up

Although the planar imaging shows evidence of ventricular reflux and slow/delayed CSF ascent, it fails to detect CSF leak. SPECT CT imaging, however, clearly demonstrates evidence of CSF leak into the posterior right nasal cavity.

To further increase the detection sensitivity, nasal and pharyngeal pledgets were placed. A pledget to serum radioactivity ratio of 2–3:1 is generally considered to be positive for CSF leak. The abnormal findings suggest CSF leak through the right cribriform plate, draining into right posterior pharynx and extending into the right posterior/anterior cribriform plates and the left posterior pharynx regions.

The constellation of the SPECT CT findings and abnormal nasal/pharyngeal pledgets to serum radioactivity ratio is diagnostic of RIGHT rhinorrhea secondary to CSF leak through the right cribriform plate.

The patient was treated with IV antibiotics during his hospital stay and was discharged home on oral penicillin. Subsequently, he underwent surgical repair of his right posterior cribriform plate. During the follow-up for more than 4 years, there has been no new episode of bacterial meningitis.

Case Summary

The history of prior brain base surgeries and recurrent bacterial meningitis is suspicious for cranial or skull base CSF leak. Although planar CSF imaging has a suboptimal sensitivity for detecting CSF leak, both SPECT CT imaging and the use of nasal/pharyngeal pledgets have improved sensitivity and accuracy. Constellation of the SPECT CT findings and abnormal pledgets/serum radioactivity ratio is diagnostic of right rhinorrhea secondary CSF leak through the right cribriform plate.

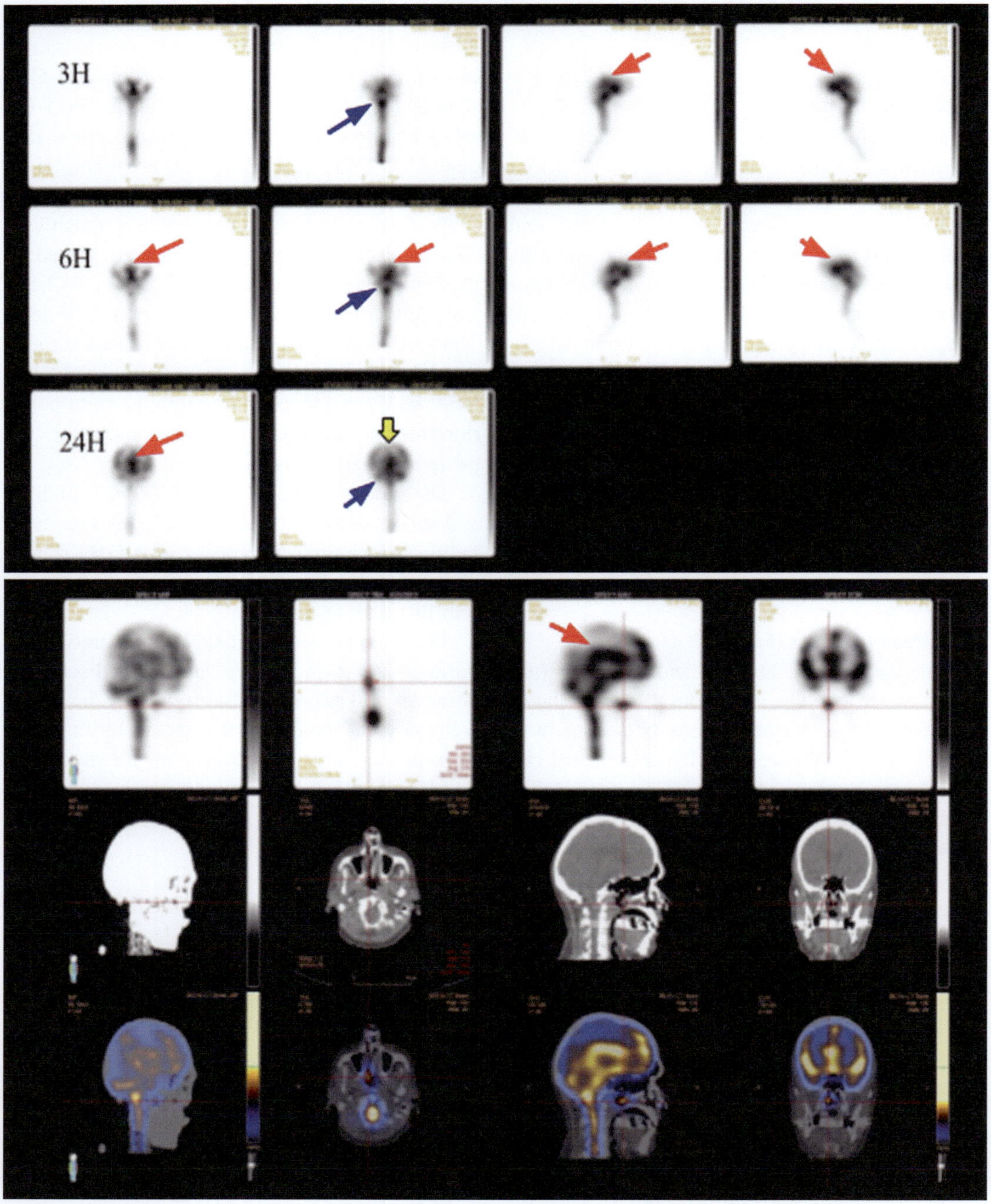

Fig. 7.9 A 78-year-old male with right posterior rhinorrhea

Case 7.10 Positive CSF Leak Imaging and Negative Follow-Up After Multiple Blood Patches

Clinical Information

Chief Complaint *Chronic postural headache*

The patient is a 46-year-old female presenting with persistent postural headache and migraine for several years. She described that the headache gets worse while upright. She also reports floaters in eyes. She had an MR imaging of the brain recently, which was normal.

She had a lumbar puncture 2 months ago, with opening CSF pressure of 100 mm H_2O (normal 100–180 mm H_2O. Subsequently she received an epidural blood patching the next day for the treatment of severe headache at an outside institution, but the symptoms were persistent.

The patient has a complex past medical history, including bipolar disorder, OCD (obsessive compulsive disorder), anxiety disorder, seizure disorder, GERD (gastroesophageal reflux disease), chronic back pain, hypothyroidism, hypoglycemia, and morbid obesity status post Roux-en-Y gastric bypass.

She denies history of head trauma or meningitis/encephalitis.

Imaging Findings (Fig. 7.10)

On the initial CSF imaging [top panel], early imaging at 0.75-hour post tracer administration was unremarkable [top panel, first row]. However, asymmetric and abnormal tracer activities are identified at right T10 to L1 at 3 hours, which are persistent at 5 hours [top panel, second and third rows], suspicious for CSF leakage (red arrows). The abnormal findings subsided at 24 hours, however [top panel, fourth row].

Despite the CSF leak, normal CSF ascent is noted, reaching the basal cisterns at 3–5 hours and substantially cleared by 24 hours (blue arrows). Meanwhile, there is complete CSF ascent over the top cerebral convexities (hatched yellow arrows). These findings indicate an essentially normal CSF flow.

There is faint tracer activity in the right kidney at 24 hours (green arrow), likely due to normal In-111 distribution after entering the blood stream. Mild tracer activity is noted in the urinary bladder, likely due to free In-111 for the early imaging and/or renally excreted tracer activity at 24 hours.

After approximately 1.5 years, repeat CSF imaging (bottom panel) showed no evidence of CSF leakage from 0.75 to 24 hours following the tracer administration, with a special reference to the right T10–L1. Again, there is a normal CSF flow. Faint tracer activity is noted in both kidneys (green arrows) at 24 hours, likely due to normal renal tracer excretion.

Discussion and Follow-Up

This patient's clinical presentation of chronic postural headache is classical for spontaneous intracranial hypotension likely secondary to CSF leak. Two months prior to the first CSF imaging study in our clinic, she received empiric epidural blood patching at an outside institution, but her symptoms persisted.

The initial CNS imaging study clearly demonstrates CSF leak at multiple levels, involving at least right T10 to L1, a common site for spontaneous CSF leak [4, 6], which subsides by 24 hours. Additional findings indicate a normal CSF flow.

The patient underwent multiple epidural blood patching, including three treatments at the level of T12–L1, and two treatments at C7–T1, and finally achieved sustained symptom relief. One and a half years later, she had a repeat CSF imaging, which showed no evidence of CSF leak (Fig. 7.10, the bottom panel), indicating effective treatment with multiple blood patching. During the follow-up for 3 years, the patient did not report recurrent headache.

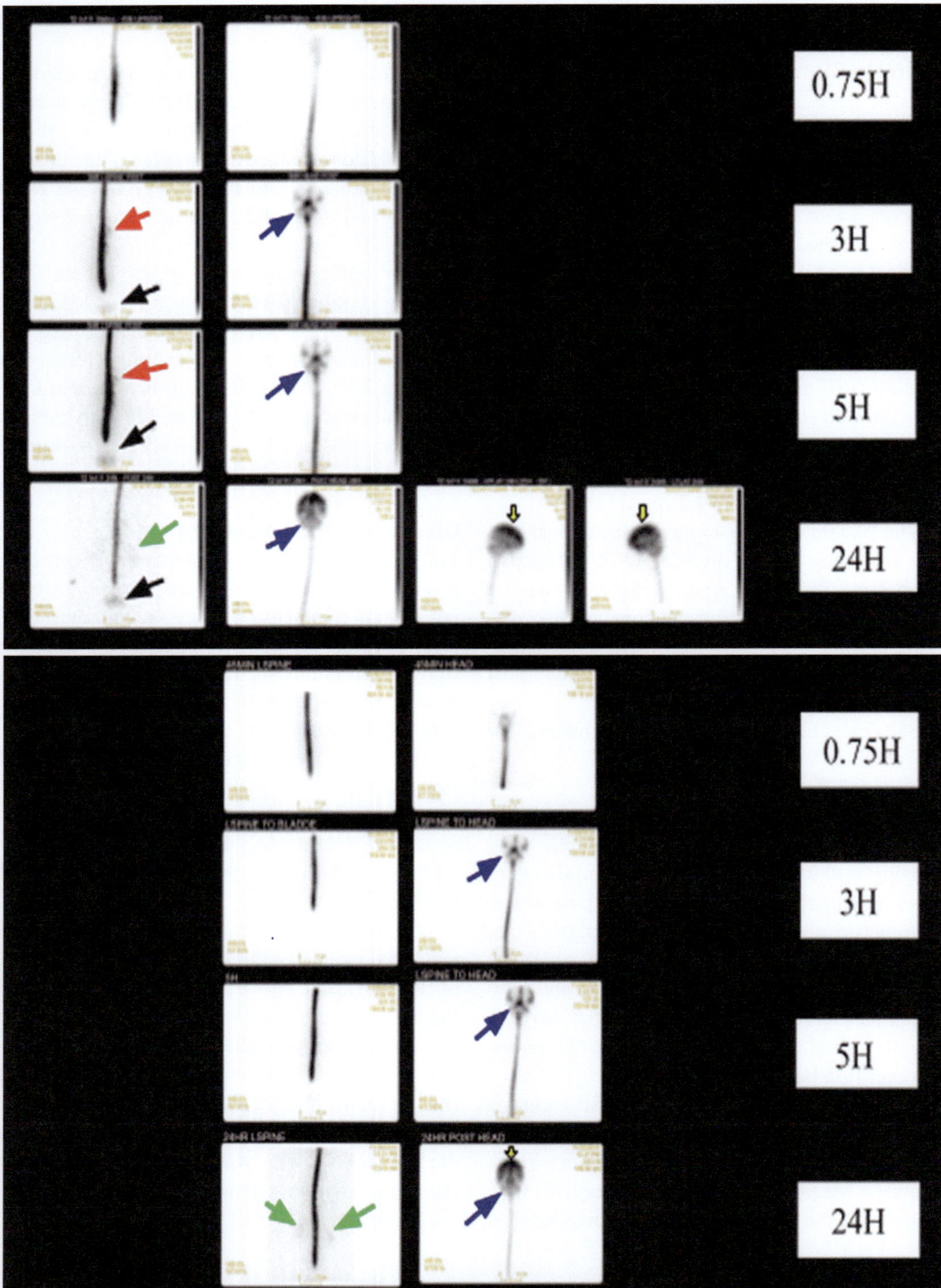

Fig. 7.10 A 46-year-old female with a positive CSF leak imaging and a negative followup imaging after received multiple rounds of blood patching

Case Summary

Chronic postural headache in this middle-aged patient is suspicious for CSF leak leading to spontaneous CNS hypotension. She received one-time empiric epidural patching at an outside institution about 2 months ago, without symptom relief. The initial CSF imaging clearly demonstrated right-sided thoracolumbar CSF leak, despite an essential normal CSF flow. The abnormal CSF imaging findings guided multiple epidural blood patching at the level of T12–L1. Additionally, she had empiric epidural blood patching at C7–T1, although CSF imaging and CT myelogram were negative for leakage in the region. A repeat CSF imaging 1.5 years later confirmed no evidence of leak, and the patient has achieved sustained symptom control for 3 years.

CSF Imaging in the Evaluation of Shunt Patency

Case 7.11 Patent Lumboperitoneal (LP) Shunt

Clinical Information

Chief Complaint *Headache, abdominal pain, and history of LP shunting*

The patient is a 6-year-old male with past medical history of cerebral palsy, Chiari malformation status post multiple decompression surgeries, and lumboperitoneal shunt placement. In addition, he has developmental delay and autism spectrum disorder. He presents with frequent headache, nausea, and abdominal pain. LP shunt survey showed disruption of lumbar peritoneal catheter and valve at the level of the abdominal wall.

Imaging Findings (Fig. 7.11)

Imaging at 0.5 hours (top panel), in anterior, posterior, right lateral, and left lateral views, respectively, shows CSF tracer activity widely dispensed in the entire abdomen (blue arrows), with accumulation at the base of the pelvis (red arrows).

Imaging at 3 hours (bottom panel) shows tracer clearance in the abdomen and pelvis, with tracer activity seen in kidneys and the urinary bladder as well as a soaked diaper (green arrows), which is an indirect evidence of patent lumboperitoneal shunt.

Discussion and Follow-Up

This pediatric patient has a complex neurological history, and his lumboperitoneal shunt survey showed disruption of shunt catheter and valve at the level of the abdominal wall. In contrast to the anatomic imaging findings, the CSF imaging reveals direct and indirect evidence of a patent lumboperitoneal shunt, thus avoiding unnecessary shunt removal [7]. In-hospital workup showed evidence of appendicitis, for which the patient underwent appendectomy and was discharged a few days later. During the follow-up for 2 years, the patient did not have any recurrent symptoms.

Case Summary

LP shunt placement is a less commonly used approach for patients with increased intracranial pressure compared to the use of ventriculoperitoneal (VP) shunting [7]. However, the advantage of LP shunting is that this is an extracranial surgical procedure with minimal intracranial complications. This case shows that CSF imaging is a short-duration study that could reveal direct (abdominopelvic tracer activity) and indirect (renal and bladder tracer activity) evidence of LP shunt patency, avoiding unnecessary shunt removal.

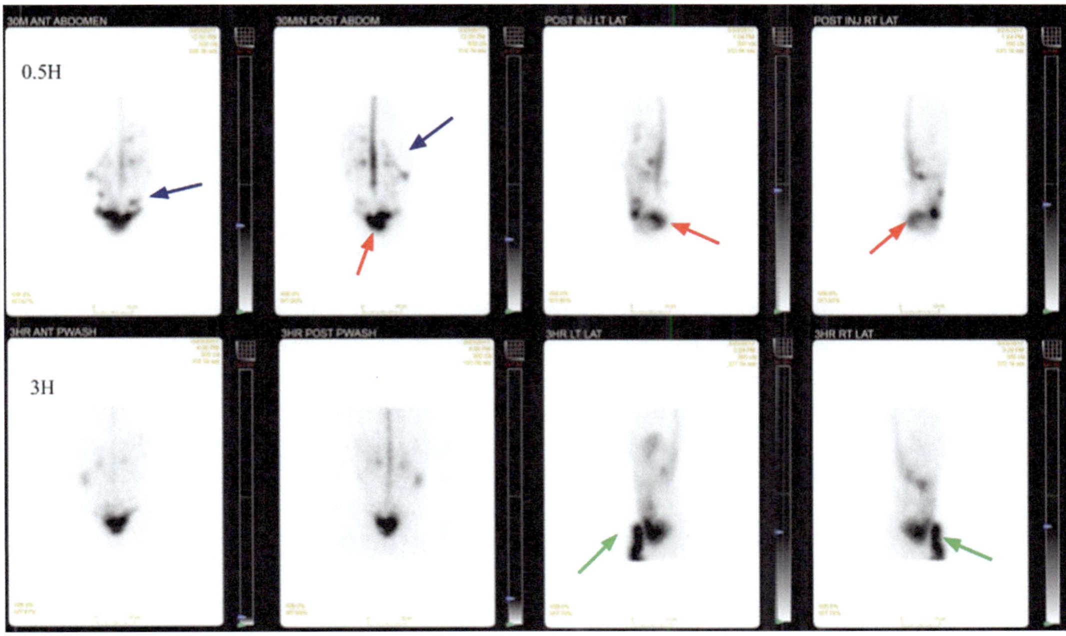

Fig. 7.11 A 6-year-old male with patent lumboperitoneal (LP) shunt

Case 7.12 Essentially Normal Ommaya Shunt Study

Clinical Information

Chief Complaint *Newly diagnosed leptomeningeal metastasis and Ommaya shunt placement*

The patient was a 48-year-old female with history of non-small-cell lung cancer and known brain metastases status post Gamma-knife treatment of multiple lesions in the left brain, now presenting with a new headache. Brain MRI showed extensive leptomeningeal enhancement suspicious for leptomeningeal metastasis. After two negative LP and CSF analyses, the third CSF cytology was positive for leptomeningeal carcinomatosis. In preparation for intrathecal chemotherapy, an Ommaya shunt was placed.

Imaging Findings (Fig. 7.12)

Imaging 4 hours post radioactive tracer administration (top panel, upper row) shows tracer deposition at the Ommaya reservoir (blue arrow) and intense tracer activity in the lateral ventricles (red arrow), indicating patent Ommaya shunt. CSF flow reaches the basal cisterns (green arrow) and spinal canal.

Imaging at 24 hours (top panel, middle row) shows clearance of the ventricular tracer activity and partially complete ascent over the convexities (yellow hatched arrows). The tracer activity in the urinary bladder (black arrow) is indirect evidence of CSF tracer clearance. There is complete CSF ascent over the convexities on the 48-hour imaging, along with further tracer clearance from the entire brain (the top panel, lower row).

The SPECT imaging at 24 hours (bottom panel) confirms partially complete CSF ascent over the convexities and also shows a small area of lack of tracer distribution in the left forefrontal lobe (red triangles) of unknown etiology. Nevertheless, this appears improved on the 48-hour planar imaging (top panel, lower row), when compared to the 24-hour planar image (top panel, middle row), indicating a transient nature.

Discussion

Ommaya shunt is a surgically implanted device through which intrathecal chemotherapy can be delivered repeatedly for the treatment of leptomeningeal carcinomatosis. Prior to CSF imaging, radioactive tracer is injected into the Ommaya reservoir which is located underneath the scalp. The injected tracer immediately reaches the cerebral ventricles through a connected catheter and then distributes along CSF flow. In this particular case, tracer distribution is essentially normal in the brain and spinal subarachnoid space, although there is a moderately delayed CSF flow. The underlying cause of delayed CSF flow is most likely due to leptomeningeal metastatic tumors. Also, there is transient lack of CSF distribution to the left forefrontal lobe of unknown etiology, and probably uncertain clinical significance, given the small area and the transient nature.

There was limited followup information about the intrathecal chemotherapy, which was performed in a private practice setting. Nevertheless, the patient survived more than 7 months after the diagnosis of leptomeningeal carcinomatosis, as he underwent a right liver biopsy 7 months later, which was positive for metastasis of lung origin.

Case Summary

Ommaya shunt patency needs to be verified prior to intrathecal delivery of chemotherapy. Since the tracer is directly injected into one of the lateral ventricles through reservoir and catheter, sequential planar imaging provides valuable information about a normal pattern of CSF flow and distribution into the subarachnoid spaces in the brain and spinal canal. SPECT imaging of the brain is useful to delineate any area of lack of CSF distribution. Moderately delayed CSF flow is often observed, most likely due to the underlying leptomeningeal carcinomatosis.

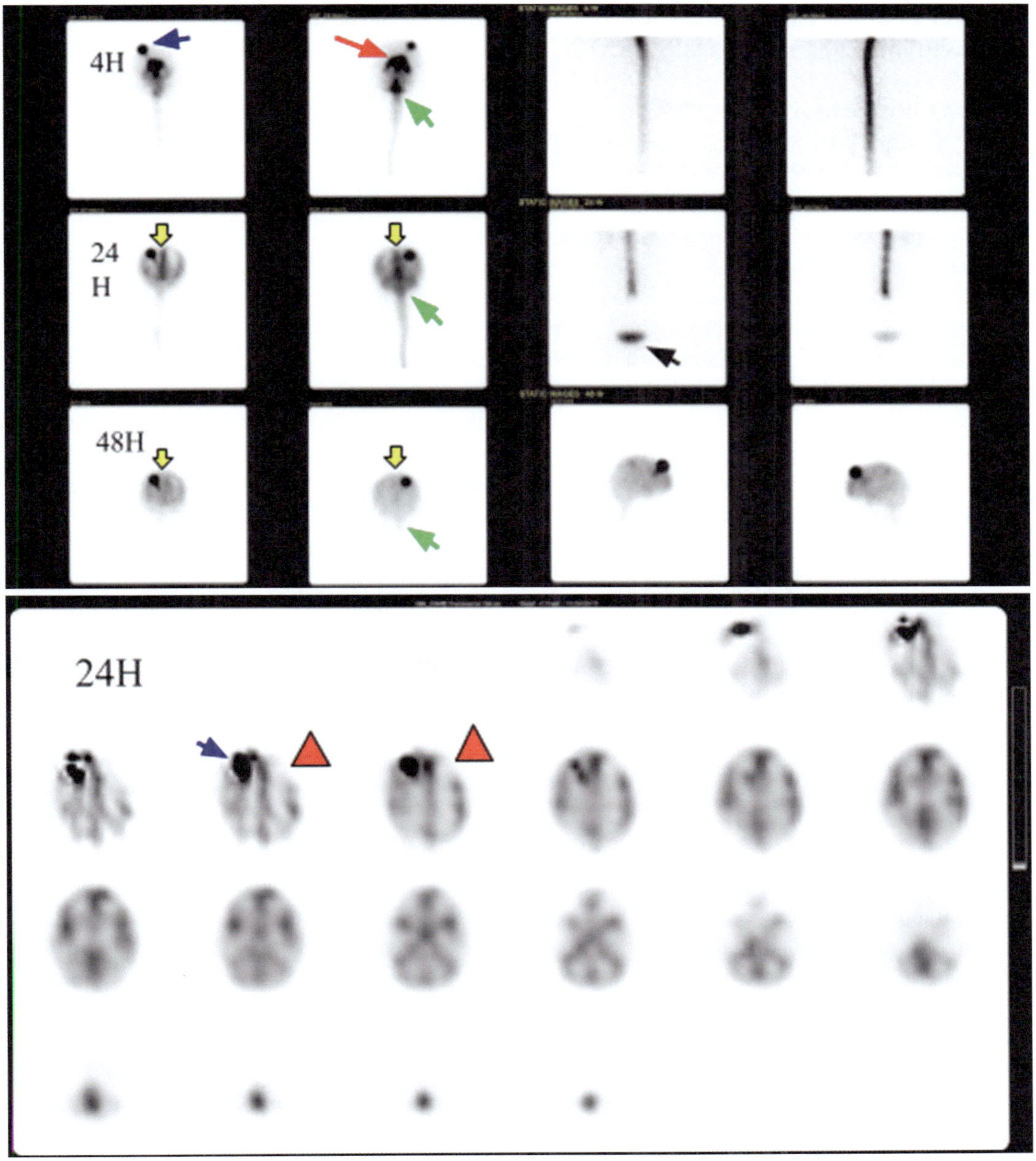

Fig. 7.12 A 48-year-old female with essentially normal Ommaya shunt patency study

Case 7.13 Patent Ommaya Shunt with Uneven CSF Flow/Distribution

Clinical Information

Chief Complaint *Worsening headache for 2 months and history of esophageal cancer*

This was a 65-year-old male patient with history of esophageal carcinoma treated at an outside institution with chemoradiation and esophagectomy a few months ago. He was admitted to our hospital with worsening headache in the occipital area radiating toward the frontal, associated with double vision, light-headedness, balance problem, sixth cranial nerve palsy, and tremor-like activity in upper extremities. He reported transient loss of vision in the right eye which recoveried without any intervention after 1 day. Additional medical history is significant for recent onset of atrial fibrillation status post pacemaker placement 3 weeks ago. The newly placed pacemaker was a contraindication for MR imaging. Initial CSF cytology was suspicious for metastatic adenocarcinoma, and a repeat CSF cytology was positive for metastatic adenocarcinoma. Ommaya shunt was placed for the delivery of intrathecal chemotherapy.

Imaging Findings (Fig. 7.13)

Imaging at 2 hours (top panel, upper row) shows tracer deposition in the Ommaya reservoir (blue arrow). Intense tracer activity is noted in the ventricles (red arrow), with normal distribution to the basal cisterns (green arrow) and the spinal canal.

At 24 hours (top panel, lower row), the planar imaging shows tracer clearance from the ventricles and basal cisterns, with complete CSF ascent over the convexities (hatched yellow arrows). This essentially normal CSF flow pattern is further supported by visualization of both kidneys and the urinary bladder (top panel, lower row). However, there is globally decreased tracer activity in the entire left brain hemisphere, especially in the left temporal region (hatched white arrows).

SPECT imaging at 24 hours (bottom panel) confirms globally decreased tracer activity in the left hemisphere and further reveals an area of absent tracer activity in the left parietal occipital region (red triangles), suspicious for focal obstruction of CSF flow/distribution.

Discussion and Follow-Up

The CSF imaging findings indicate a patent Ommaya shunt. Although the CSF flow pattern is essentially normal, asymmetric CSF distribution is noted, with lack of CSF distribution in the left parietal/occipital region in addition to globally decreased CSF flow to the entire left hemisphere. The underlying cause of the abnormalities is unknown; however, the left-sided abnormal imaging findings appear to correspond to the patient's symptom of right visual disturbance.

After the CSF imaging, the patient received two doses of intrathecal chemotherapy through Ommaya shunt. Further intrathecal treatment was stopped due to a low likelihood of response. Moreover, due to Ommaya shunt infection and meningitis, the Ommaya shunt was removed 6 days after the placement. The patient's condition further deteriorated due to development of metabolic encephalopathy. At family members' request, he was discharged to hospice.

Case Summary

This case illustrates the value of CSF imaging, not only in the verification of Ommaya shunt patency but also the CSF distribution into subarachnoid spaces and CSF flow. The asymmetric CSF distribution and decreased CSF flow/distribution in the entire left brain hemisphere, especially in the left parietal/occipital region, appear to correspond to the patient's right-sided visual disturbance, likely due to underlying leptomeningeal/subarachnoid metastasis. The abnormal CSF imaging findings predicted a poor response to intrathecal chemotherapy and a worse prognosis. In this particular case, his condition was further complicated by Ommaya reservoir infection and meningitis, for which the Ommaya shunt was surgically removed only 6 days after placement.

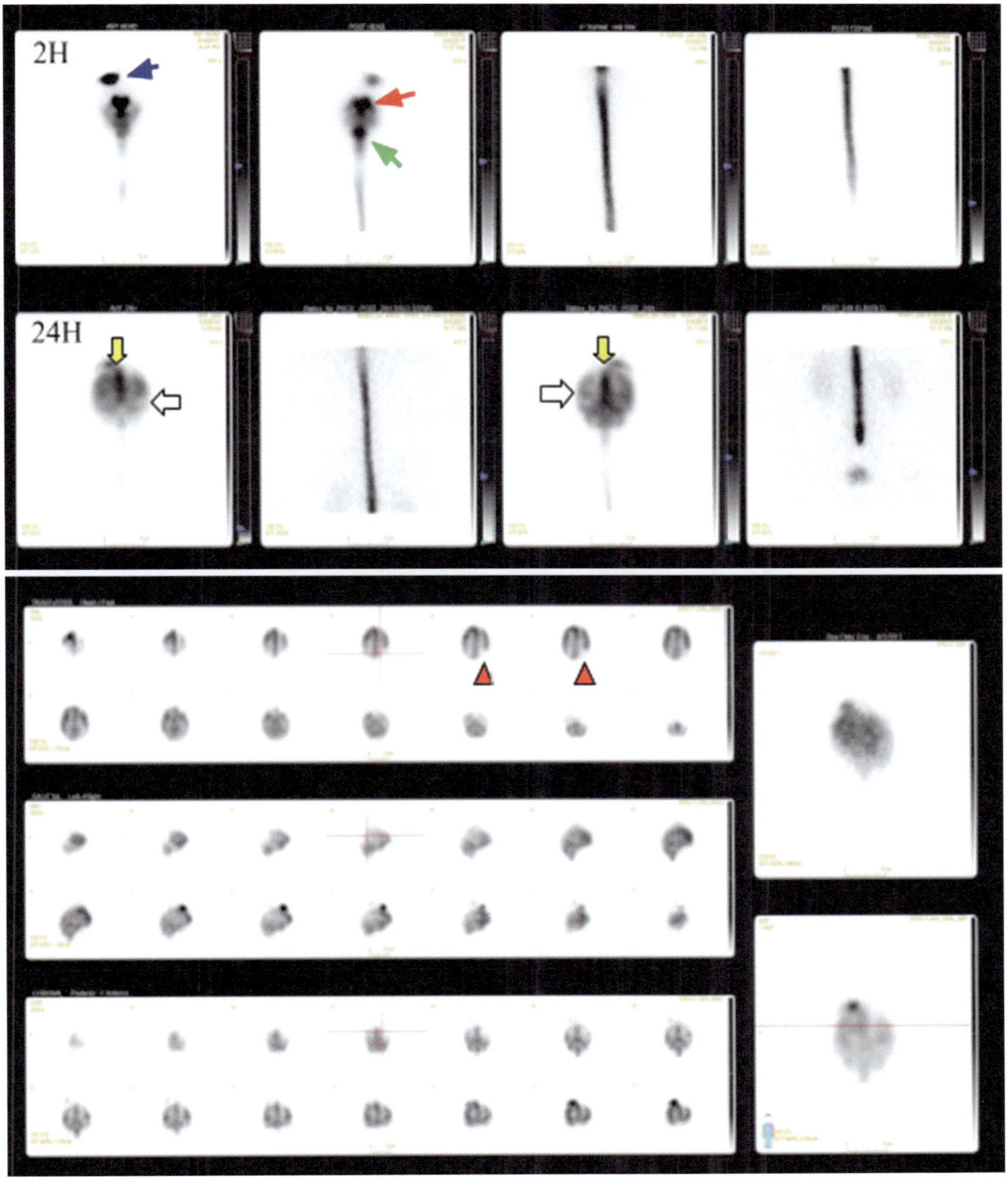

Fig. 7.13 A 65-year-old male with patent Ommaya shunt but uneven CSF flow/distribution

Case 7.14 Patent Ventriculoperitoneal (VP) Shunt

Clinical Information

Chief Complaint *Gait instability and history of VP shunt placement*

The patient is a 67-year-old right-handed female presenting with unsteady gait for weeks. She reports that her gait has been off, and she needs a wheelchair and a walker for ambulation. Her bladder control is intact. She has no double vision, blurred vision, or vision loss. She denies headache. Past medical history is notable for obstructive hydrocephalus secondary to multiple posterior cerebellar hemangioblastoma, status post multiple rounds of surgical resection or decompression. She underwent left VP shunt placement 1.5 years ago.

MR imaging of the brain revealed a left frontal approach ventriculoperitoneal shunt catheter in stable position coursing through the body of the left lateral ventricle.

Imaging Findings (Fig. 7.14)

The dynamic imaging (top panel) shows injected tracer activity at the VP shunt reservoir (blue arrow) extending into the lateral ventricle region. After approximately 10 minutes into the study, increasing tracer activity is seen within the distal catheter (red arrows), which empties into the peritoneal cavity.

Static imaging at 0.5 hours (bottom panel) confirms the aforementioned findings and further reveals CSF tracer dispersion into the abdomen (green arrow). At 1 hour, imaging shows residual activity at the reservoir (blue arrow) and the ventricles (purple arrow), with possible migrated activity at the basal cisterns. Diffusely dispersed tracer activity is noted in the abdomen at this time (green arrows). Visible tracer activity is noted in the right kidney, and accumulated tracer activity in the urinary bladder (hatched yellow arrows), both indicating peritoneal CSF tracer absorption into the bloodstream and subsequent renal excretion, with accumulation in the bladder. These findings are indirect evidence of patent VP shunting.

Discussion

The initial dynamic imaging shows tracer filling of the proximal (ventricle) catheter and then the distal (peritoneum) catheter. Further imaging shows clearance of tracer activity in the ventricles and shunt reservoir, while there is increasing tracer activity dispersion into the peritoneal cavity, without focal abnormality. The visualization of kidneys and urinary bladder indicates peritoneal tracer absorption into the bloodstream with subsequent renal excretion. The findings confirm the patency of the VP shunt and a normal pattern of CSF dispersion within the peritoneal and pelvic cavity.

Case Summary

Patency of a VP shunt on CSF imaging is indicated by the filling of both ventricular (proximal) and peritoneal (distal) catheters. Moreover, tracer clearance from the ventricles and shunt reservoir with increasing diffuse tracer activity is seen in the abdomen/pelvis on subsequent imaging, without focal abnormality.

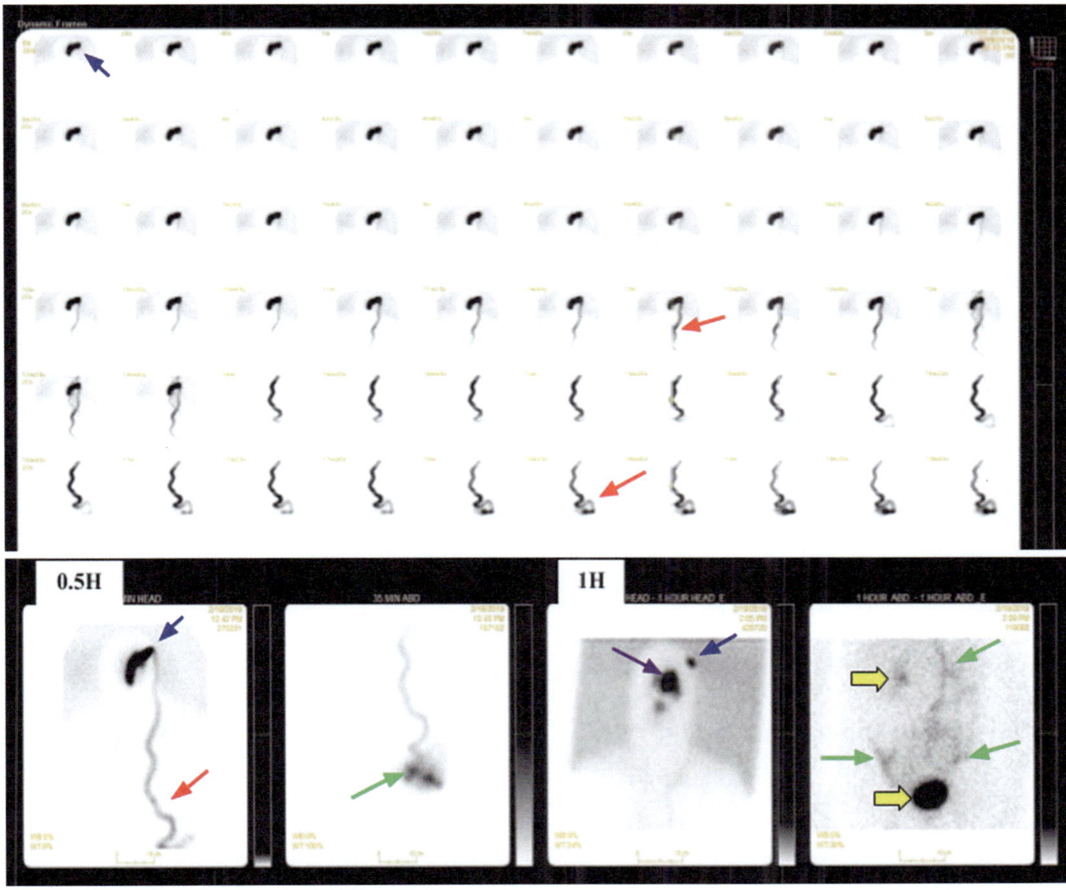

Fig. 7.14 A 67-year-old female with patent VP shunt

Case 7.15 Obstruction of the Proximal and Distal VP Shunt Catheters

Clinical Information

Chief Complaint *Headache, blurry vision, history of VP shunt placement and revision*

The patient is a 29-year-old right-handed female with history of pseudotumor cerebri, status post VP shunt placement 3 years ago and revision 1 year ago. She reports recent new-onset blurry vision in her right eye, intermittent headache, and nausea/vomiting for several weeks. VP shunt re-obstruction was suspected.

Imaging Findings (Fig. 7.15)

Both the dynamic (upper panel) and static images (lower panel) show injected tracer activity in the shunt reservoir only (red arrows), without evidence of ventricular activity throughout the study, indicating a complete obstruction of the proximal (ventricular) catheter.

The static images (lower panel) show no visible tracer activity filling the distal (peritoneal) catheter. However, faint activity is noted in the kidneys (blue arrows), with accumulated tracer activity in the urinary bladder (black arrows), following the tracer administration, suggestive of a high-grade, but incomplete obstruction of the distal (peritoneal) catheter.

Discussion and Follow-Up

The imaging findings indicate complete obstruction of the proximal (the ventricle portion) catheter, as there is no appreciable tracer activity seen within the ventricles and catheters throughout the study. The obstruction of the distal (peritoneal portion) catheter is high-grade, but incomplete, given the minimal renal activity and accumulted bladder activity. This suggests limited CSF drainage through the VP distal catheter into the peritoneum and absorbance into blood stream.

Two days after the abnormal CSF imaging study, the patient underwent VP shunt revision, during which both proximal (ventricular) and distal (peritoneal) catheters were replaced. One day after the shunt revision, the patient reported that her symptoms had resolved. She was discharged home 2 days later.

Case Summary

High-grade or complete obstruction of both proximal and distal VP shunt catheters is indicated by persistent tracer activity confined within the reservoir, without evidence of ventricular activity and no filling of the distal catheter nor appreciable tracer activity dispersed within the peritoneal cavity. Shunt revision is the treatment of choice [7]. This patient reported that all the symptoms resolved immediately after her VP shunt revision.

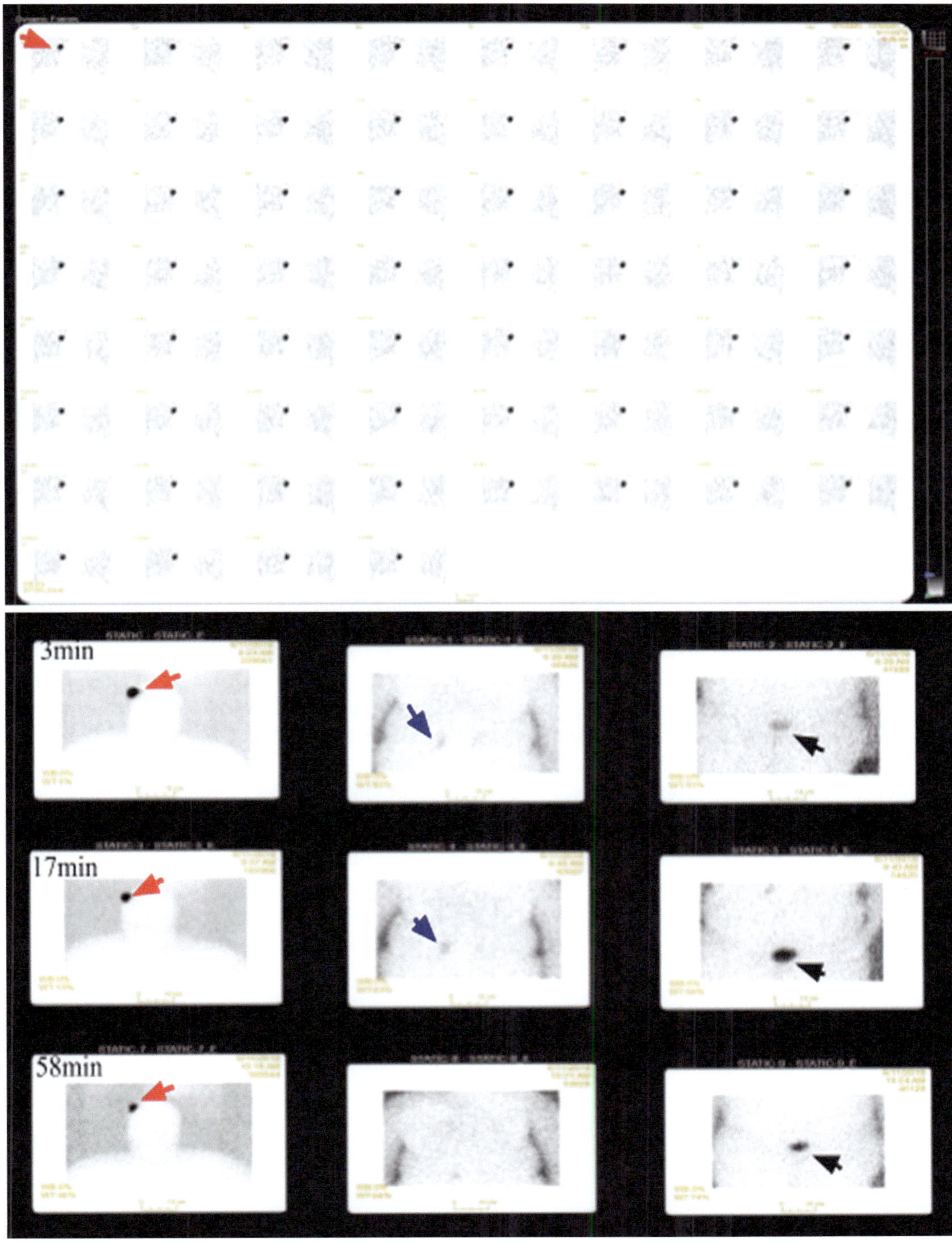

Fig. 7.15 A 29-year-old female with obstruction of the proximal and distal VP shunt catheters

Case 7.16 Obstruction of the Distal VP Shunt Catheter

Clinical Information

Chief Complaint *Persistent headache and history of VP placement*

The patient is a 26-year-old female with history of pseudotumor cerebri treated with VP placement 5 years ago in the state of Georgia. She now complains of recurrent intractable headaches, blurry vision, nausea, and vomiting for a few weeks. She denies any history of fever or chills. Neuro-ophthalmology examinations showed no papilledema. CT of the head/brain showed no acute hemorrhage or evidence of ventriculomegaly.

Imaging Findings (Fig. 7.16)

The dynamic imaging obtained after tracer administration (upper panel) shows injected tracer activity within the shunt reservoir (blue arrow), which instantly fills the ventricular catheter and the lateral ventricle (red arrow) despite intermittent motion artifacts.

The static imaging from 0.5 h to 2.0 h (lower panel) shows migration of tracer activity along CSF flow at the basal cisterns, ascent through the Sylvian fissures and filling of the spinal canal (green arrows). Minimal tracer activity is noted in the urinary bladder (black arrows), suggesting tracer absorption at the cerebral convexities into bloodstream with subsequent renal excretion, or it could be due to free In-111 in the preparation. However, throughout the study, there is no appreciable tracer activity in the VP shunt distal catheter or within the peritoneal cavity.

Discussion and Follow-Up

The imaging findings indicate a patent proximal VP shunt catheter and a normal CSF flow pattern in the ventricles, basal cisterns, and the spinal canal. However, there was no appreciable tracer activity in the VP shunt distal (peritoneal) catheter throughout the study, highly suggestive of high-grade obstruction.

One week after the abnormal CSF imaging study, her VP shunt was removed, during which the distal catheter obstruction was confirmed.

Case Summary

Obstruction of the VP shunt distal (peritoneal) catheter is the most common VP shunt failure in adult patients [7]. CSF imaging shows no tracer filling the distal catheter and no appreciable tracer activity within the peritoneal cavity, although there is tracer activity in the lateral ventricles indicating patency of the proximal catheter. Conventional treatment of VP shunt failure includes shunt revision or shunt removal at discretion of the neurosurgeon and preference of the patient.

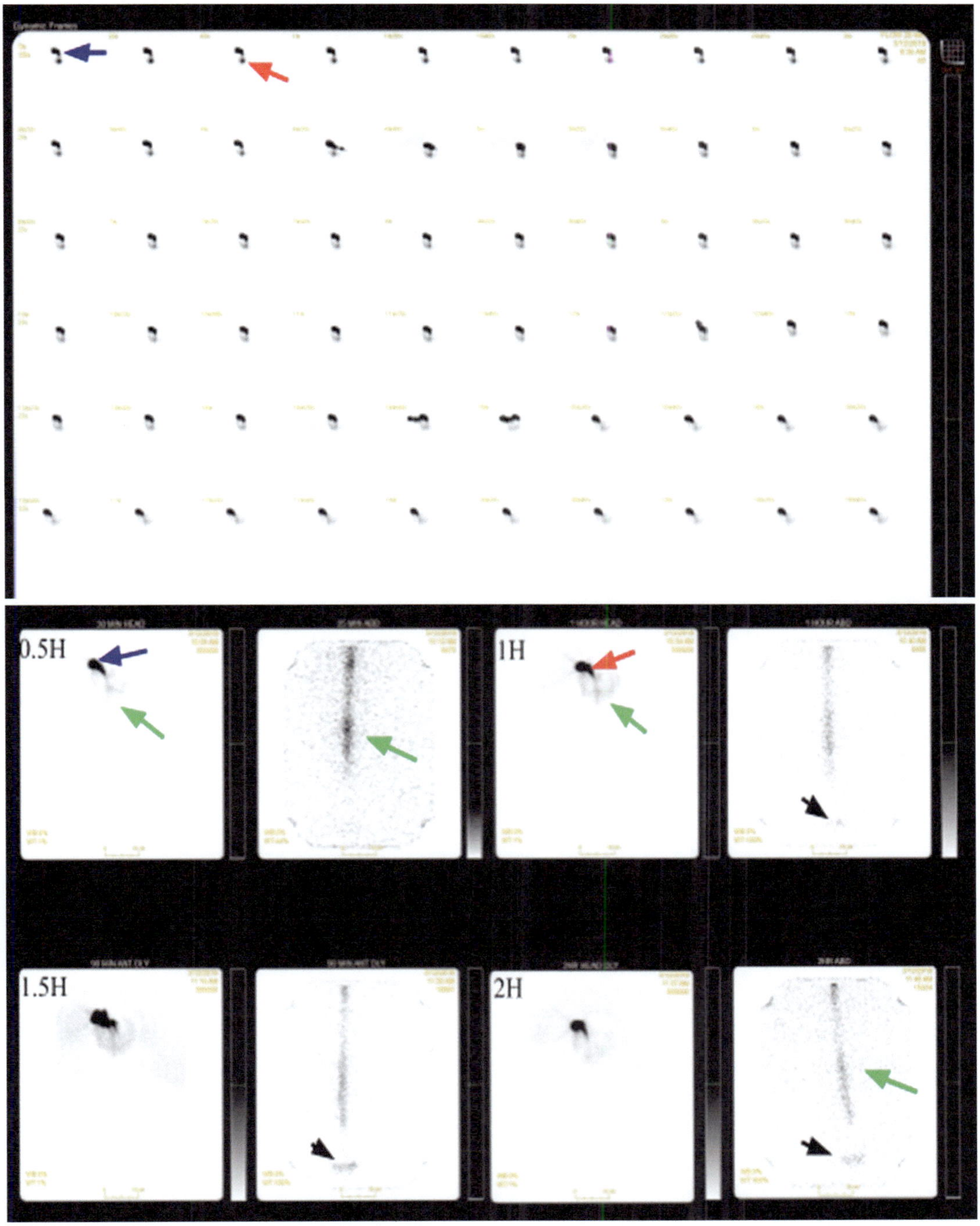

Fig. 7.16 A 26-year-old female with obstruction of VP shunt distal catheter

References

1. Jacobs L, Conti D, Kinkel WR, et al. "Normal-pressure" hydrocephalus. Relationship of clinical and radiographic findings to improvement following shunt surgery. JAMA. 1976;235(5):510–2.
2. Kitami K, Suzuki A, Hadeishi H, et al. Normal pressure hydrocephalus after subarachnoid hemorrhage – with regard to pathogenesis and factors influencing the efficacy of shunt surgery. No ToShinkei. 1986;38(8):781–8.
3. Klassen BT, Ahlskog JE. Normal pressure hydrocephalus, how often does the diagnosis hold water? Neurology. 2011;77:1119–25.
4. Ali SA, Cesani F, Zuckermann JA, et al. Spinal-cerebrospinal fluid leak demonstrated by radiopharmaceutical cisternography. Clin Nucl Med. 1998;23(3):52–155.
5. Limaye K, Samant R, Lee RW. Spontaneous intracranial hypotension: diagnosis to management. Acta Neurol Belg. 2016;116(2):119–25.
6. Eljazzar R, Loewenstern J, Dai JB, et al. Detection of CSF leaks: is there a radiological standard of case? A systematic review detection of CSF leaks: a systematic review. World Neurosurg. 2019;127:307–15.
7. Chiewvit S, Nuntaaree S, Kanchaanapiboon P, et al. Assessment lumboperitoneal or ventriculoperitoneal shunt patency by radionuclide technique: a review experience cases. World J Nucl Med. 2014;13(2):75–84.

8 Miscellaneous Clinical Nuclear Medicine Neuroimaging Studies

Brain Death Scintigraphy

Case 8.1 Positive Study Consistent with Brain Death

Clinical Information

Chief Complaint *Status post aortic dissection repair, new onset of strokes, and cardiac arrest*

The patient was a 46-year-old male admitted due to acute thoracic aortic type A dissection, status post repair 2 weeks ago. Over the last few days, he developed multi-organ failure including acute-on-chronic kidney failure, toxic metabolic encephalopathy, and acute respiratory failure with hypoxia. Also, there was new onset of multiple embolic strokes. He underwent a tracheostomy and was on a ventilator. One day prior to the SPECT brain perfusion study, the patient had acute changes in neurological status with fixed and dilated pupils. He no longer moved his legs to pain stimulation. EKG showed a wide complex bradycardia and then went into cardiac arrest. Chest compressions were immediately performed, and medications were administered. The patient achieved return of spontaneous circulation (ROSC). CT of the head/brain revealed diffuse brain edema, for which mannitol was started. Neurological consultation and exam confirmed brain death by neurological criteria.

Imaging Findings (Fig. 8.1)

The dynamic imaging (Fig. 8.1a) showed no appreciable tracer activity in the entire brain parenchyma. Subsequently, the static imaging (Fig. 8.1b) in anterior/posterior and right and left lateral views, respectively, further revealed no perfusion to the brain parenchyma, while moderate tracer activity was noted in the skull and neck, indicating perfusion in the peripheral. Finally, the SPECT images (Fig. 8.1c) confirmed no appreciable perfusion to the brain parenchyma including the brain stem, although perfusion was noted in the skull and the base of the skull.

Discussion and Follow-Up

Prior to brain death scintigraphy, the patient was diagnosed with brain death by neurological criteria. Additionally, CT of the head/brain showed diffuse brain edema. The brain perfusion study including flow, static, and SPECT imaging with Tc-99 m neurolite (a highly lipid soluble radioactive tracer) consistently revealed no appreciable brain parenchymal perfusion, while there was perfusion in the peripheral. The scintigraphic findings, in line with the clinical diagnosis and anatomic neuroimaging results, were consistent with brain death [1].

Following the positive brain perfusion study for brain death, the patient was evaluated by Gift of Life. Family was updated, and decision was made to withdraw care 2 days later.

D. Wu, *Clinical Nuclear Medicine Neuroimaging*, https://doi.org/10.1007/978-3-030-40893-0_8

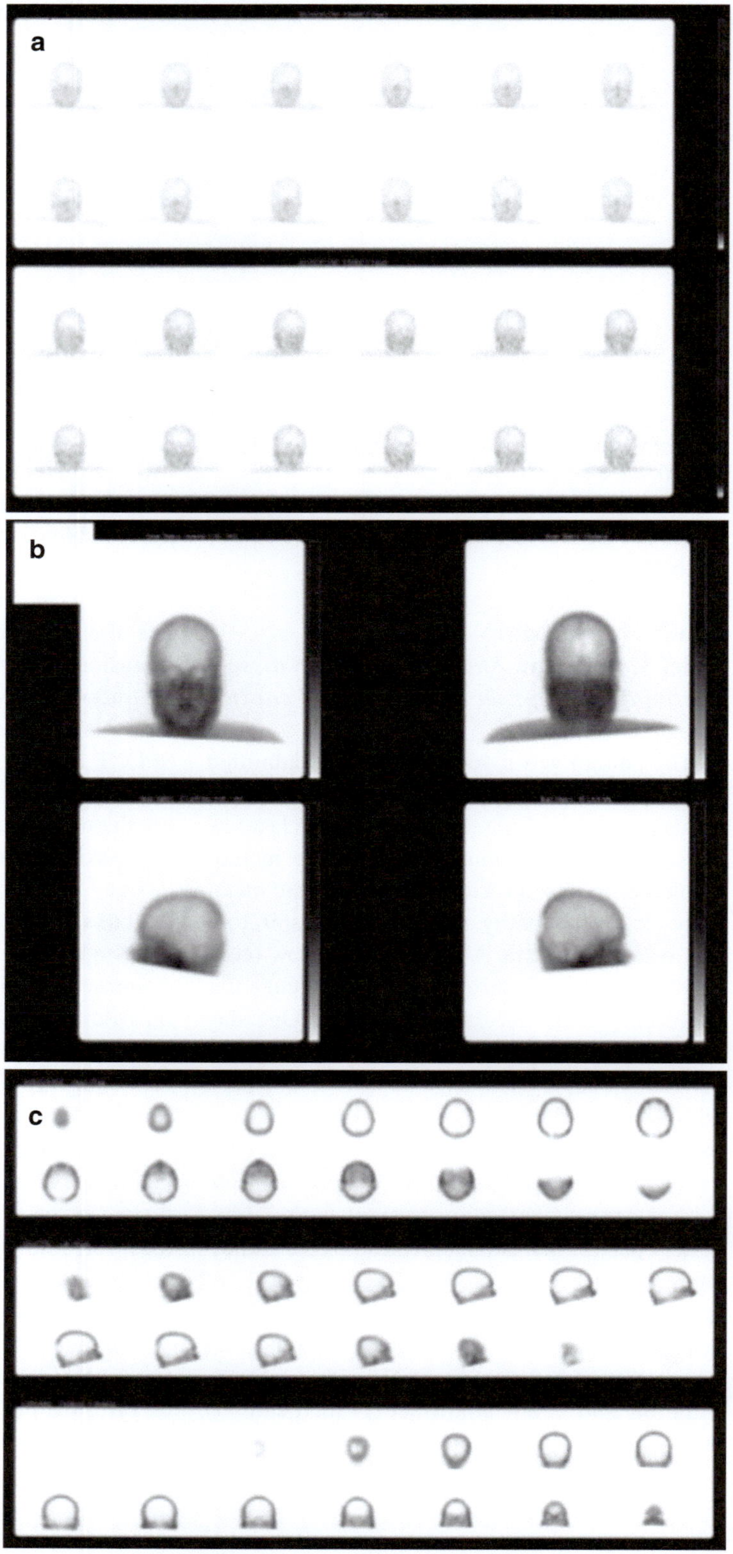

Fig. 8.1 A 46-year-old male with positive brain death scintigraphy

Case Summary

Brain death is often diagnosed by clinicians mainly using neurological criteria. Nuclear medicine brain death scintigraphy is an adjunctive neuroimaging approach for confirmation of the clinical diagnosis [1]. Scintigraphic findings consistent with brain death are characterized by no appreciable flow to or perfusion of the entire brain parenchyma, while perfusion is seen in the peripheral. Dynamic and static imaging of the head/brain is very informative, and SPECT imaging makes the study more conclusive.

Case 8.2 Positive Brain Death Scintigraphy with a "Hot Nose Sign"

Chief Complaint *Cardiac arrest and no neurological response for 3 days*

The patient was a 33-year-old male with cardiac arrest 3 days ago due to heroin overdose per reports from police officers and EMS responders. Since admission, he was intubated and started on a cooling protocol which was discontinued due to severe hypotension despite treatment with several pressors. Past medical history was notable for polysubstance abuse (including abuse of alcohol, marijuana, and heroin), alcoholic pancreatitis, and drug abuse-related pericarditis. Neurological exam showed no purposeful or nonpurposeful movements. Pupils were fixed and dilated. There was no reaction to verbal or painful stimuli. CT of the head/brain showed "no acute intracranial process." In-hospital EEG revealed findings indicating severe diffuse encephalopathy.

Imaging Findings (Fig. 8.2)

Due to the patient's unstable vital signs, the brain perfusion study was performed using a single-head mobile gamma camera. Despite the technical limitations, the flow/dynamic imaging (a) showed no appreciable tracer activity in the entire brain parenchyma, while there was increased tracer activity in the vertical elongated pattern in the nasal region (red arrows). The limited static scan (b) with anterior, right lateral and left lateral views confirmed focally increased perfusion to the nasal region (red arrows), again, no appreciable perfusion to the brain parenchyma.

Discussion and Follow-Up

This was a technically limited brain perfusion study without SPECT imaging. The study was performed using a single-head mobile gamma camera due to patient's unstable condition. Despite the limitations, the flow/dynamic imaging and limited static imaging showed no appreciable blood flow to the entire brain parenchyma, which was direct imaging evidence of brain death. In contrast, perfusion was seen in the skull and the remainder of the head and neck, more prominent in the nasal region. The latter is referred to as "hot nose sign," which is indirect imaging evidence of brain death [1]. This finding was also confirmed on static lateral views (see Fig. 8.2b, red arrows), although the anterior views may not be distinguishable from brain stem perfusion. The underlying mechanism of a "hot nose sign" is likely due to shutdown of internal carotid artery flow due to brain death leading to increased external carotid artery flow, with subsequent increased perfusion of the nasal region.

Following the positive brain perfusion study for brain death, the patient was evaluated and transferred to surgical service for organ procurement for Gift of Life.

Case Summary

Due to the patient's unstable condition, the brain perfusion study was performed with a single-head mobile gamma camera. Despite the technical limitations, *e.g.*, limited static views and lack of SPECT imaging, the images showed absent perfusion of entire brain parenchyma that was direct scintigraphic evidence of brain death. In contrast, there was increased perfusion to the nasal region, often referred to as "hot nose sign," which is indirect imaging evidence of brain death.

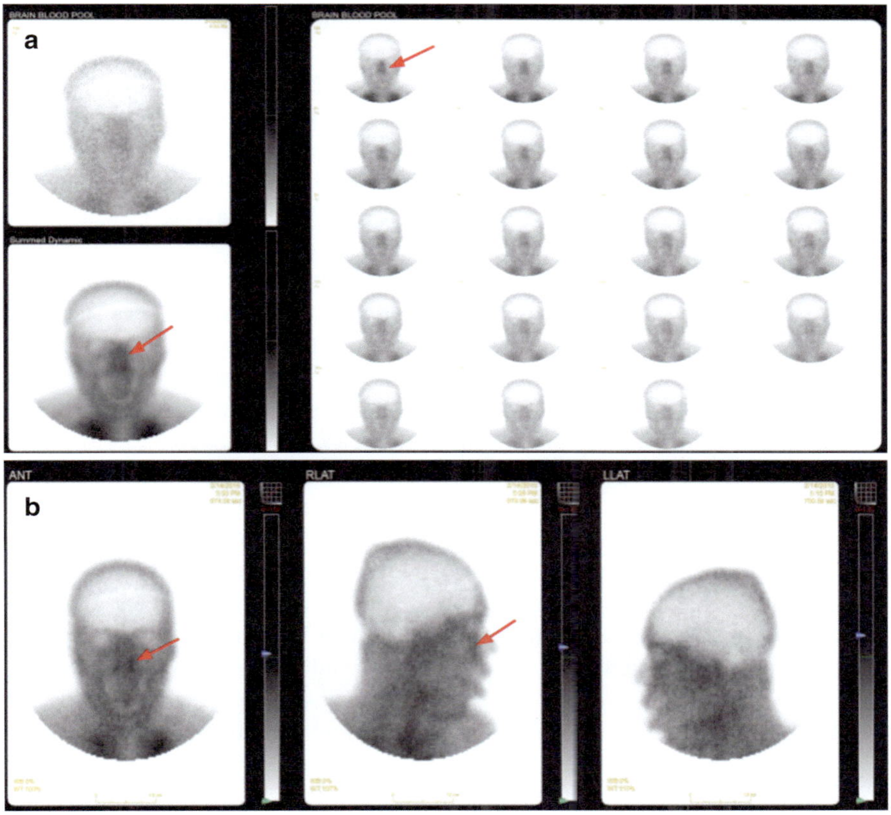

Fig. 8.2 A 33-year-old male with direct and indirect imaging evidence of brain death

Brain Perfusion SPECT of Chronic Lyme Encephalopathy

Case 8.3 Negative Study without Scintigraphic Evidence of Lyme Encephalopathy

Chief Complaint *Chronic pain, memory loss, and equivocal Lyme testing*

The patient is a 70-year-old female with a complex history of chronic pain and memory loss. She states that her Lyme testing was equivocal at an outside institution. In addition, she complains of word retrieval difficulty, numbness, weakness, imbalance, and urinary/fecal incontinence. She was diagnosed with fibromyalgia. MR imaging of the brain at an outside institution showed small white matter changes. Two months ago, she underwent lumbar laminectomy (L2–L5) for the treatment of lumbar stenosis. However, her neck pain is persistent.

Imaging Findings (Fig. 8.3)

Images show mildly decreased tracer activity in bilateral forefrontal and anteroinferior temporal lobes, right slightly more prominent than left (white arrows). Similarly, tracer activity in bilateral anterior cingulate gyri is also decreased, right > left. In contrast, tracer activity is well preserved in the posterior cingulate gyri and the precuneus regions (hatched red arrows). Tracer activity in primary visual cortices is increased likely due to visual stimulation during the tracer uptake period. Tracer activity in the remainder of the cerebral cortices, bilateral basal ganglia, thalami, and cerebella is overall within normal limits.

Discussion and Follow-Up

Lyme disease is caused by tick-borne spirochete *Borrelia burgdorferi*, often involving multiple systems including CNS [2]. Lyme disease is an essentially clinical diagnosis based on (1) clinical criteria, (2) positive Lyme serological testing results, and (3) response to treatment of appropriate antibiotics [2]. This patient has equivocal Lyme testing results, per report, without clinically established diagnosis. Therefore, the pretest likelihood of Lyme encephalopathy is low.

The imaging findings indicate mild hypoperfusion in the forefrontal lobes and anteroinferior temporal lobes, which are common cortical areas affected by brain atrophy. Although there is slight prominence on the right, the overall pattern of the mild abnormality is essentially symmetric. There is no discrete focal abnormality to suggest cortical defects. All the features are suggestive of brain atrophy, rather than Lyme encephalopathy.

Four months after the cerebral perfusion study, the patient had a new MR imaging of the brain, which confirmed “generalized loss of parenchymal volume, more prominent in the bilateral frontal and anterior temporal lobes.” During the follow-up for 5 years, the patient’s symptoms are stable, except for one admission to an outside institution due to acute chronic neck pain and new left jaw pain. In-hospital workup revealed cervical spine degenerative changes; she was discharged with final diagnosis of cervicalgia.

Case Summary

This patient has a low likelihood of Lyme encephalopathy based on clinical data despite her complex medical history. The imaging findings of mild cortical hypoperfusion in forefrontal and anterior temporal lobes, in an essentially symmetric and diffuse pattern, are suggestive of brain atrophy, rather than Lyme encephalopathy. The brain perfusion imaging impression of brain atrophy has been confirmed or supported by follow-up MR imaging and clinical data.

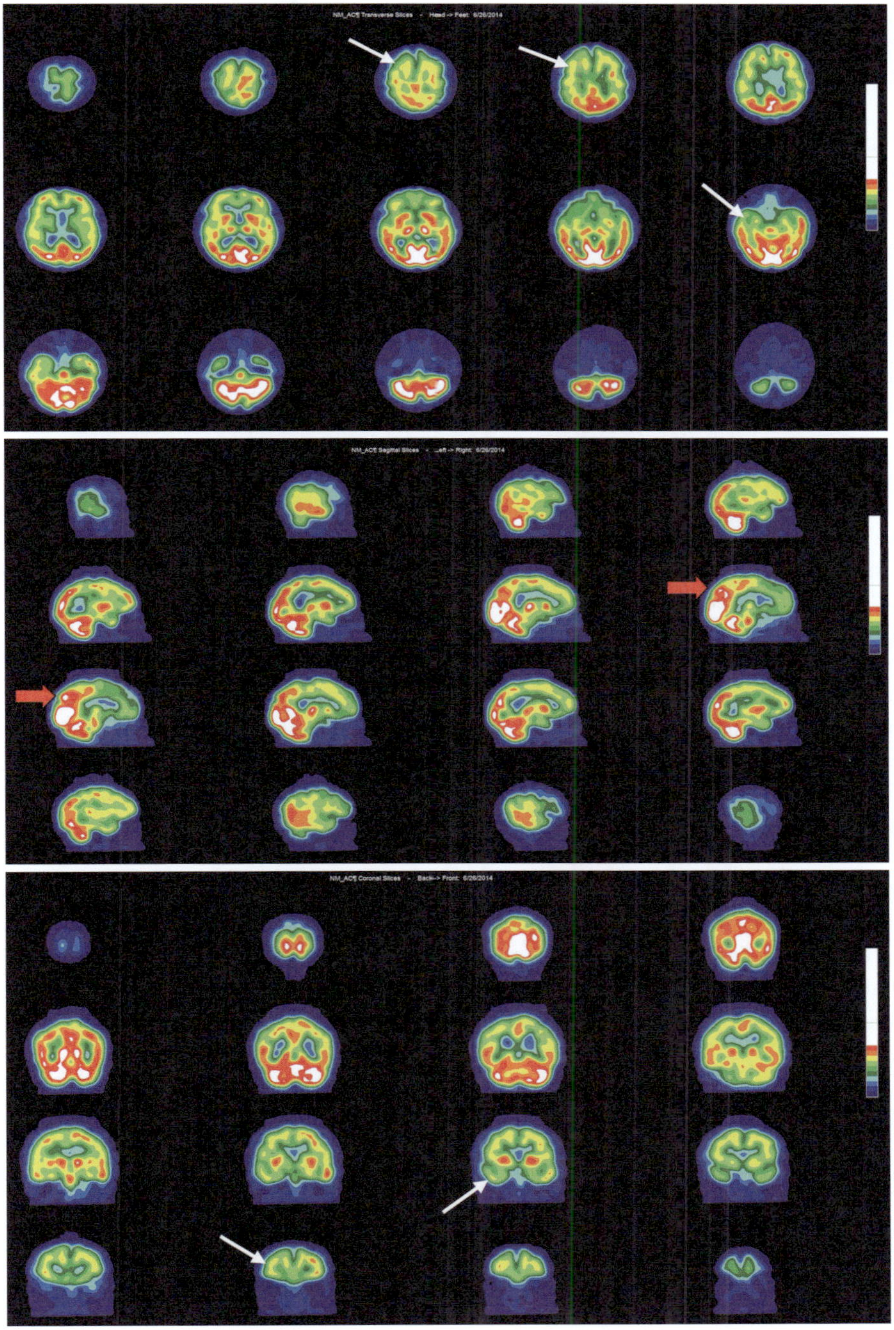

Fig. 8.3 A 70-year-old female with scintigraphic findings suggestive of brain atrophy but no definite evidence of Lyme disease

Case 8.4 Abnormal Brain Perfusion Study Suspicious for Lyme Encephalopathy

Chief Complaint *Chronic fatigue, neck/back pain, and history of Lyme disease*

The patient is a 46-year-old female with history of Lyme disease diagnosed 6 years ago and treated with doxycycline. However, she complains of chronic fatigue and neck/back pain over the last years but denies history of stroke/seizure. There was no history of head injury.

Past medical history is notable for asthma, fatigue, depression, low back pain, anxiety, cervical spinal stenosis, insomnia, chronic sinusitis status post multiple times of functional endoscopic sinus surgery, obstructive sleep apnea (OSA) on CPAP (continuous positive airway pressure), and morbid obesity.

Brain MRI at an outside institution was normal, per report.

Imaging Findings (Fig. 8.4)

Images show multiple areas of cortical hypometabolism (red arrows) involving at least the frontoparietal lobes and the occipitotemporal lobes. Additionally, there are multiple small or punctate cortical defects (white arrows) involving at least the right frontal lobe and bilateral parieto-occipital lobes. However, tracer activity in bilateral posterior cingulate gyri and the precuneus regions is well preserved (hatched red arrows).

Tracer activity in bilateral primary visual cortices, basal ganglia, thalami, and cerebella is overall within normal limits.

Discussion and Follow-Up

The patient has a history of Lyme disease treated with antibiotics 6 years ago. The imaging findings of multifocal/asymmetric cortical hypoperfusion in addition to multiple tubular-like defects are suggestive of cortical sclerotic changes, while preserved perfusion to the cerebella, in conjunction with the history and clinical presentation, is suggestive of chronic Lyme encephalopathy [2, 3].

During the follow-up for 2 years, the patient underwent another endoscopic maxillary sinus surgery, and laparoscopic sleeve gastrectomy for weight control, with reported more energy and decreased back pain.

Case Summary

This case demonstrates multifocal/asymmetric cortical hypoperfusion in addition to multiple tubular-like cortical defects suggestive of cortical sclerotic changes, but preserved perfusion to the cerebella in a middle-aged female patient with history of Lyme disease treated with antibiotics. Constellation of the scintigraphic findings, the history of treated Lyme disease, and the current clinical presentation, is consistent with chronic Lyme encephalopathy.

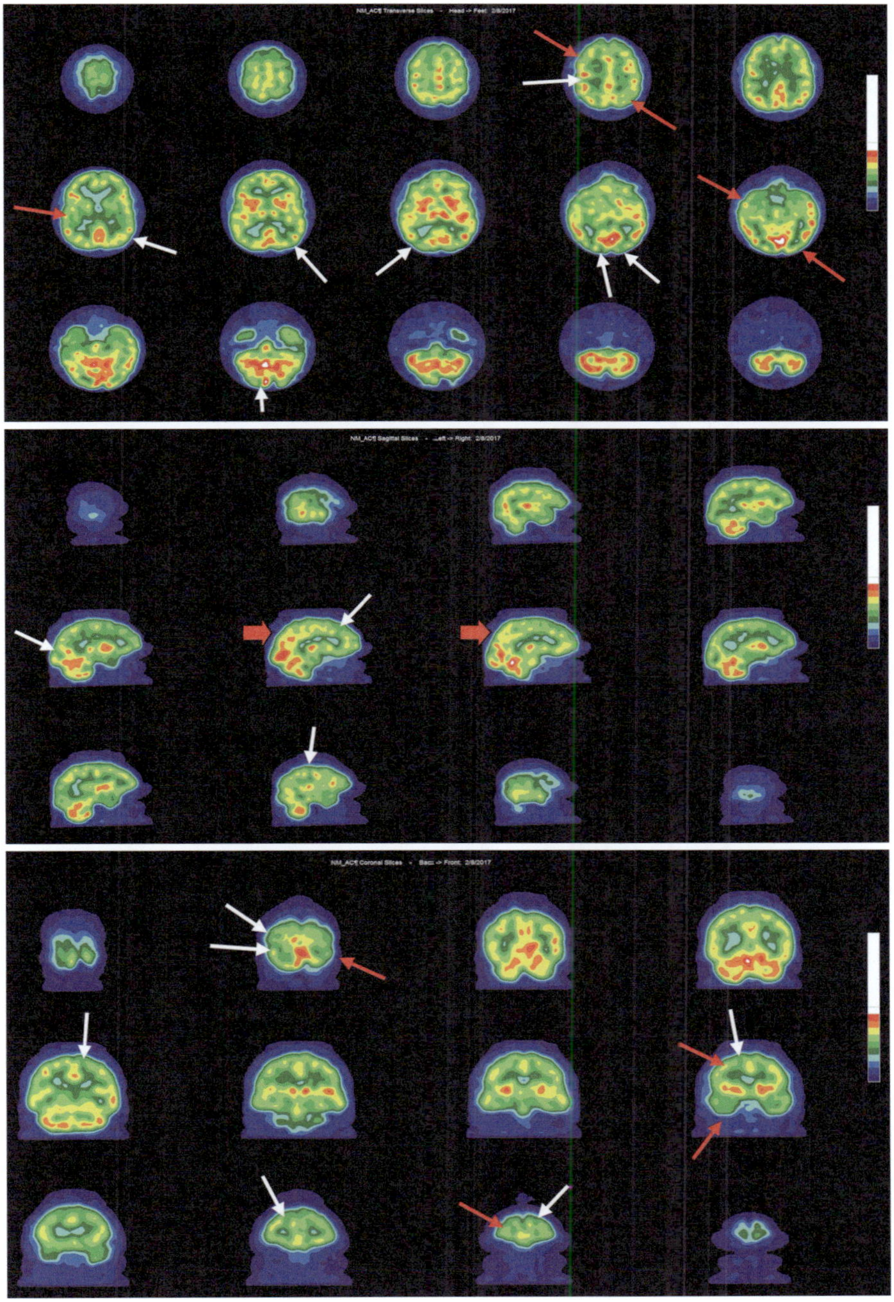

Fig. 8.4 A 46-year-old female with an abnormal study consistent with chronic Lyme encephalopathy

Case 8.5 Positive Study for Chronic Lyme Encephalopathy with Improvement on Follow-Up Imaging

Chief Complaint *Cognitive and behavioral changes, hallucinations, and history of Lyme disease*

The patient is a 26-year-male presenting with intermittent headache since 2009. Family members notice that he has had cognitive and behavioral changes and hearing and visual hallucinations. He was diagnosed with Lyme disease in 2011. He denies history of stroke, head injury, or seizures. He states that he underwent brain MRI and CT studies at an outside institution 3 months ago, both with no abnormal findings. Current medications include lorazepam 1 mg, three times a day; clonazepam 400 mg, nightly; citalopram 20 mg, nightly; and minocycline 100 mg, twice a day.

The first brain perfusion SPECT study was performed, with the patient's MMSE (mini-mental state examination) score of 21/30.

Nine months later, the patient underwent a follow-up brain perfusion SPECT study, with an improved MMSE (mini-mental state examination) score of 24/30.

Imaging Findings

The first scan (Fig. 8.5a) shows diffuse cortical hypoperfusion in bilateral frontotemporal lobes, more prominent than in the right orbitofrontal and the right temporal regions (red arrows), in addition to focal areas of hypometabolism in bilateral parietal lobes, again right greater than the left (red triangles). Also, there are several small or punctuate cortical defects scattered in the bilateral frontal lobes and the left parietal lobe (white arrows). Tracer activity in the right thalamus is decreased (blue arrow), relative to the left. Tracer activity in the primary visual cortices and cerebella is within normal limits.

The follow-up scan (Fig. 8.5b) reveals much overall improved cortical perfusion in the frontotemporal and parietal lobes, with some residual hypoperfusion confined to the right orbitofrontal (red arrows) and the right parietal regions (red triangle), now right more prominent than the left. All the previously noted tubular-like cortical defects have resolved or nearly resolved. Tracer activity the right thalamus is nearly normalized (blue arrow). Tracer activity in the visual cortices and cerebella remains within normal limits.

Discussion and Follow-Up

This 26-year-old male patient has a history of Lyme disease diagnosed 3 years ago; however, he is currently taking antibiotics (minocycline 100 mg, twice a day) indicating chronicity of his Lyme disease [2]. The first brain perfusion SPECT study shows diffuse cortical hypoperfusion, frontotemporal lobes being more affected than the parieto-occipital lobes, with preserved perfusion of the primary visual cortices and the cerebella. Hypoperfusion is also noted in the right thalamus. There are multiple tubular-like small or punctuate cortical defects involving at least the frontal lobes and the left parietal lobe. These findings are suggestive of chronic Lyme encephalopathy in this young patient.

Nine months later, the follow-up brain scan does reveal overall improved perfusion to cortices, and the right thalamus, corresponding to the patient's improved MMSE score.

Case Summary

This case demonstrates that in patients with chronic Lyme disease, SPECT brain perfusion scan could be utilized not only for confirmation of Lyme encephalopathy characterized by heterogeneity and multifocal hypoperfusion/defects but also for monitoring antibiotic treatment response, *e.g.,* effective therapy leading to improved brain perfusion.

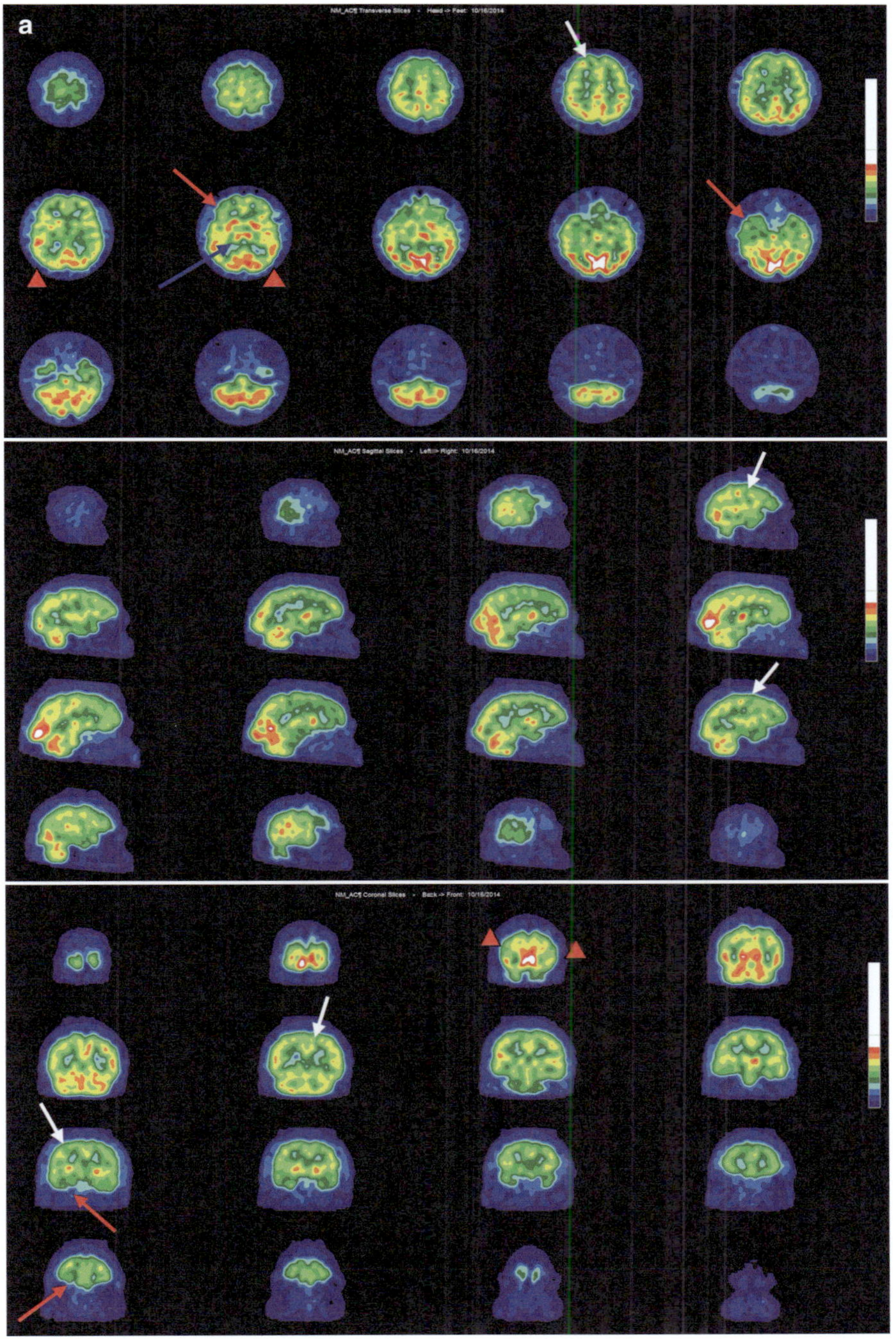

Fig. 8.5 (**a**) A 26-year-old male with an abnormal study consistent with chronic Lyme encephalopathy. (**b**) A follow-up scan showing interval improvement

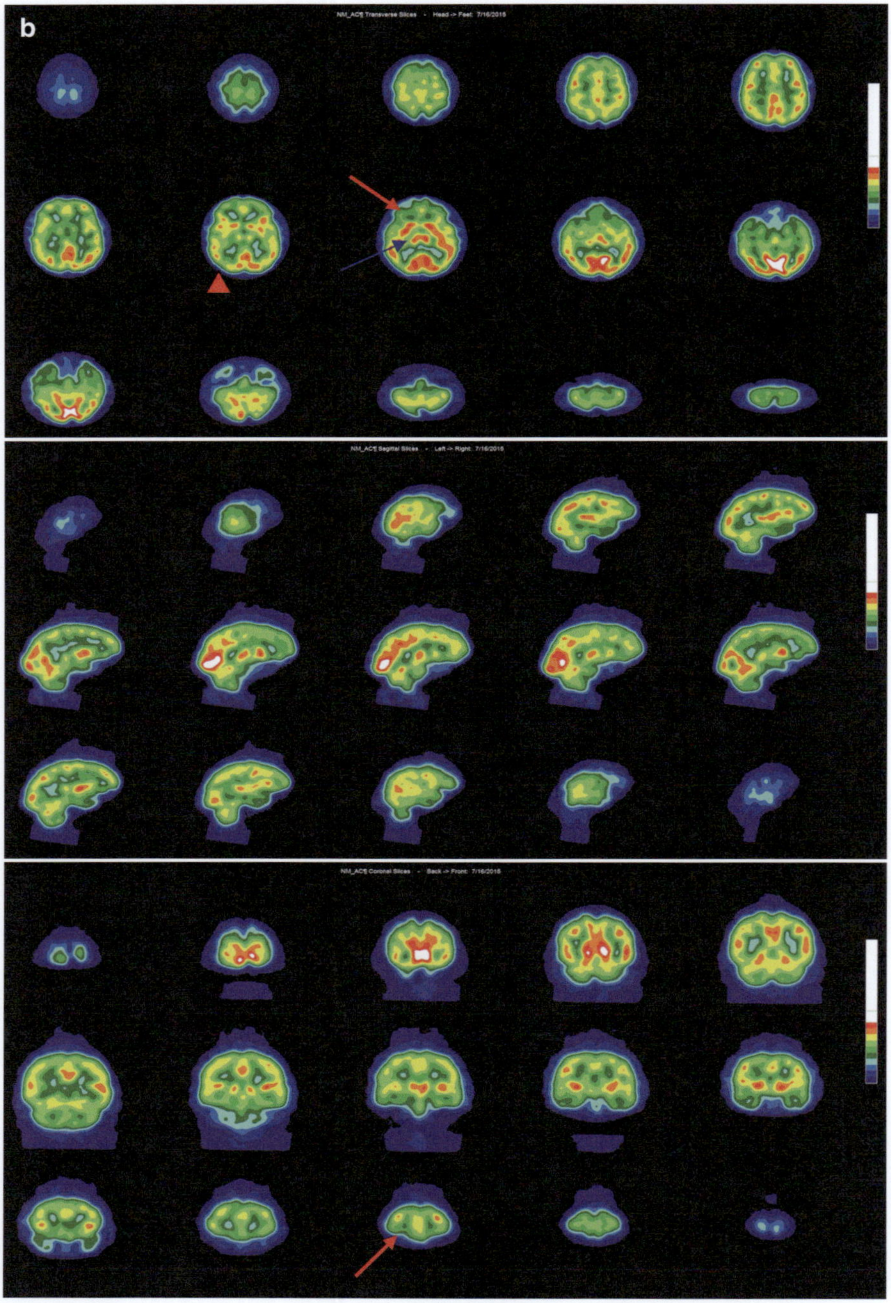

Fig. 8.5 (continued)

Case 8.6 Positive Study Consistent with Lyme Encephalopathy Without Interval Improvement on Follow-Up Imaging

Clinical Information

Chief Complaint *Chronic back pain, cognitive dysfunction, and history of Lyme disease*

The patient is a 22-year-old female presenting with chronic back pain for approximately 5 years. Spine MRI showed congenital partial fusion of T10–T11 associated with perineural cyst on the right causing expansion of the neural foramen. Neurosurgery evaluation recommended no intervention, however. She was diagnosed with Lyme disease 1 year ago and had received IV antibiotics for 9 months. The patient denies history of head injury; there is no history of stroke or seizure. She scored 26/30 on MMSE.

Past medical history is notable for anxiety, bladder incontinence, chronic fatigue, depression, gastroesophageal reflux disease (GERD), chronic tension-type headache, hyperthyroidism, and osteoarthritis.

The first brain perfusion SPECT study was performed, with the patient's MMSE score of 26/30.

Nearly 1.5 years later, the patient underwent a follow-up brain perfusion SPECT study, when the patient reported persistent fatigue, continuous cognitive dysfunction, and memory loss. Her MMSE score remained at 26/30.

Imaging Findings

The first SPECT brain scan (Fig. 8.6a) shows heterogeneous, mild to moderate hypoperfusion in bilateral orbitofrontal lobes and bilateral temporal lobes (red arrows). Tubular-like cortical defects are noted in the left frontal and right parietal lobes (white arrows). Tracer activity in the remainder of the cerebral cortices, bilateral basal ganglia, thalami, and cerebella is within normal limits.

The follow-up scan (Fig. 8.6b) reveals similar cortical hypoperfusion in the orbitofrontal lobes and temporal lobes bilaterally (red arrows). The tubular-like cortical defect in the left frontal is not evident; however, the defect in the right parietal lobe remains (white arrows). Additionally, there is a new cortical defect in the left parietal region (green arrow).

Discussion and Follow-Up

This young patient has a history of Lyme disease treated with a course of 9 months of antibiotics, indicating severity of the disease. Clinically, her symptoms persist with unchanged MMSE score of 26/30 between the two brain perfusion SPECT studies with 1.5 years apart. The follow-up brain perfusion study shows similar cortical hypoperfusion and defects, without significant interval improvement. The overall stable imaging finding of heterogeneity and asymmetric/multifocal hypoperfusion, in conjunction with persistent clinical symptoms, is consistent with chronic Lyme encephalopathy.

Case Summary

Prior to brain perfusion SPECT studies, this young patient has had severe Lyme disease for which she received IV antibiotics for 9 months. In line with the persistent clinical symptoms and unchanged MMSE score of 26/30, the two SPECT brain perfusion studies with 1.5 years apart consistently show multifocal/asymmetric hypoperfusion and cortical defects, without significant interval changes. Constellation of the scintigraphic findings and clinical presentation is consistent with chronic Lyme encephalopathy.

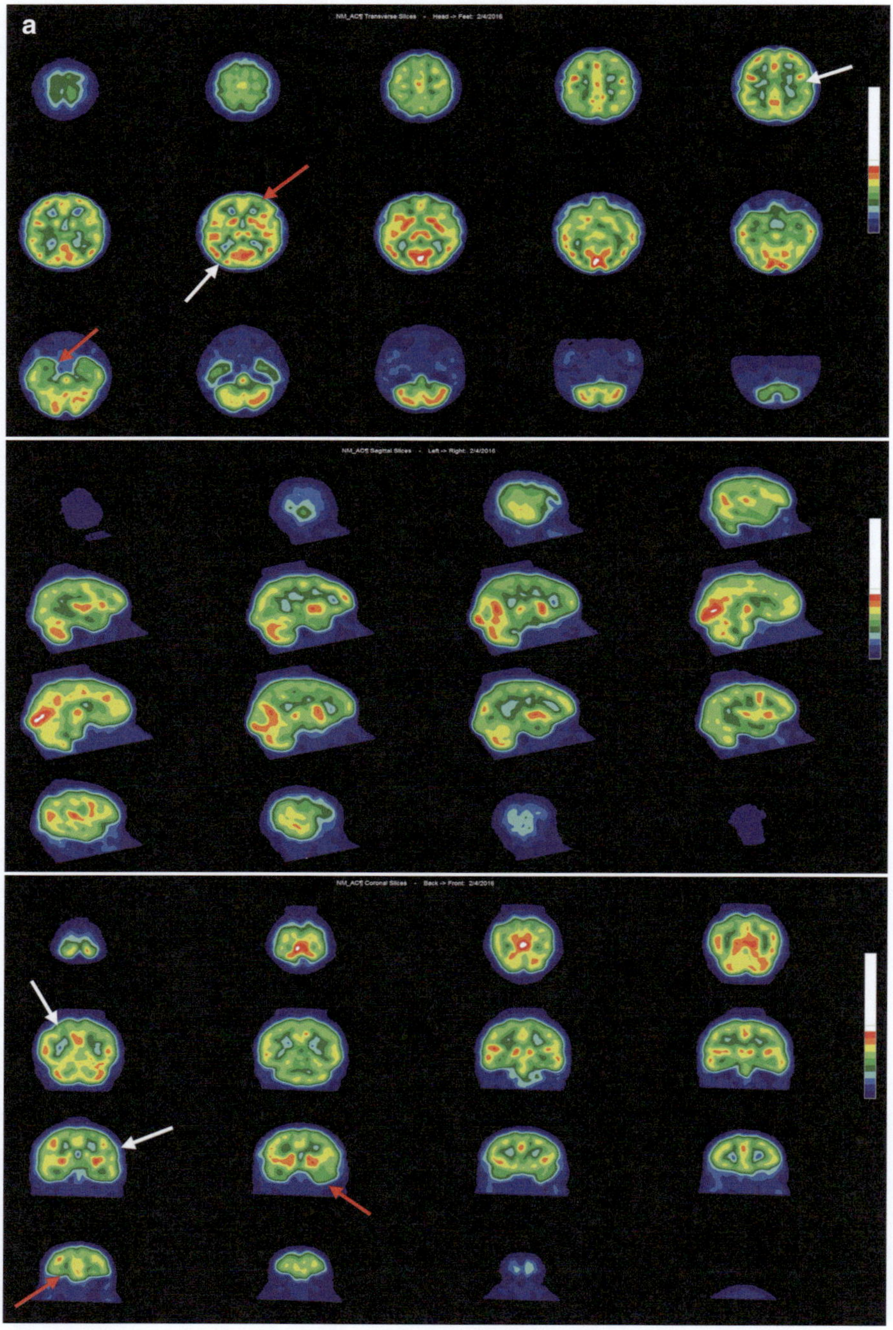

Fig. 8.6 (**a**) A 22-year-old female with abnormal study consistent with chronic Lyme encephalopathy. (**b**) A follow-up scan showing no significant interval improvement

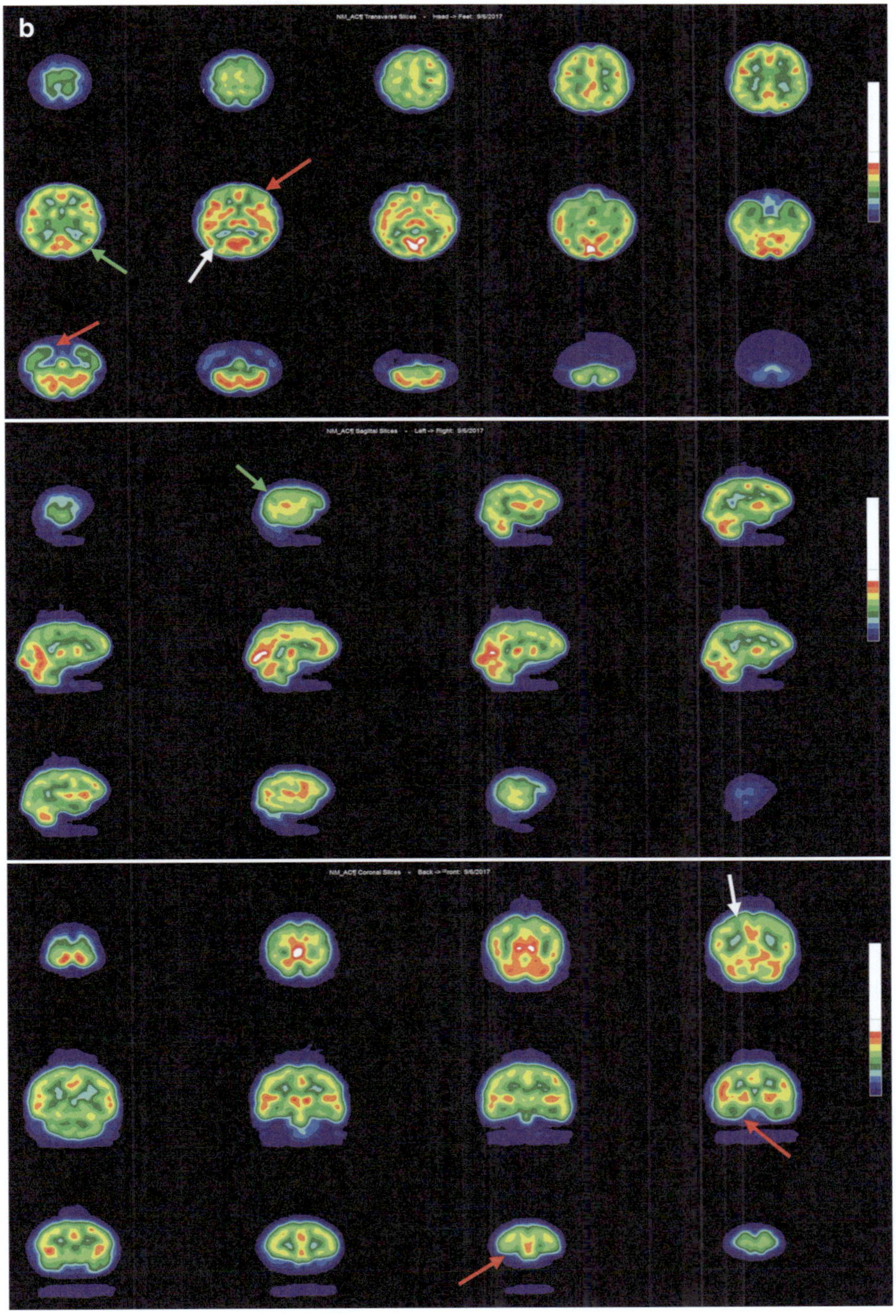

Fig. 8.6 (continued)

Others

Case 8.7 Brain Perfusion SPECT Study as Part of the Wada Test

Chief Complaint *History of drug-resistant seizures*

The patient is a 21-year-old right-handed female with medically refractory epilepsy and is referred for pre-surgical evaluation. MR imaging of the brain revealed left mesial temporal sclerosis. Brain FDG PET showed hypometabolism in left mesial temporal region, suspicious for an interictal epileptogenic focus/zone. Functional MRI (fMRI) demonstrated bilateral language representation. Magnetoencephalography (MEG) suggested right dominance, but lack of visual spatial deficits, while neuropsychiatric (NP) profile was most suggestive of left dominance. Given the lack of congruence between MEG/fMRI/NP results, the Wada test was performed to further assess functional dominance and reserve.

Imaging Findings (Fig. 8.7)

Brain perfusion SPECT images show globally decreased perfusion to the entire left brain hemisphere as expected, including all the left cerebral cortices (red arrows), but more prominent in the left temporal lobe, and the left basal ganglia and thalamus (white arrows). In contrast, perfusion of the right brain hemisphere is well preserved.

Perfusion of the right cerebellum (hatched yellow arrows) is diffusely decreased relative to the left, indicating crossed cerebrocerebellar diaschisis.

Discussion and Follow-Up

The Wada test is named after Dr. Juhn Atsushi Wada, MD, who performed the first test in the late 1940s [4]. The test is also known as intracarotid sodium amobarbital procedure (ISAP) that helps establish brain hemispheric language and memory representation.

The brain perfusion SPECT images show expected global hypoperfusion to the entire left brain hemisphere secondary to anesthetic/sedative effects of intracarotid administration of sodium amobarbital. The more prominent hypoperfusion in the left temporal lobe is likely due to intrinsic temporal lobe's baseline low perfusion relative to other cerebral cortices or due to underlying disease (*e.g.,* intractable left temporal epilepsy) or both. Hypoperfusion is also observed in the left basal ganglia and thalamus. The crossed cerebrocerebellar diaschisis in the right cerebellum is likely sequelae of intractable left temporal epilepsy. It's important to note that there is no area of hypoperfusion in the entire right brain hemisphere, indicating no surgical contraindications.

Approximately 14 months after the Wada test, the patient underwent left anterior temporal lobectomy at an outside institution. One year later, the patient was admitted to our hospital for an updated postsurgical diagnostic evaluation, during which no seizures or spells were recorded. She was discharged with seizure medication adjustments.

Case Summary

Wada test, also known as the intracarotid sodium amobarbital procedure (ISAP), is performed as part of pre-neurosurgical evaluation of language and memory representation/dominance. This case demonstrates expected post-amobarbital global left brain hemisphere hypoperfusion and crossed cerebrocerebellar diaschisis on the right. In contrast, perfusion of the right brain hemisphere and the left cerebellum is preserved. The scintigraphic findings, as part of the Wada test, not only confirm the left language and memory dominance in this patient, but also demonstrate the perfusion/functional integrity of the contralateral brain hemisphere, indicating no surgical contraindications.

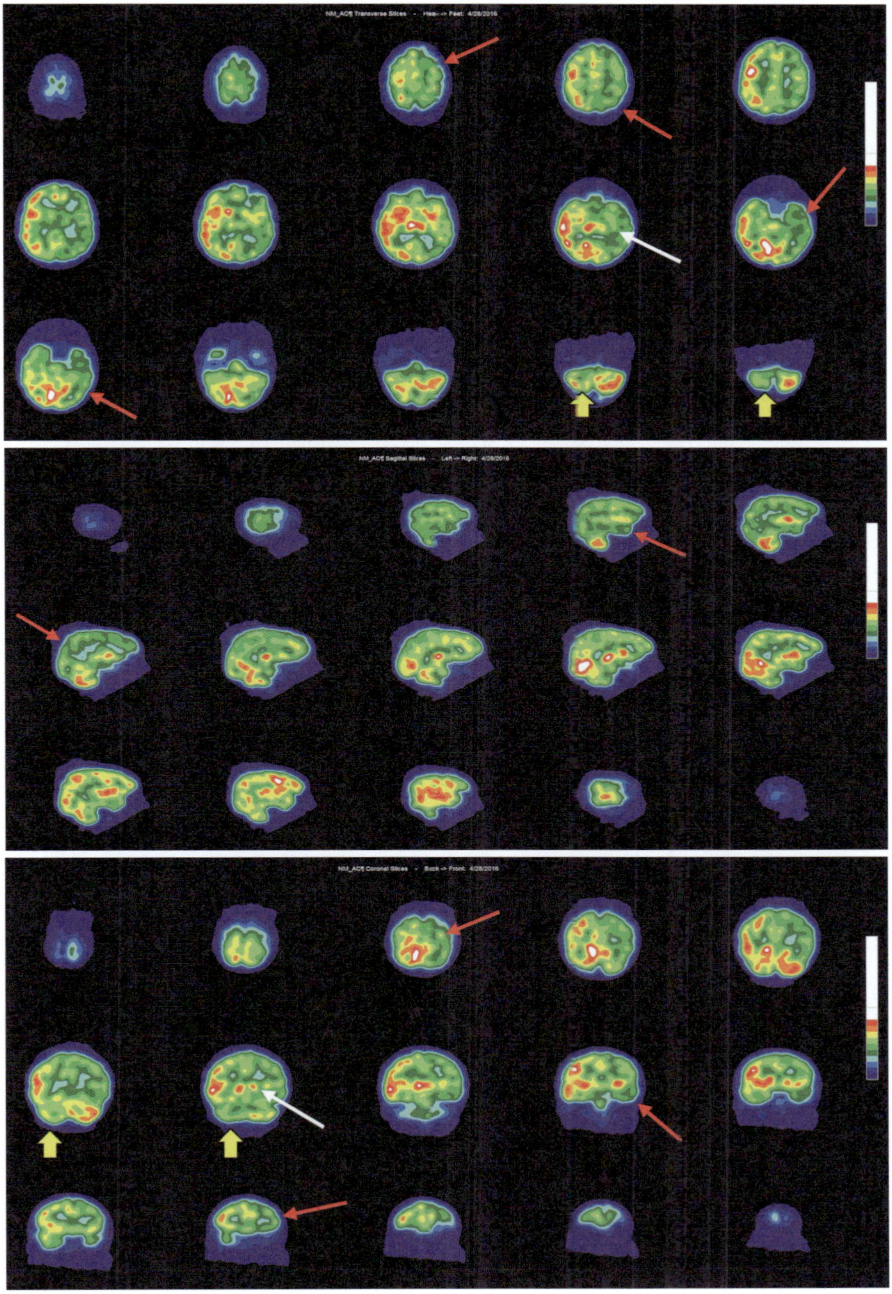

Fig. 8.7 A 21-year-old female undergoing the Wada test

Case 8.8 Intracerebral Steal Phenomenon (ISP) on Brain Perfusion SPECT with Diamox Challenge

Chief Complaint *History of stroke and seizure secondary to known left MCA occlusion*

The patient is a 50-year-old female with history of stroke and seizure occurred approximately 14 months ago. A recent diagnostic cerebral angiogram revealed diffuse atherosclerotic changes, occlusion of the proximal left middle cerebral artery (MCA), and 75% stenosis of the left vertebral artery. Past medical history is significant for hyperlipidemia and known coronary artery disease. He scored 27/30 on the Mini-mental state examination (MMSE).

Current medications include levetiracetam, 500 mg twice a day; alprazolam, 0.5 mg twice a day; aspirin, 81 mg once a day; clopidogrel, 75 mg once a day; atorvastatin, 80 mg once a day; cyclobenzaprine, 10 mg three tablets a day; hydrocodone-acetaminophen, 10–325 mg four tablets a day; and ranitidine, 150 mg twice a day.

Imaging Findings

The baseline brain perfusion SPECT (Fig. 8.8a) shows subtle hypoperfusion in the left orbitofrontal, the left superior superior parietal, and the left lateroinferior temporal lobes (red arrows). There is no focally decreased or absent tracer activity to suggest a cortical or lacunar infarct. Tracer activity in bilateral basal ganglia, thalami, and cerebella, as well as the entire right brain hemisphere, is overall within normal limits.

The repeat brain perfusion SPECT with Diamox challenge, a cerebral vascular dilating agent (Fig. 8.8b), however, shows profound hypoperfusion, diffusely involving nearly entire left cortices (red arrows), including the left basal ganglia and thalamus (white arrow), except for the left medial frontal and the left medial parietal lobes. Again, tracer activity in the entire right brain hemisphere and bilateral cerebella is within normal limits.

Discussion and Follow-Up

Although the patient reports a history of stroke and known left middle cerebral artery (MCA) occlusion, the baseline SPECT brain scan shows subtle hypoperfusion scattered in the left frontoparietal and temporal lobes, suggestive of substantial collateral perfusion and underlying vascular autoregulation, suggestive of mild, watershed area ischemia. There was no scintigraphic evidence of a cortical or lacunar infarct. The repeat scan with premedication of Diamox, however, reveals profound hypoperfusion in the entire left MCA territory, which is referred to as "intracerebral steal phenomenon (ISP)", indicating a poor cerebral vascular reserve (CVR) in the left MCA territory with critically reduced perfusion [5].

After the brain perfusion SPECT study with Diamox challenge, the patient underwent MR imaging of the brain, which showed subtle T2 and FLAIR signal hyperdensity in subcortical white matter of the left frontal lobe and no evidence of acute ischemia. Follow-up brain MRI performed 3 years later again showed a few white matter foci, stable since the prior brain MRI study.

Case Summary

This case demonstrates that, due to substantial collateral perfusion and cerebral vascular autoregulation, only minimal to mild watershed area hypoperfusion can be appreciated on a baseline SPECT brain scan, although the patient has known left middle cerebral artery (MCA) occlusion. With premedication of Diamox (acetazolamide), a potent cerebral vascular dilating agent, however, a repeat brain perfusion SPECT revealed profound hypoperfusion, diffusely involving the entire left MCA territory. This finding is referred to as "intracerebral steal phenomenon (ISP)", indicating a poor cerebral vascular reserve (CVR) in the left MCA territory with critically reduced perfusion.

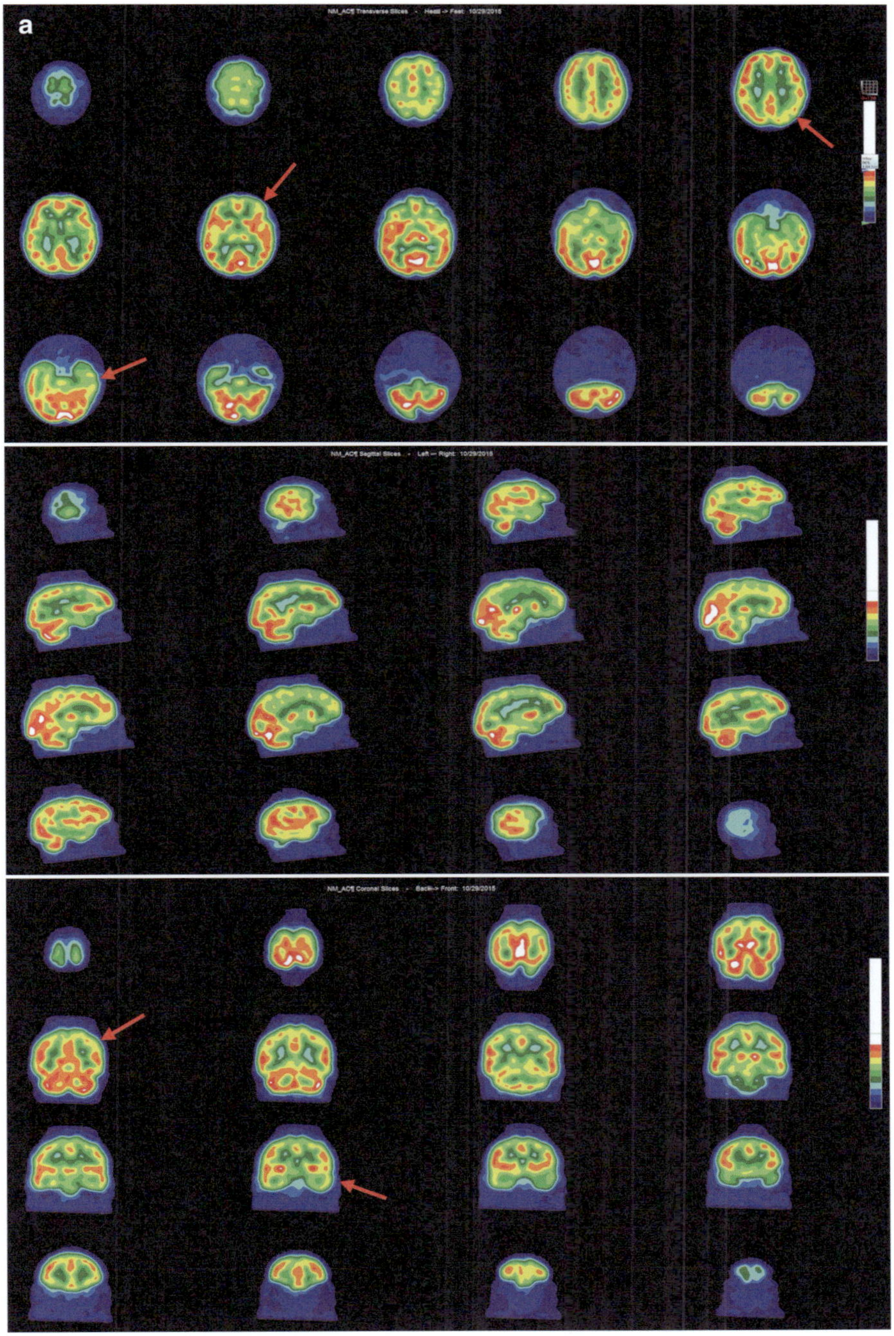

Fig. 8.8 (**a**) A 50-year-old female with known left MCA occlusion undergoing a baseline brain perfusion SPECT. (**b**) The same patient with known left MCA occlusion undergoing a brain perfusion SPECT with Diamox challenge

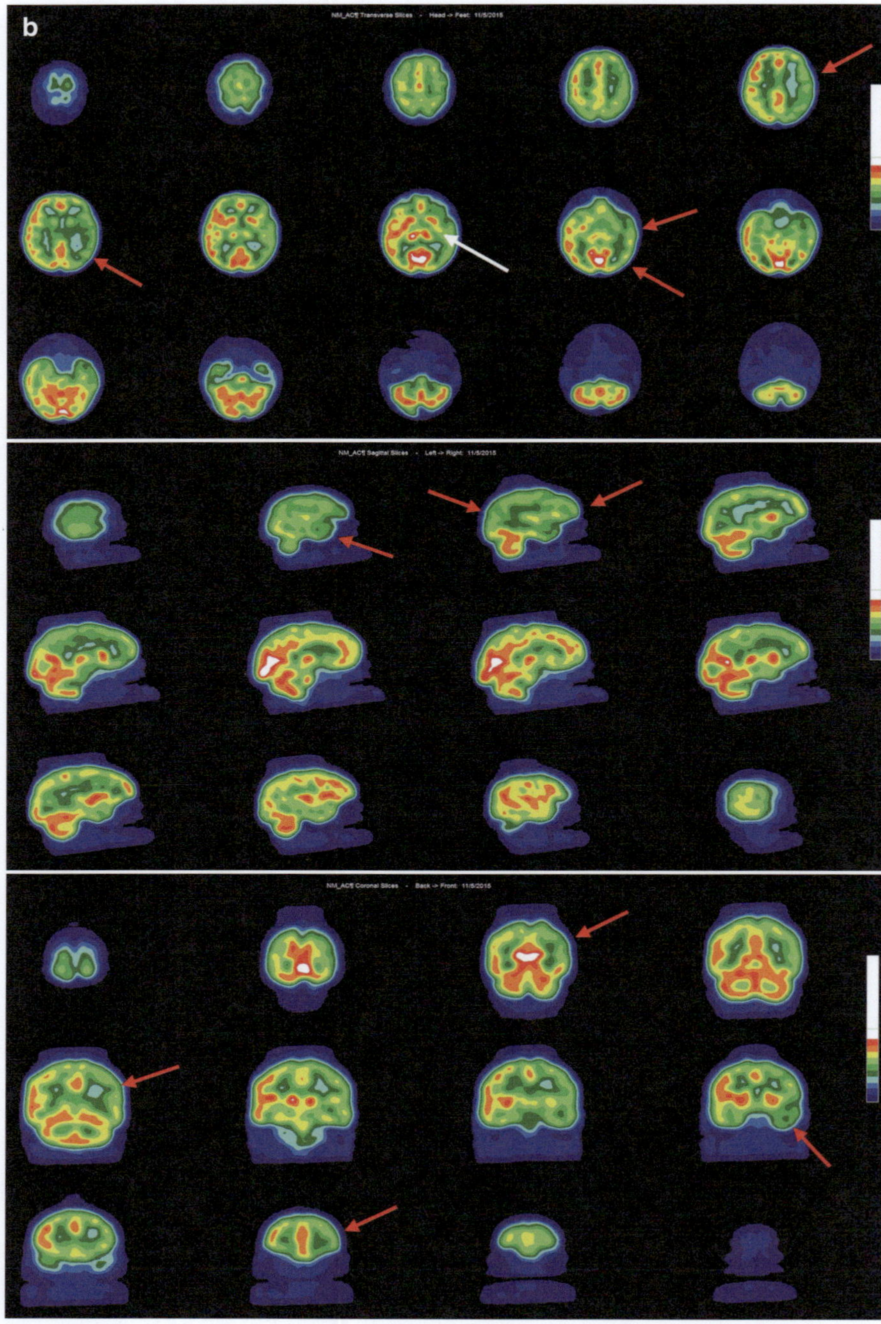

Fig. 8.8 (continued)

Case 8.9 Brain FDG PET of Possible *Mycoplasma* Encephalitis

Clinical Information

Chief Complaint *Altered mental status/nonverbal*

This is a 14-year-old male presented to the emergency room due to altered mental status. His parents stated that for the past 3 days, their son has not been feeling well, and he was not acting normal and not talking all the time. He had headache, cough, and decreased appetite. He once was getting up in the midnight and attempting to leave home for school. The parents recalled that the patient attended camp a month ago, during which he did not sleep well at camp.

The patient does not have history of any autoimmune disease. He does not take any drugs or medications at this time. There is no reported syncope or notable seizure. There are no rashes on physical examination. In-hospital workup revealed low-grade fever (100.9 °F), mildly elevated C-reactive protein, and ESR, but all other tests were negative, including normal CT scan of the head/brain, normal chest x-ray, normal brain MRI, normal EEG, normal white count and hemoglobin, essentially normal chemistry panels, normal lumbar puncture with normal CSF analysis, normal thyroid function tests, negative rapid influenza, negative Lyme titers, and negative meningitis/encephalitis panel. The patient was initially treated with IV vancomycin, ceftriaxone, and acyclovir. Further tests showed positive *Mycoplasma* titers. The symptoms subsided quickly, and the patient was discharged at the request of parents. Take-home medications included oral azithromycin for 1 week, because of the positive *Mycoplasma* titers.

FDG brain PET was performed 4 days after the discharge, with the patient's blood glucose level of 78 mg/dL prior to FDG administration. In our nuclear medicine clinic, the patient was asymptomatic except for left arm discomfort due to an IV line.

Imaging Findings (Fig. 8.9)

The FDG PET images show cortical hypermetabolism in bilateral frontal lobes, left greater than the right (red arrows), and in the bilateral insular regions, right more prominent than the left (white arrows). In contrast, diffuse and symmetric hypometabolism is noted in bilateral thalami, the temporal lobes, and the cerebella (green arrows). FDG activity in the remainder of the cerebral cortices and bilateral basal ganglia is within normal limits.

In the region of the fossa of Rosenmuller, there is intense FDG uptake (hatched red arrows), suggestive of upper respiratory infection or inflammatory/reactive changes.

Discussion and Follow-Up

Although the FDG PET imaging was performed after the patient was treated with IV vancomycin, ceftriaxone, and acyclovir in the emergency department and with 4-day oral azithromycin at home, the study demonstrates increased cortical metabolism in bilateral frontal and insular lobes, while diffuse and symmetric hypometabolism is identified in bilateral thalami, temporal lobes, and cerebella. In addition to the abnormal findings in the brain, there is focal intense FDG activity in the fossa of Rosenmuller, suggestive of upper respiratory infection or inflammatory/reactive changes. These PET findings, although obtained after the patient's symptoms had resolved, are suspicious for encephalitis or encephalopathy in the clinical setting [6].

The patient completed a course of azithromycin by mouth for 7 days. Three weeks later, a follow-up doctor's office visit by the patient and his father showed that patient has normal behavior, sleeping well and eating well, with stable school performance. The father did not appreciate any seizure-like activity, no hallucinations, and altered speech patterns. There was no fever, or rashes, no cough, or no difficulty in breathing. Physical examination was normal as well. The unifying diagnosis for this patient's recent illness is likely *Mycoplasma* encephalitis, in retrospect.

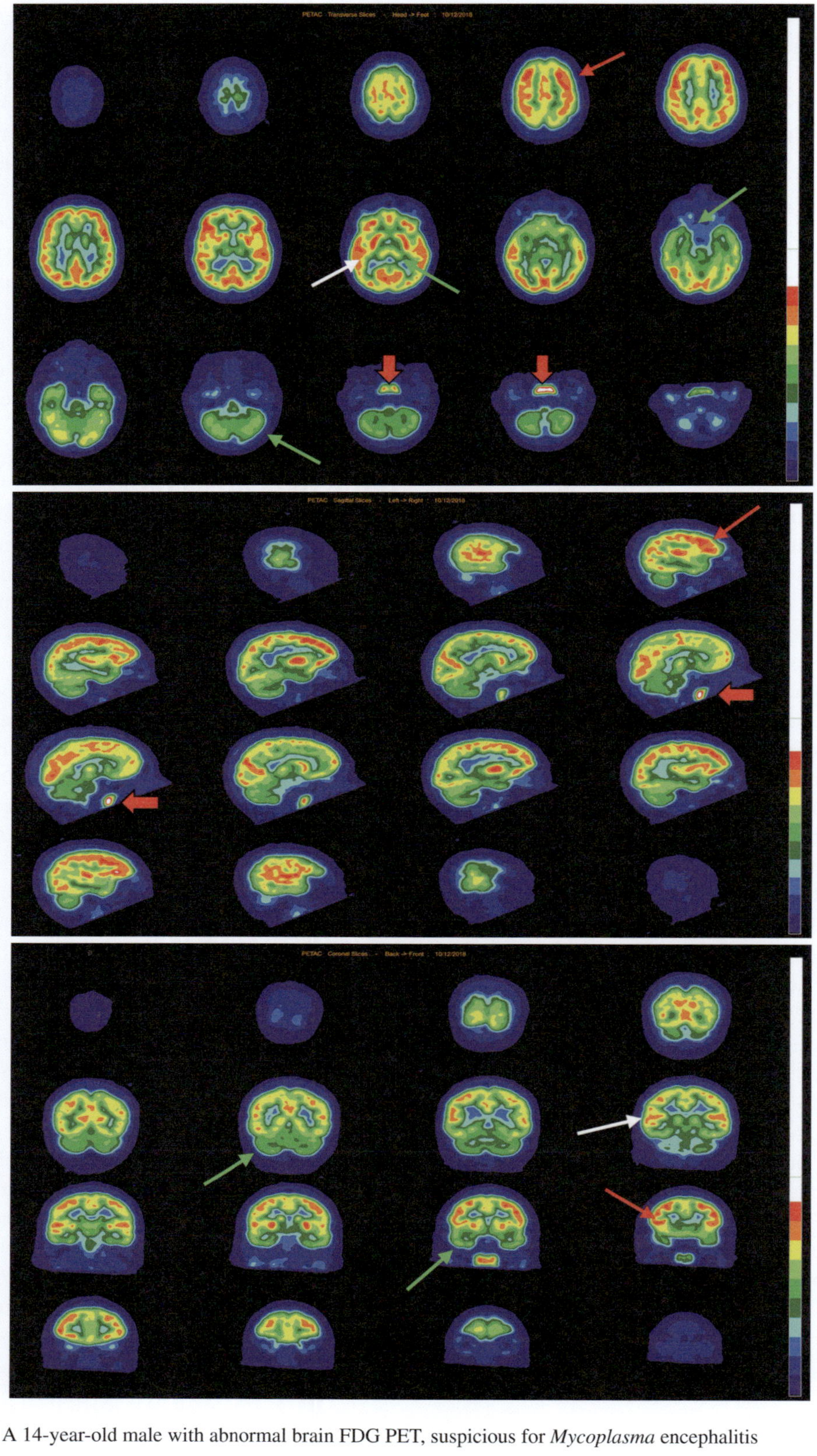

Fig. 8.9 A 14-year-old male with abnormal brain FDG PET, suspicious for *Mycoplasma* encephalitis

Case Summary

This 14-year-old male was admitted to our hospital for altered mental status and atypical measles-like syndrome. Although anatomic neuroimaging studies and multiple other tests were negative except for positive *Mycoplasma* titers, brain FDG PET demonstrates diffuse cortical hypermetabolism in bilateral frontal and insular lobes, and hypometabolism in bilateral thalami, temporal lobes, and cerebella, in addition to focal hypermetabolism in the fossa of Rosenmuller after the patient's symptoms had resolved. These FDG PET findings, in conjunction with positive *Mycoplasma* titers, make *Mycoplasma* encephalitis as the unifying diagnosis, in retrospect.

References

1. Donohoe KJ, Agrawal G, Frey KA, et al. SNM practice guideline for brain death scintigraphy 2.0. JNMT. 2012;40(3):198–203.
2. Logigian EL, Kaplan RF, Steere AC. Successful treatment of Lyme encephalopathy with intravenous ceftriaxone. J Infect Dis. 1999;180(2):377–83.
3. Sumiya H, Kobayashi K, Mizukoshi C, et al. Brain perfusion SPECT in Lyme neuroborreliosis. J Nucl Med. 1997;38:1120–2.
4. Wada JA. A new method for the determination of the side of cerebral speech dominance. A preliminary report of the intra-carotid injection of sodium amytal in man (article in Japanese). Igaku to Seibutsugaki, Tokyo. 1949;14:221–2.
5. Vagal AS, Leach JL, Fernandez-Ulloa M, et al. The acetazolamide challenge: Techniques and applications in the evaluation of chronic cerebral ischemia. AJNR. 2009;30(5):876–84.
6. Turpin, et al. ^{18}F-Flurodeoxyglucose positron emission tomography with computed tomography (FDG PET/CT) findings in children with encephalitis and comparison to conventional imaging. Euro J Nucl Med Mol Imaging. 2019;46(6):1309–24.

Appendix I: Self-Assessment Quiz

Quiz #1

This is a 65-year-old male patient presenting with memory loss and behavioral changes for 1 year. Additionally, the patient reports recently developed paranoia for the past 2 months. He denies history of stroke, head injury, or seizures. He is a non-smoker and has no history of alcohol or drug abuse. Brain MRI revealed prominent sulci and ventricles with frontal lobe predominance as well as nonspecific T_2 hyperintensity with periventricular white matter also with frontal predominance, suspicious for Pick's disease. Brain FDG PET images are displayed in Fig. Q1. According to the clinical presentation and neuroimaging findings, which is the most likely imaging impression for this patient?

A. Alzheimer's disease (AD)
B. Frontotemporal dementia (FTD)
C. Dementia with Lewy bodies (DLB)
D. Corticobasal degeneration (CBD)
E. Vascular dementia (VD)

D. Wu, *Clinical Nuclear Medicine Neuroimaging*, https://doi.org/10.1007/978-3-030-40893-0

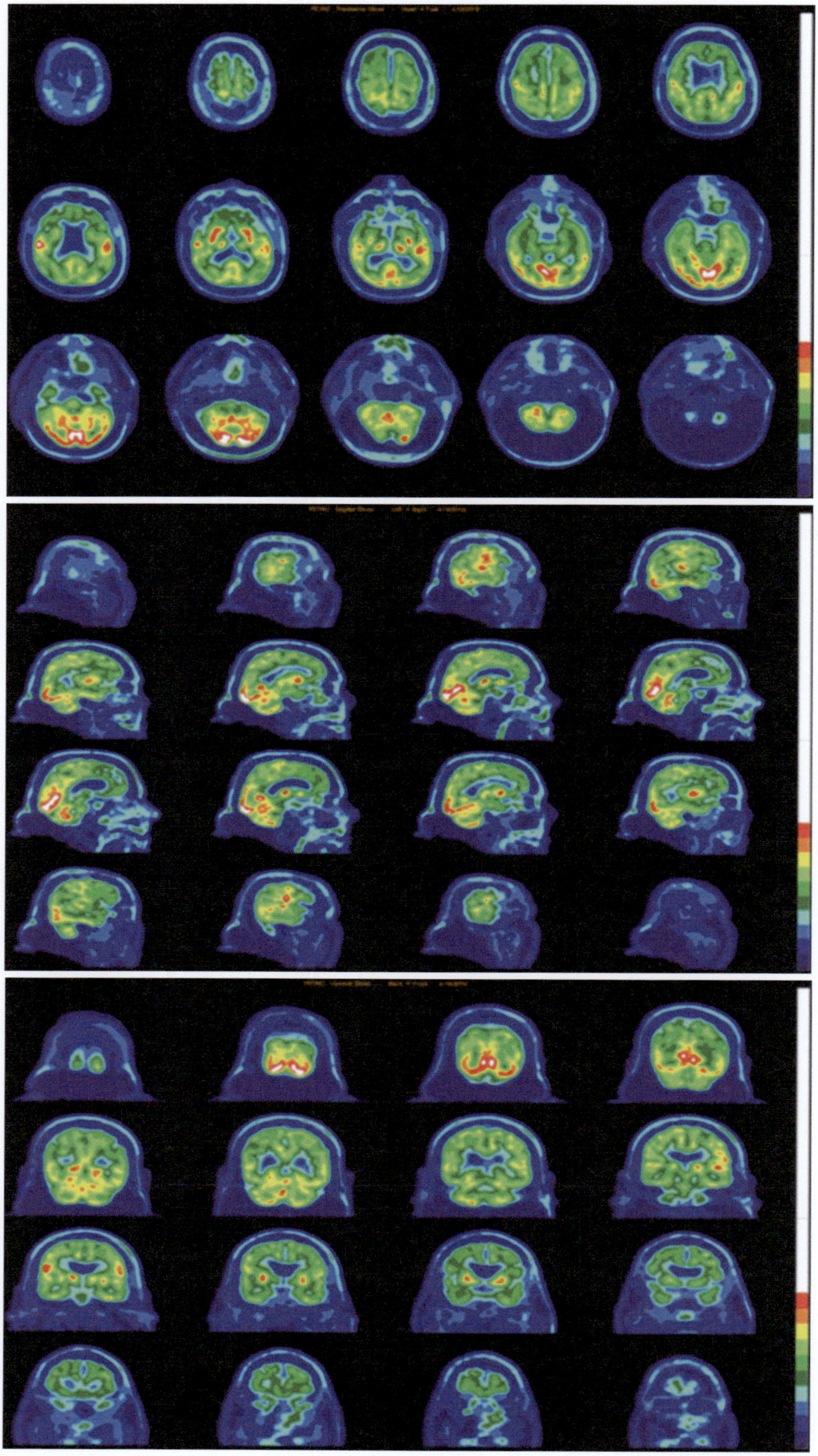

Fig. Q1

Quiz #2

The patient is an 88-year-old female who has had difficulty with her memory, attention, and word finding over the last 2 years. After the death of her husband recently, she has had increased word finding difficulty and has become more confused. She especially has short-term memory loss and difficulty maintaining new information, for which she could no longer pay her bills and stopped driving. A recent CT of the head/brain revealed diffuse chronic small vessel disease and an age-indeterminate large chronic infarct involving the left basal ganglia. Brain FDG PET images are shown in Fig. Q2. According to the clinical presentation and neuroimaging findings, which is the most likely imaging impression for this patient?

A. Alzheimer's disease (AD)
B. Frontotemporal dementia (FTD)
C. Dementia with Lewy bodies (DLB)
D. Corticobasal degeneration (CBD)
E. Vascular dementia (VD)

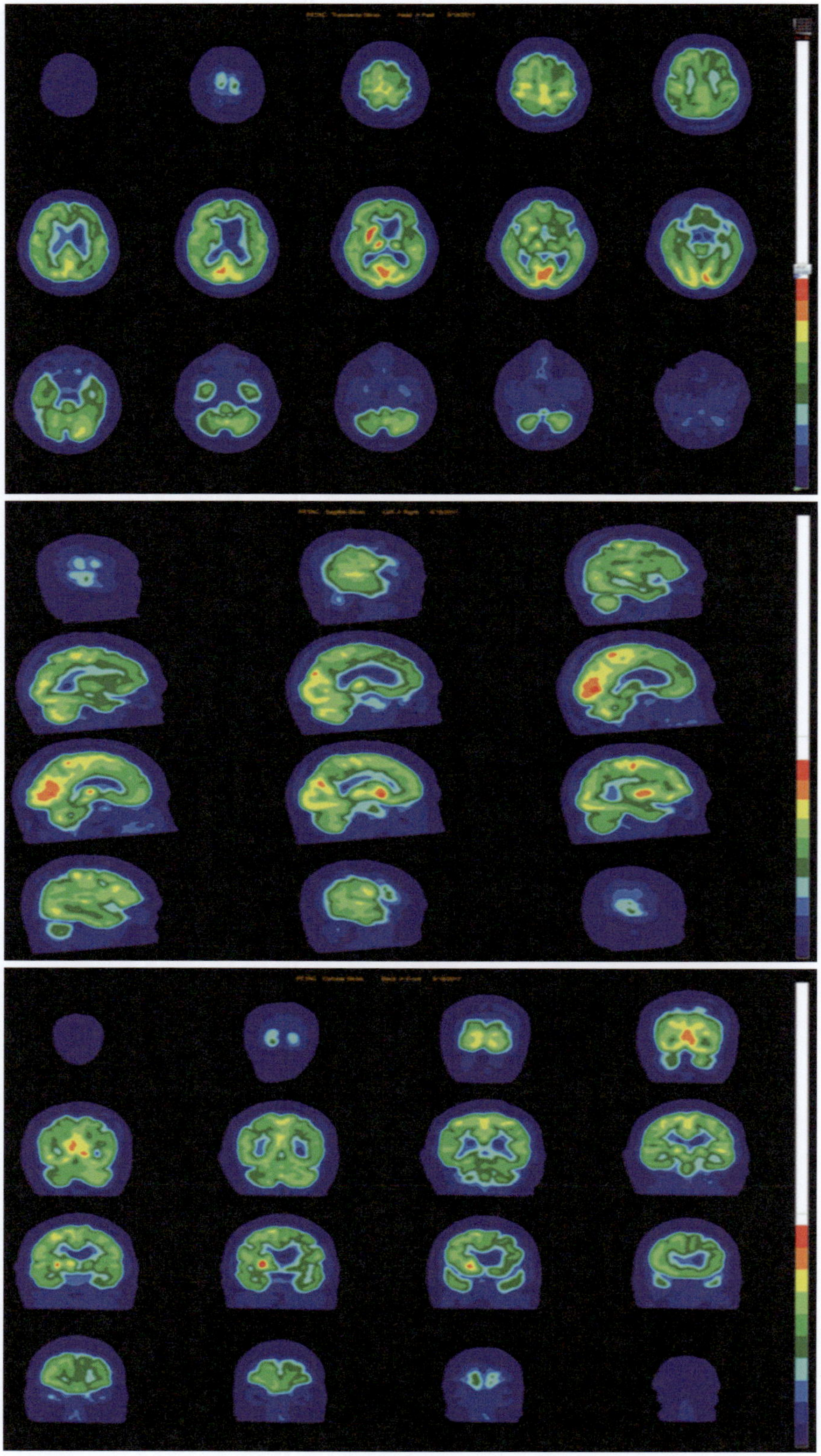

Fig. Q2

Quiz #3

The patient is a 69-year-old female presenting with progressive short-term memory loss for 13 months. On dementia screening interview, the patient had problems with judgment, demonstrated decreased interest in hobbies, and repeated the same things over and over. She had trouble learning and often forgot the date. She also had trouble remembering appointments and could not manage her personal finances. Laboratory tests showed no reversible causes of dementia. Brain MRI was essentially unremarkable. Brain FDG PET was performed, and the images are shown in Fig. Q3.

According to the clinical presentation and neuroimaging findings, which is the most likely imaging impression for this patient?

A. Alzheimer's disease (AD)
B. Frontotemporal dementia (FTD)
C. Dementia with Lewy bodies (DLB)
D. Corticobasal degeneration (CBD)
E. Vascular dementia (VD)

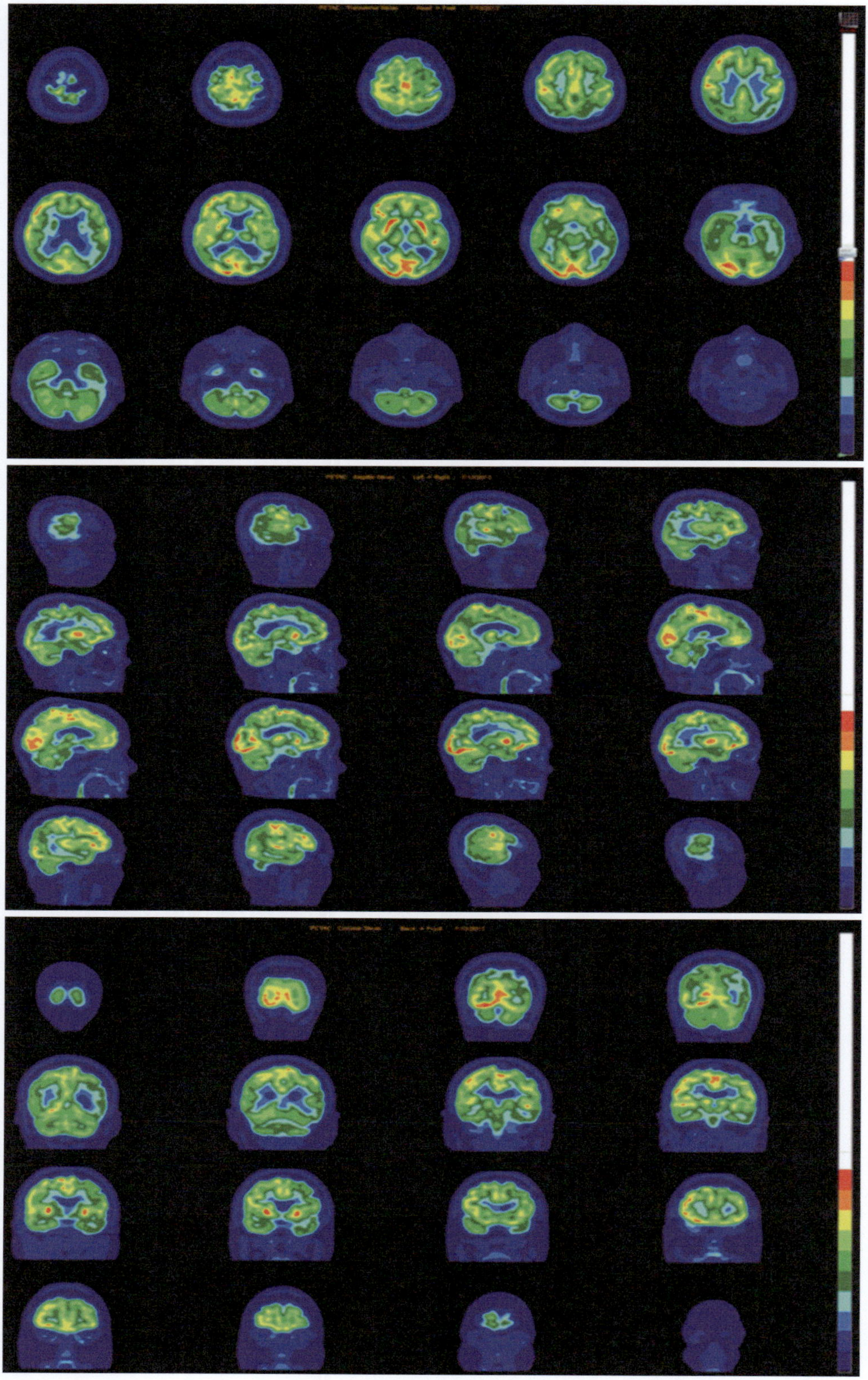

Fig. Q3

Quiz #4

This is a 76-year-old right-handed female patient with chief complaint of short-term memory loss and hallucinations for more than 1 year. Her hallucinations were often associated urinary tract infections, but no urgency. She states that her hallucinations were getting worse, now occurring throughout the day and at night. For example, she described seeing rats in her house even on the ceiling fan. She also reported seeing relatives who died many years ago. Past medical history includes hypertension and hyperlipidemia, but no history of diabetes or eye disease.There is no history of liver, kidney, lung, or thyroid disease. She denies any history of psychiatric or psychological intervention. There is no history of drug or alcohol abuse. Brain MRI showed mild to moderate cerebral atrophy and chronic white matter ischemic changes. Laboratory tests revealed no reversible causes of dementia. Brain FDG PET images are shown in Fig. Q4. Which is the most likely imaging impression for this patient?

A. Alzheimer's disease (AD)
B. Frontotemporal dementia (FTD)
C. Dementia with Lewy bodies (DLB)
D. Corticobasal degeneration (CBD)
E. Vascular dementia (VD)

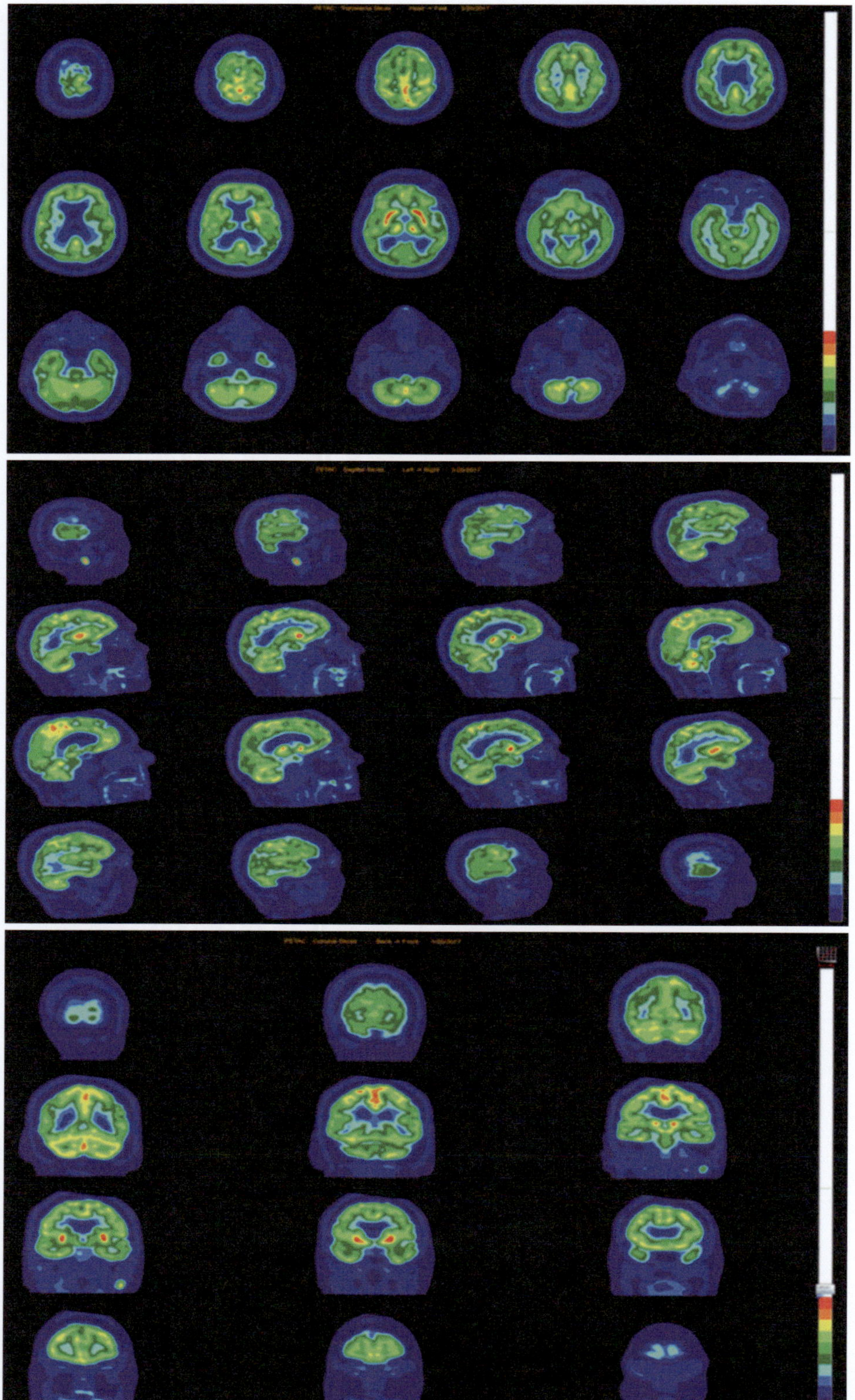

Fig. Q4

Quiz #5

The patient is a 56-year-old male with history of glioblastoma multiforme (GBM), status post left craniotomy with stereotactic debulking in 2005, whole-beam radiotherapy, and chemotherapy with last treatment in 2009. He developed recurrent disease in 2012 which was treated with avastin (bevacizumab). Following the chemotherapy, he developed headaches and seizures for which he is on levetiracetam and valproic acid. Medical oncology history is notable for prostate cancer status post prostatectomy in 2015 and recently diagnosed chronic lymphocytic leukemia (CLL). A recent brain MRI revealed increasing irregular solid enhancement along posteromedial aspect of the known cystic surgical cavity in the left occipitoparietal lobe and a new 1.3 cm ring-enhancing focus in the medial precentral gyrus of the left frontal lobe. Both findings were concerning for recurrent GBM. What's the best impression of the brain FDG PET/CT findings in Fig. Q5?

A. Essentially negative study without PET evidence of FDG-avid brain tumor.
B. Findings are concordant with the MRI, suspicious for recurrent GBM in both left medial frontal lobe and the left occipitoparietal region.
C. Findings are suspicious for recurrent or new GBM in the right medial parietal region.
D. Findings are suspicious for recurrent or new GBM in the left forefrontal lobe.
E. Findings are suspicious for recurrent GBM in the left medial frontal lobe and likely necrosis in the left occipitoparietal region.

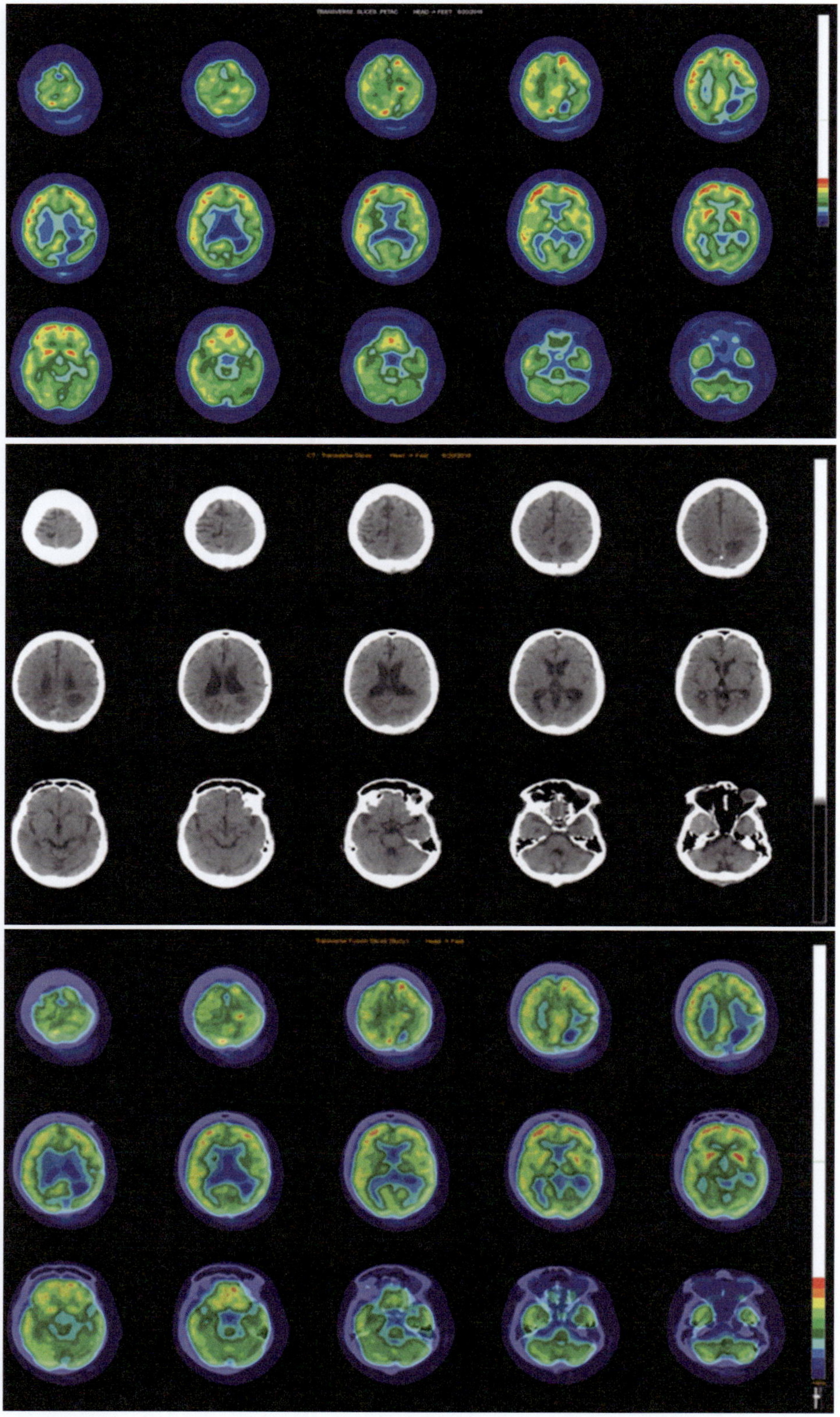

Fig. Q5

Quiz #6

The patient is a 50-year-old female with history of stroke and seizure occurred approximately 14 months ago. A recent diagnostic cerebral angiogram revealed diffuse atherosclerotic changes, occlusion of the proximal left middle cerebral artery (MCA), and 75% stenosis of the left vertebral artery. Past medical history is significant for hyperlipidemia and known coronary artery disease. He scored 27/30 on the mini-mental state examination (MMSE). Brain perfusion SPECT studies without and with Diamox challenge were performed, with images displayed in Fig. Q6a, b, respectively. Which is the best impression of the SPECT studies?

A. The studies confirm ischemia in the left MCA territory with a good cerebral vascular reserve (CVR).
B. The studies confirm ischemia in the left MCA and left vertebral artery territories with a good cerebral vascular reserve (CVR).
C. The studies confirm ischemic disease in the left MCA territory with good collateral perfusion and a poor cerebral vascular reserve (CVR).
D. The studies confirm ischemia in the left MCA territory and in the watershed areas.
E. The studies indicate a poor cerebral vascular reserve (CVR) in the left MCA and left vertebral artery territories.

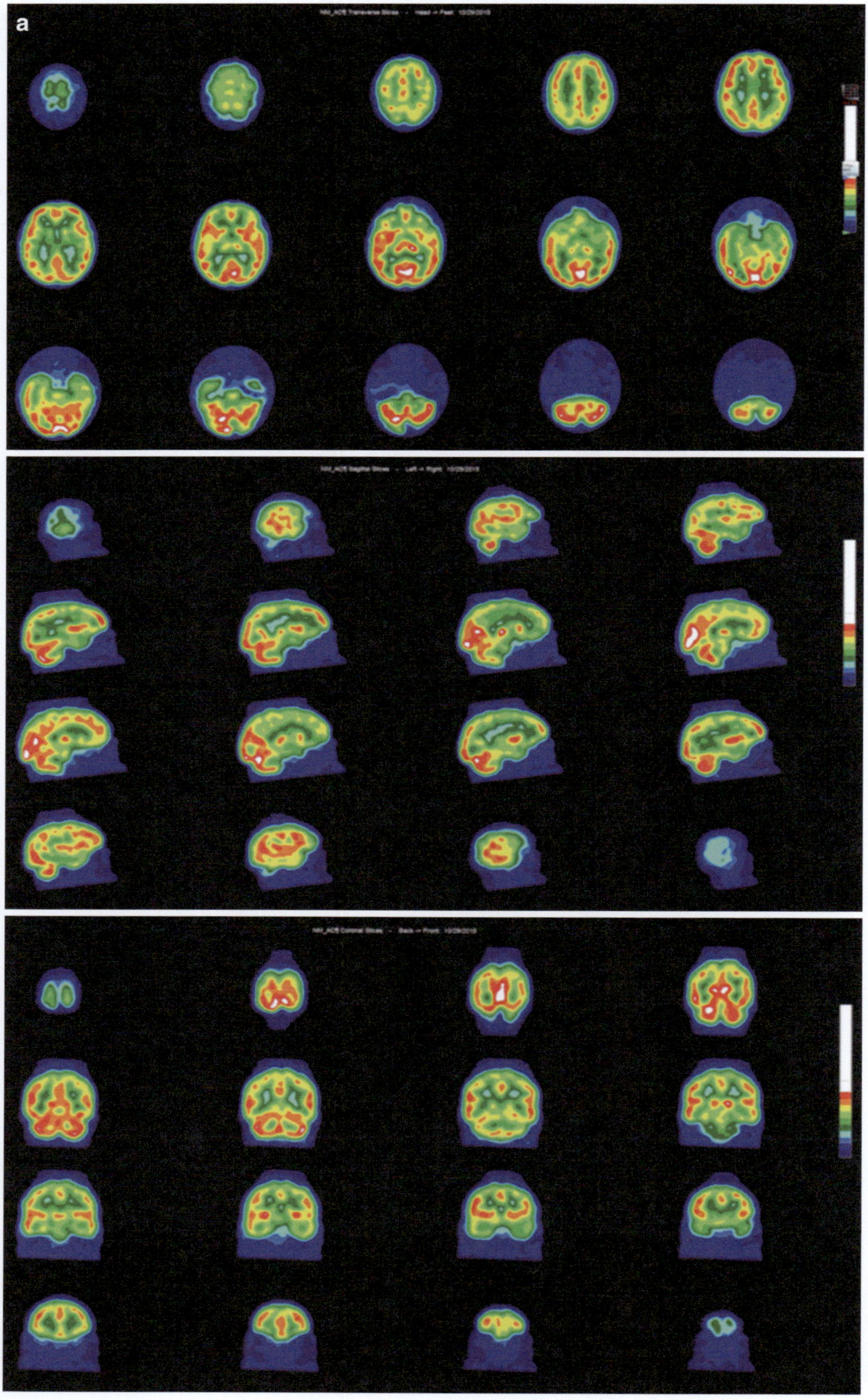

Fig. Q6 (**a**, **b**)

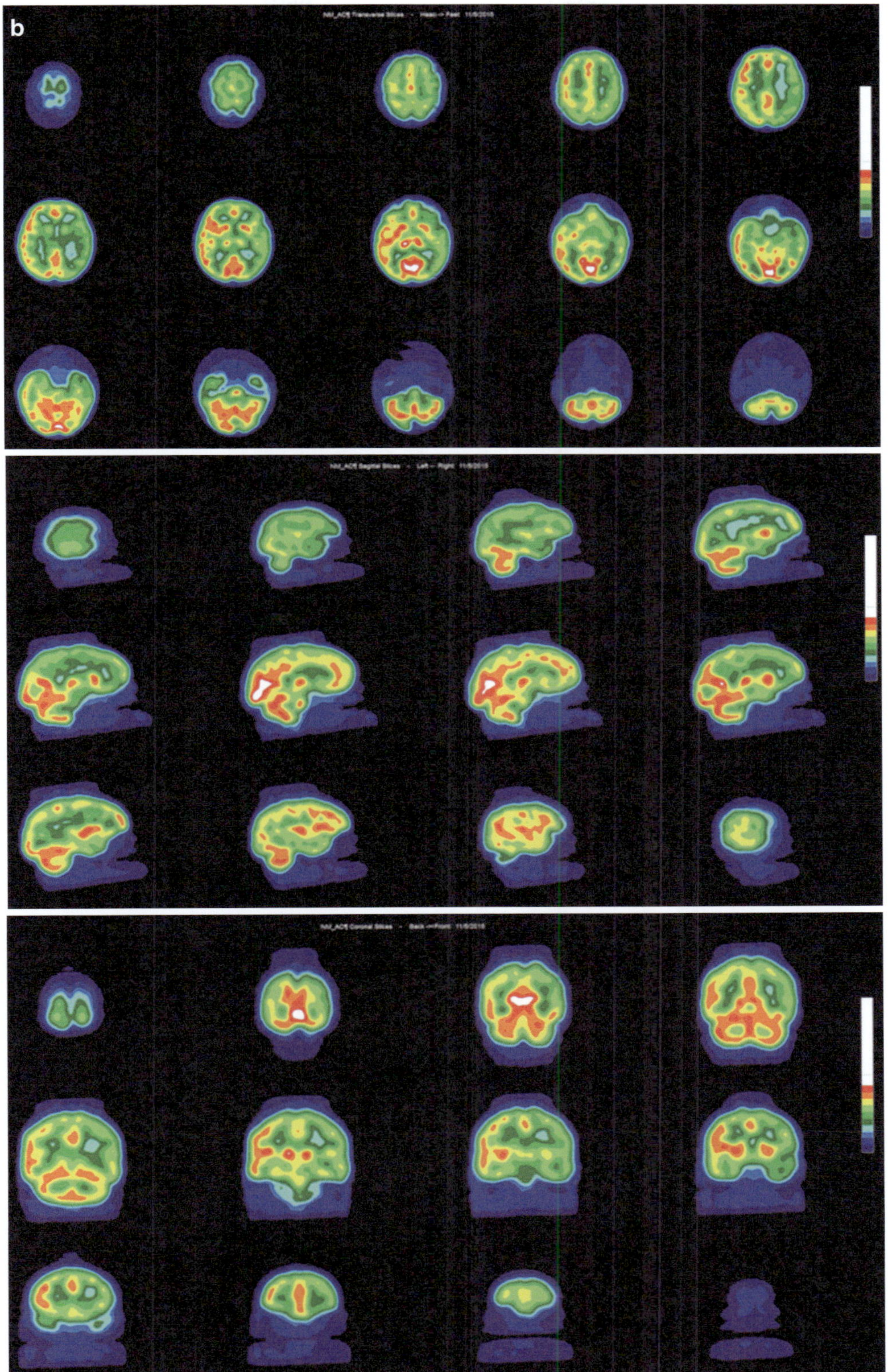

Fig. Q6 (continued)

Quiz #7

The patient is a 21-year-old right-handed female with known complex partial epilepsy that started at age of 2. She was treated at multiple institutions/hospitals with several antiepileptic medications; however, her seizures have been poorly controlled. The seizures are often preceded by a "rush" sensation over her body, followed by impaired awareness and unresponsiveness lasting approximately 30–60 seconds. No oral or manual automatisms are reported. Postictally, she often has trouble verbalizing or understanding speech for several minutes. In addition, she has a history of focal to bilateral tonic-clonic seizures. Multiple EEG studies showed epileptogenic activities in the left temporal region. Three recent MR imaging studies revealed "reduced volume and increased T2 FLAIR signal of the head, neck, and body of the left hippocampal formation and blurring hypointense T2 signal at the associated white matter, consistent with left mesial temporal sclerosis." Based on the seizure semiology, MRI results, and brain FDG PET findings in Fig. Q7, what is the most likely epilepsy this patient may have?

A. Left mesial temporal lobe epilepsy (MTLE)
B. Left lateral temporal lobe epilepsy (LTLE)
C. Left temporal lobe epilepsy (TLE)
D. Left temporoparietal lobe epilepsy
E. Bilateral temporal lobe epilepsy

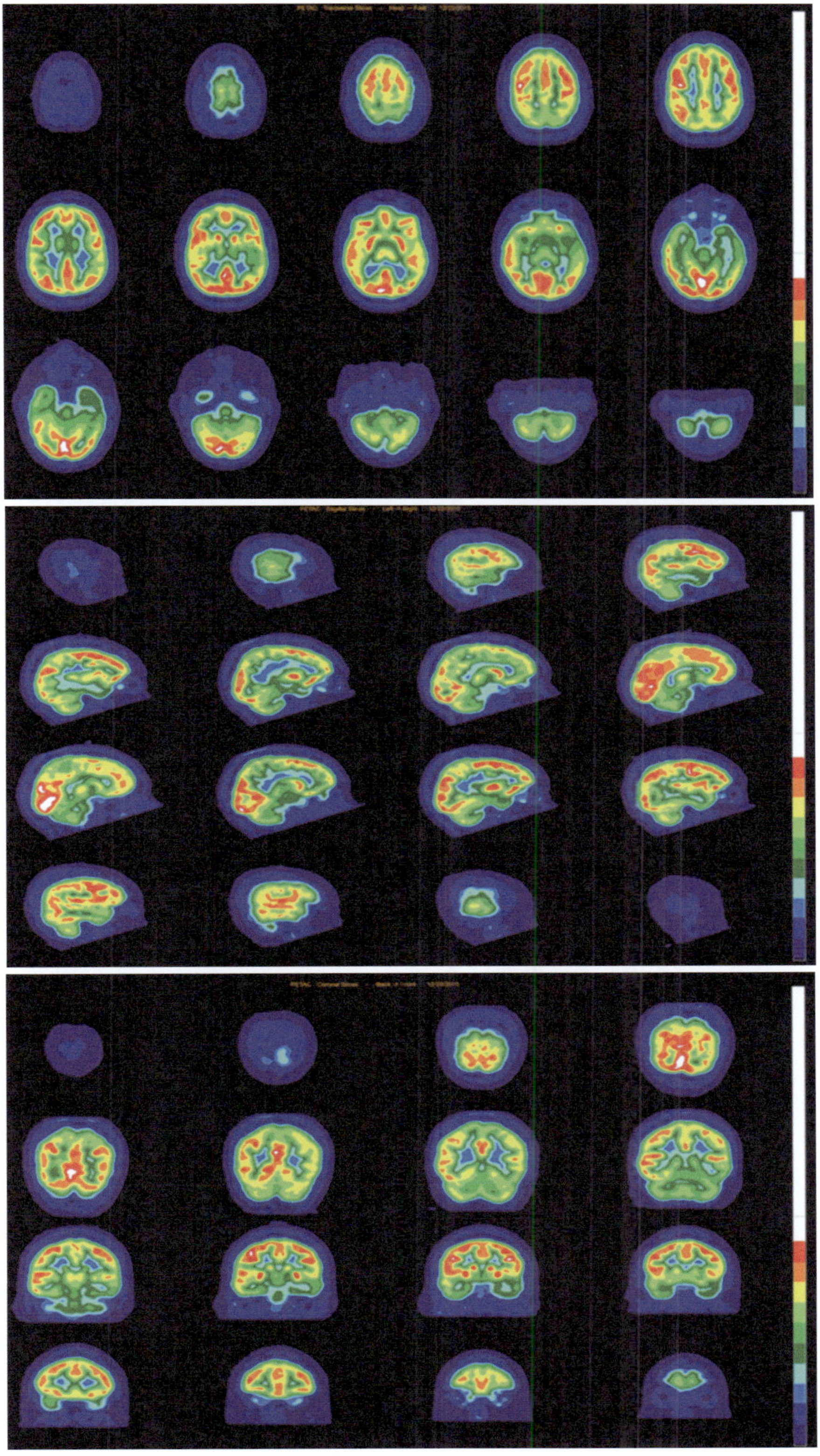

Fig. Q7

Quiz #8

The patient is a 76-year-old male presenting with progressive weakness and ataxia. In addition, he has dysarthria (difficulty speaking) and dysphagia for more than 10 years. There is no tremor. The patient denies history of head injuries, and there is no history of being exposed to chemicals or toxins or endemic infections. Past medical history is notable for known cerebellar/pontine degeneration, hypothyroidism, dysphonia, anemia, urinary retention, coronary artery disease, bradycardia, erectile dysfunction, and dyspnea. MRI brain showed "cerebellar and pontine atrophy," with a representative sagittal view attached, suspicious for multiple system atrophy (MSA). What is the best impression of the DaTscan study findings in Fig. Q8?

A. Essentially normal DaTscan with head tilting to the left
B. Abnormal DaTscan study with findings suspicious for early Parkinson's disease
C. Abnormal DaTscan study showing depletion of dopamine transporters in left striatum
D. Abnormal DaTscan study with findings likely secondary to MSA
E. Abnormal DaTscan study showing depletion of dopamine transporters in bilateral putamen

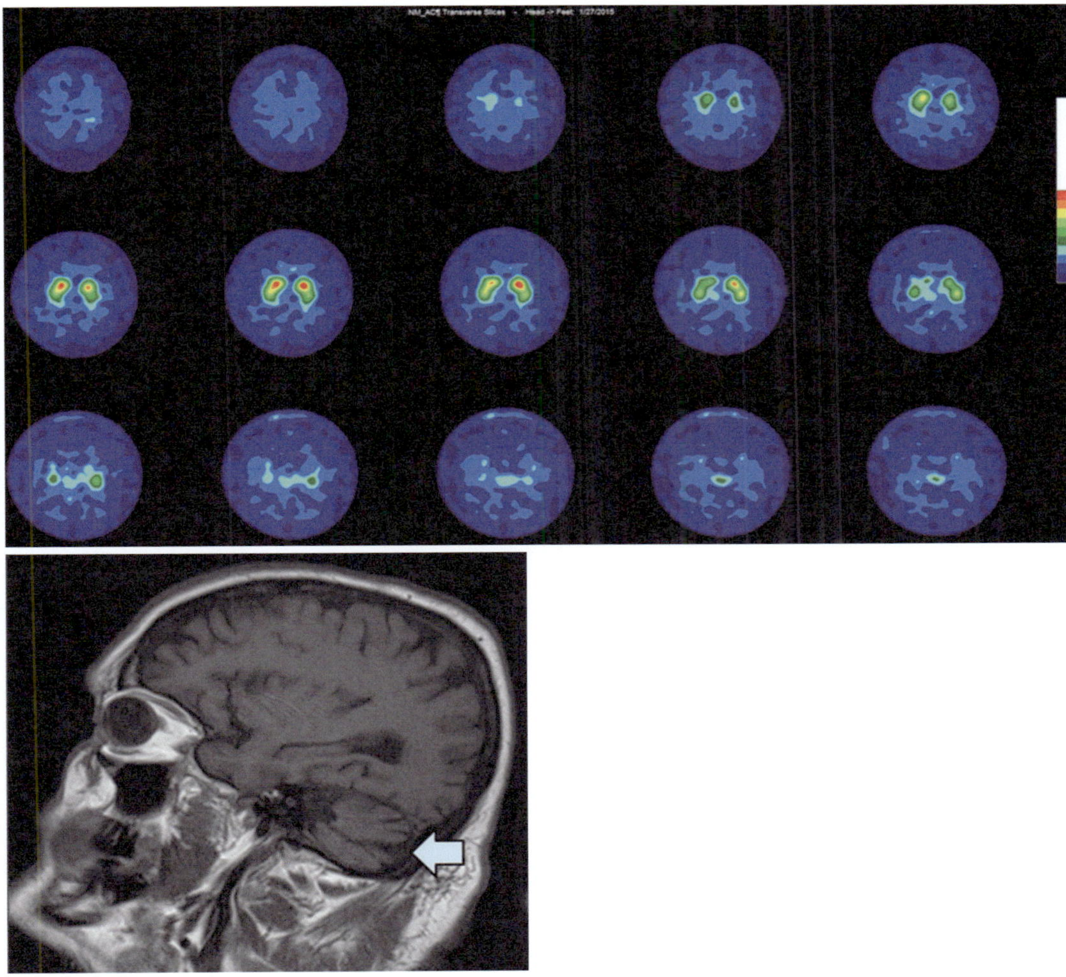

Fig. Q8

Quiz #9

This is a 65-year-old male patient with history of esophageal carcinoma treated at an outside institution with chemoradiation and esophagectomy. He was admitted to our hospital with worsening headache in the occipital area radiating toward the frontal region, associated with double vision, light-headedness, balance problem, the 6th cranial nerve palsy, and tremor-like activity in his upper extremities. He reported 1-day, transient loss of vision in the right eye which recovered without any intervention. Past medical history is significant for recent onset of atrial fibrillation status post pacemaker placement 3 weeks ago. The newly placed pacemaker is contraindicative for MR imaging. Initial CSF cytology was suspicious for metastatic adenocarcinoma, and a repeat CSF cytology 1 week later was positive for metastatic adenocarcinoma. Ommaya shunt was placed subsequently for delivery of intrathecal chemotherapy. Which is the most appropriate statement for the Ommaya shunt study as shown in Fig. Q9?

A. Patent Ommaya shunt with essentially normal CSF flow and distribution
B. Partially blocked Ommaya shunt, especially to the left brain
C. Patent Ommaya shunt with decreased CSF flow to the left brain and absent CSF distribution to the left parietal region
D. Patent Ommaya shunt with global markedly decreased CSF flow
E. Patent Ommaya shunt with uneven CSF flow/distribution but no significant impacts on intrathecal treatment response or prognosis

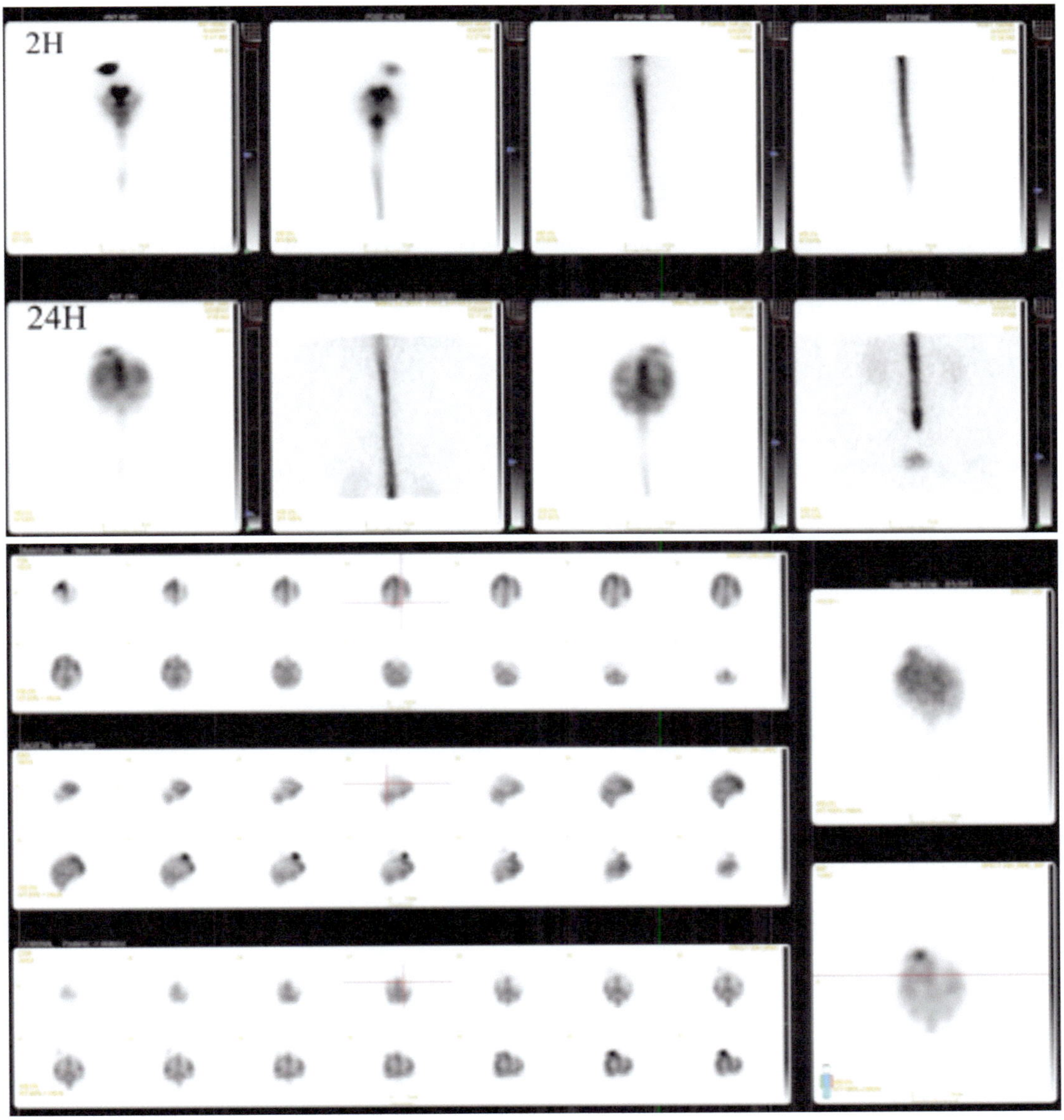

Fig. Q9

Quiz #10

The patient is a 72-year-old female complaining of occasional tremors of both hands for 3 years. Neurological examination has been unremarkable, although there is a clinical concern for conversion disorder. Past medical history is significant for hypertension, non-insulin-dependent diabetes, peripheral vascular disease, paroxysmal atrial fibrillation, uterine cancer, and stroke in 2011. What is the most likely impression of this DaTscan (Fig. Q10)?

A. Abnormal study with findings typical for a neurodegenerative process affecting the left striatum
B. Abnormal study with findings likely due to prior a left-sided stroke
C. Abnormal study with findings typical for Parkinson's disease
D. Abnormal study suggestive of severe depletion of dopamine transporters in left striatum and moderate depletion of dopamine transporters in the right putamen
E. Technically limited study likely due to difficulty head positioning or technical artifact blurring left striatum or both

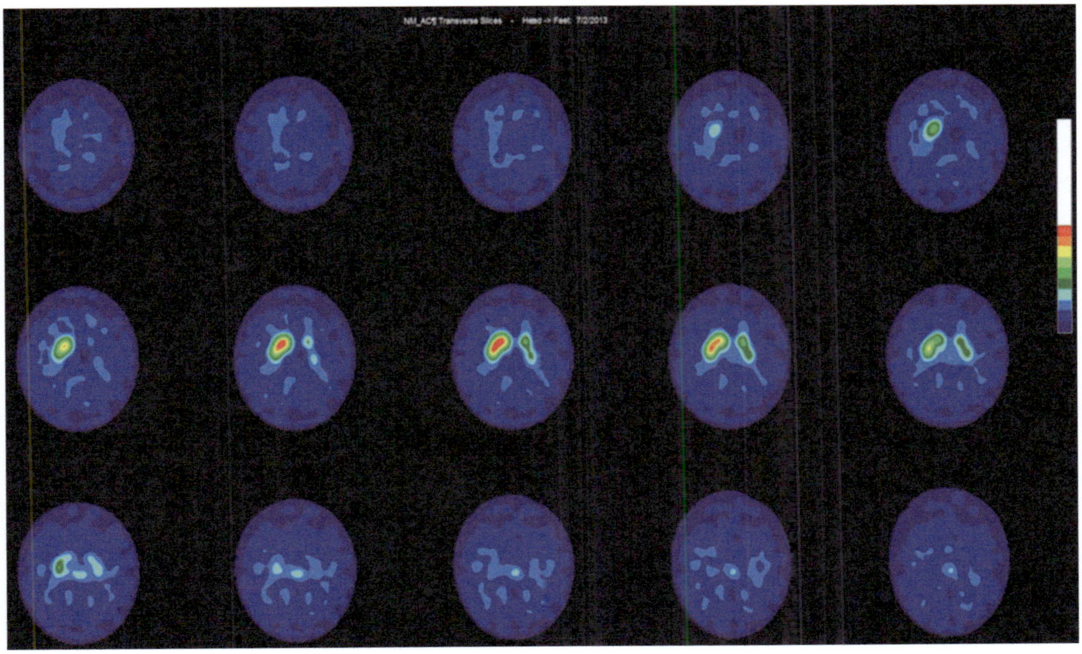

Fig. Q10

Quiz #11

The patient is a 51-year-old male presenting with progressive short-term memory loss that started 5–6 years ago. Although the patient believes his memory problem has been fairly stable, his wife noticed that he has worsening memory loss. He is a non-smoker and works as insurance agent. He is frustrated with his loss of independence and particularly with difficulty in word finding. There is no history of drug or alcohol abuse. He denies history of stroke, head injury, or seizures. Neurological examination reveals that his speech is fluent without any significant dysphasia or dysarthria. There is no tremor. Gait is steady and symmetric without any assistance. Brain MRI at an outside institution was unremarkable. Brain FDG PET images are displayed in Fig. Q11. According to the clinical presentation and FDG PET findings, what is the most likely imaging diagnosis?

A. Frontotemporal dementia (FTD)
B. Vascular dementia (VD)
C. Early-onset Alzheimer's disease (EOAD)
D. Dementia with Lewy bodies (DLB)
E. Late-onset Alzheimer's disease (LOAD)

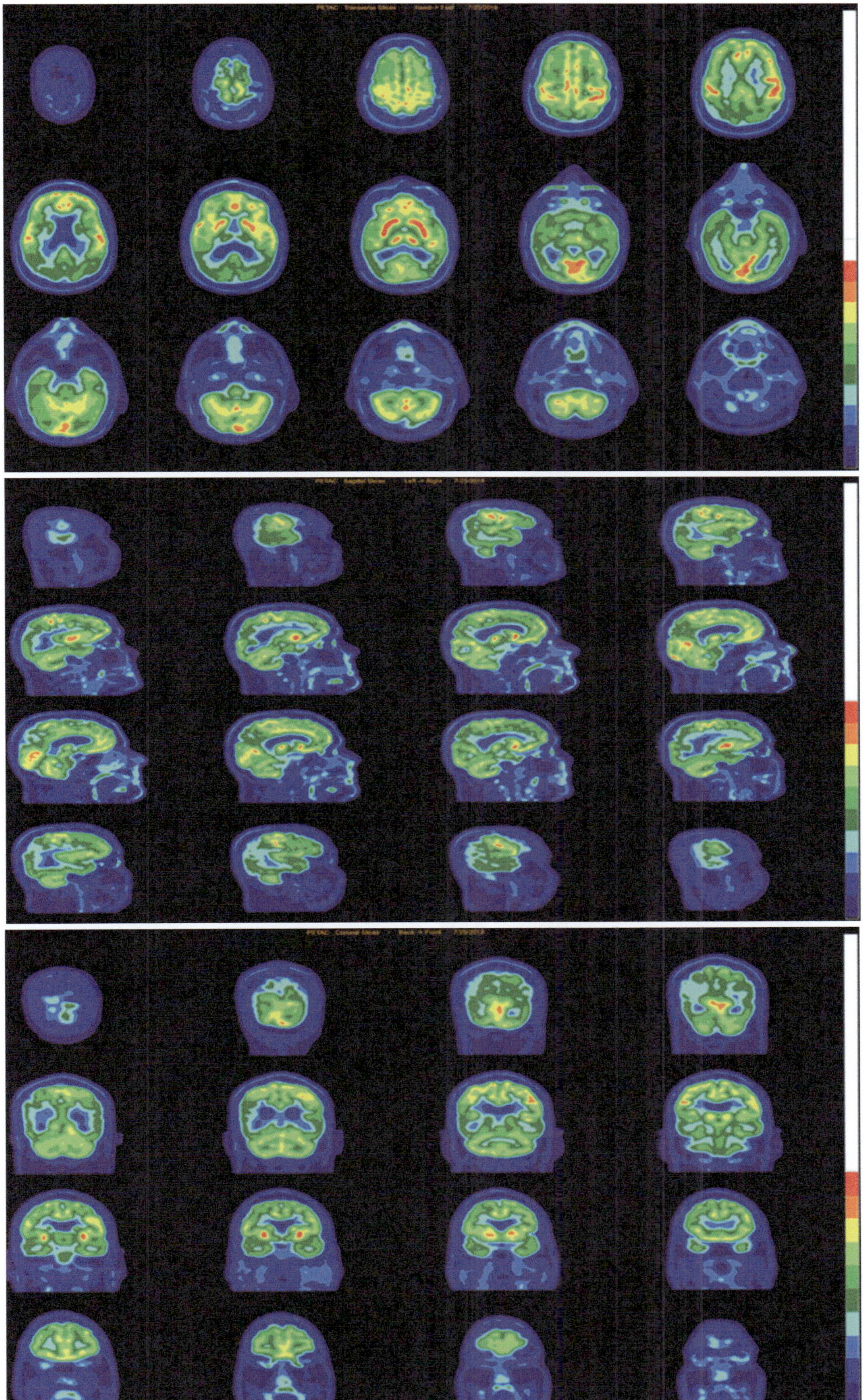

Fig. Q11

Quiz #12

The patient is a 26-year-old female with history of pseudotumor cerebri treated with VP shunt placement 5 years ago in the state of Georgia. Recently, she complains of recurrent intractable headache, blurry vision, nausea, and vomiting for a few weeks. She denies having fever or chills. Neuro-ophthalmology examinations showed no papilledema. CT of the head/brain showed no acute hemorrhage, no evidence of ventriculomegaly. VP shunt study images are shown in Fig. Q12. What is the most likely imaging diagnosis for this patient?

A. Abnormal study with findings suggestive of obstruction of proximal and distal VP shunt catheters.
B. Probably normal study as a normal CSF flow is appreciated after tracer administration.
C. Abnormal study with findings suggestive of partial obstruction as tracer activity can be seen in the urinary bladder.
D. Abnormal study with findings suggestive of patent proximal catheter but high-grade distal catheter obstruction.
E. Abnormal study with findings suggestive of a partial obstruction of the distal catheter.

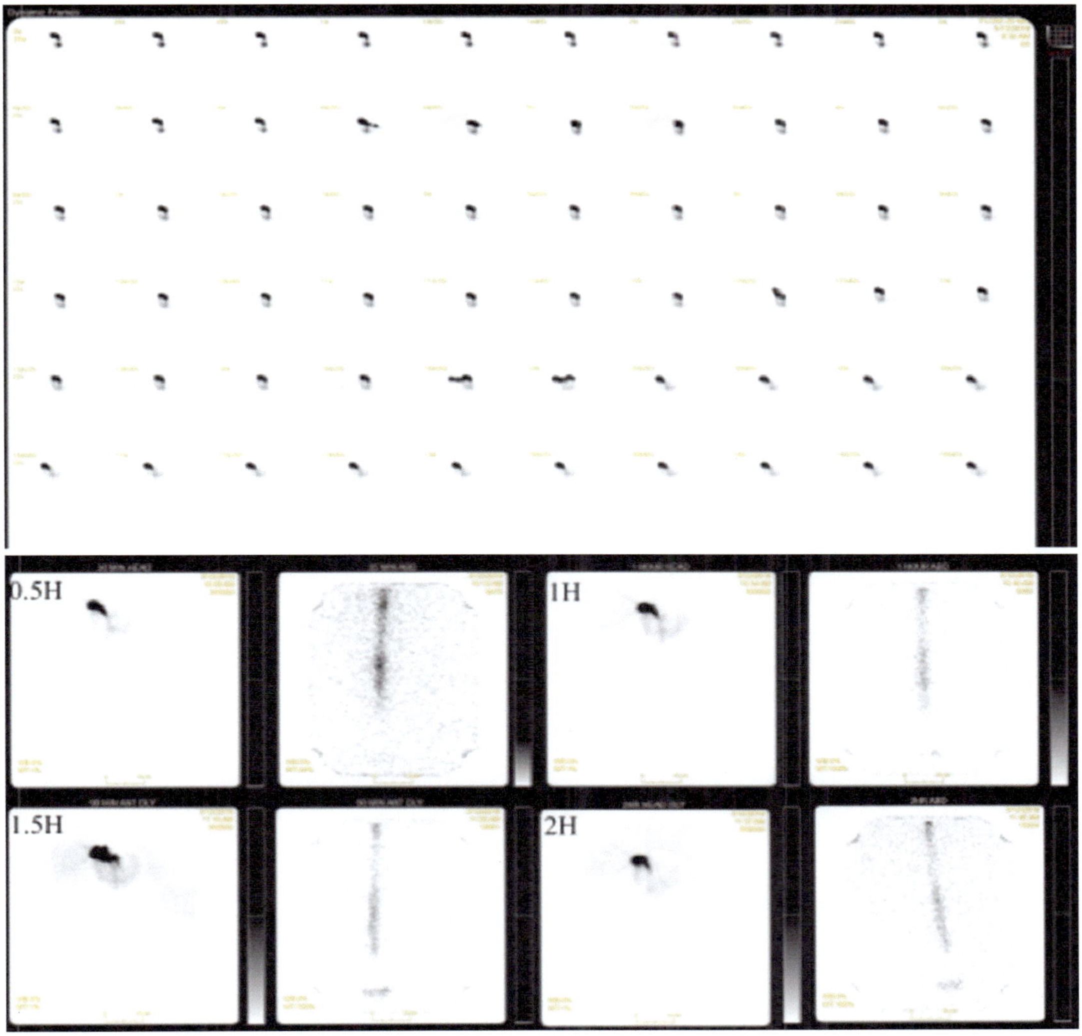

Fig. Q12

Quiz #13

The patient is a 63-year-old male complaining of tremor in left arm and hand. Past medical history is notable for essential hypertension, hyperlipidemia, cervical spinal stenosis, bipolar disorder, and depression. Current medications include Risperdal Consta (risperidone) IM injection every 2 weeks for long-term treatment of his bipolar disorder. At the request of the ordering physician, DaTscan was performed without stopping Risperdal Consta IM injection. What is the most likely imaging impression of the DaTscan results as shown in Fig. Q13?

A. Essentially normal study with head tilting
B. Essentially normal study suggestive of neuroleptic/drug-induced Parkinsonism
C. Abnormal study with findings concerning for early stage of Parkinson's disease, affecting the left striatum
D. Essentially normal study indicating essential tremor (ET)
E. Equivocal study likely due to patient's motion during imaging acquisition

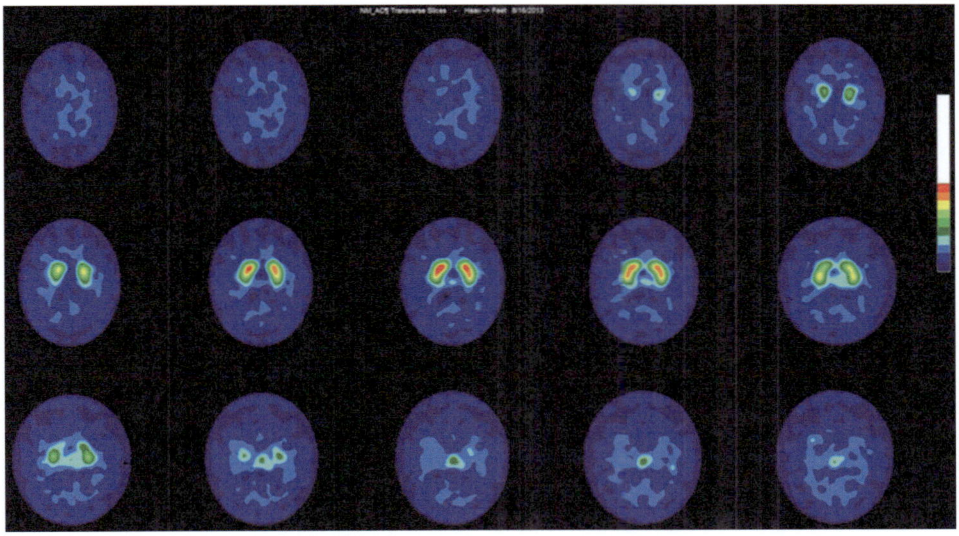

Fig. Q13

Quiz #14

The patient is a 3-year-old ambidextrous-handed (right > left) female presenting with medically refractory focal motor seizures and infantile spasms that started when she was 5-month-old. Past treatments included steroids, ACTH, and multiple antiepileptic medications. The seizures occurred at variable times, but mostly in the mornings, with triggering factor of sun exposure. No auras were reported. The seizures manifested as brief events during which she would get a blank look on her face, eyelids flutter, and arms raising up and shaking. The duration of the seizures was often a few seconds but could last 20–25 seconds. If the patient was standing when the seizure occurred, she would fall forward. She resumed her activity shortly after seizures. Two recent brain MR imaging studies were read unremarkable. EEG studies consistently showed focal epileptiform discharges from right parietal/posterior temporal/centrotemporal region. Brain FDG PET with EEG monitoring demonstrated a local cortical hypometabolism in the superolateral anterior right occipital lobe, suspicious for an interictal epileptogenic focus/zone. Subsequently, she underwent ictal, interictal brain perfusion SPECTs and SISCOM analysis, with images shown in Fig. Q14a–c, respectively. What's the most likely epilepsy this girl may have?

A. Right parietal lobe epilepsy (PLE)
B. Right occipital lobe epilepsy (OLE)
C. Right temporal lobe epilepsy (TLE)
D. Right frontal lobe epilepsy (FLE)
E. Right insular lobe epilepsy (ILE)

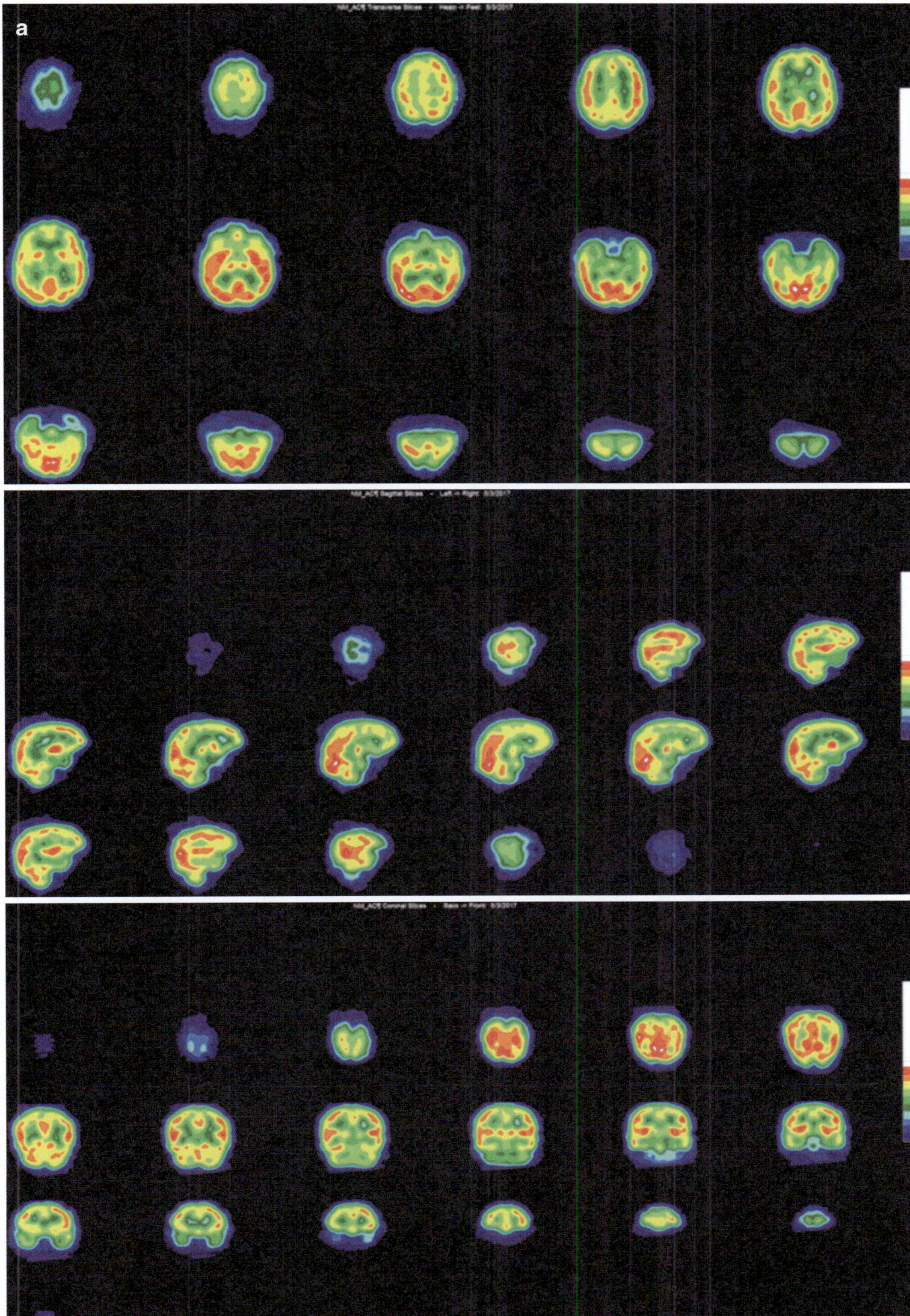

Fig. Q14 (**a**–**c**)

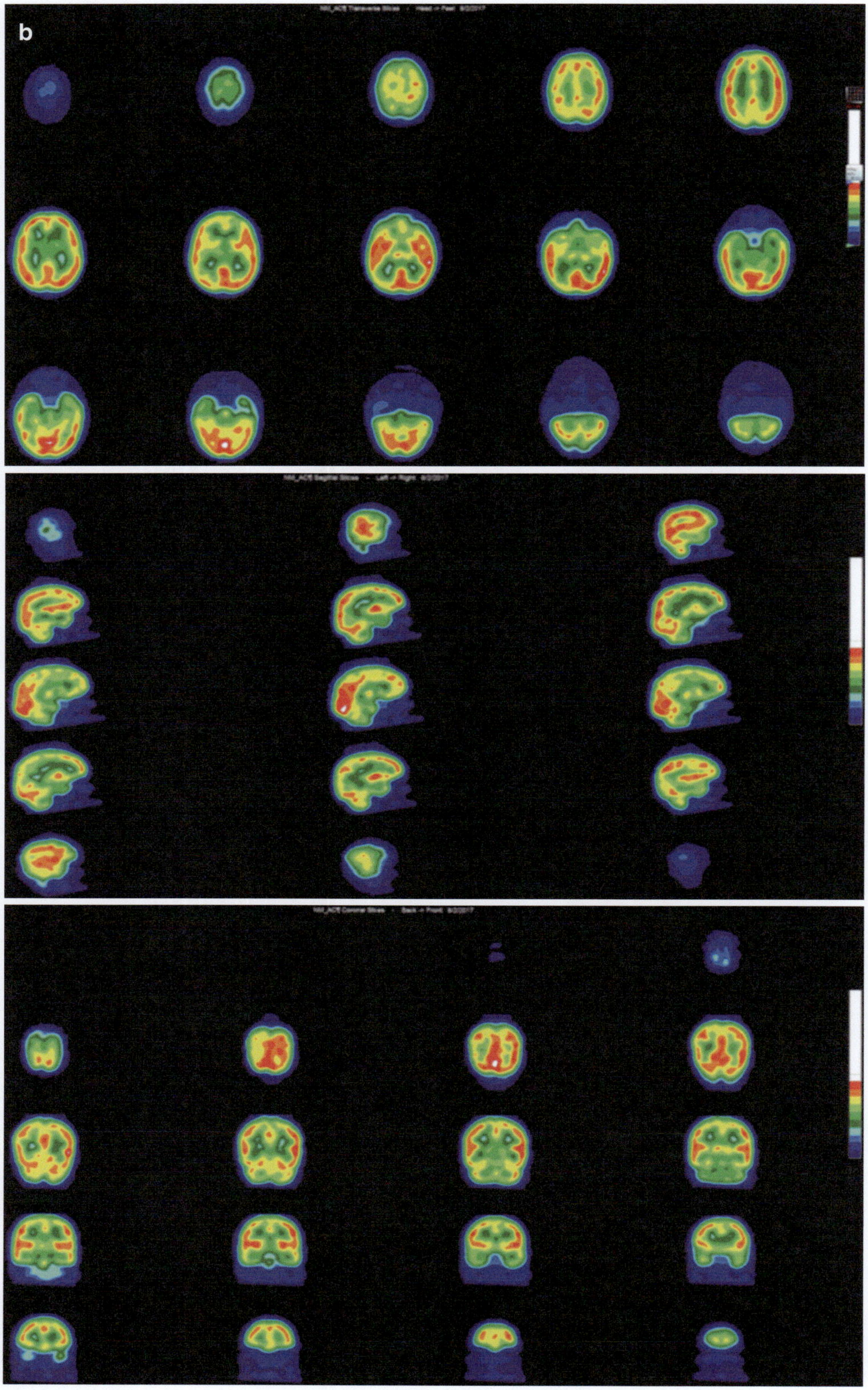

Fig. Q14 (continued)

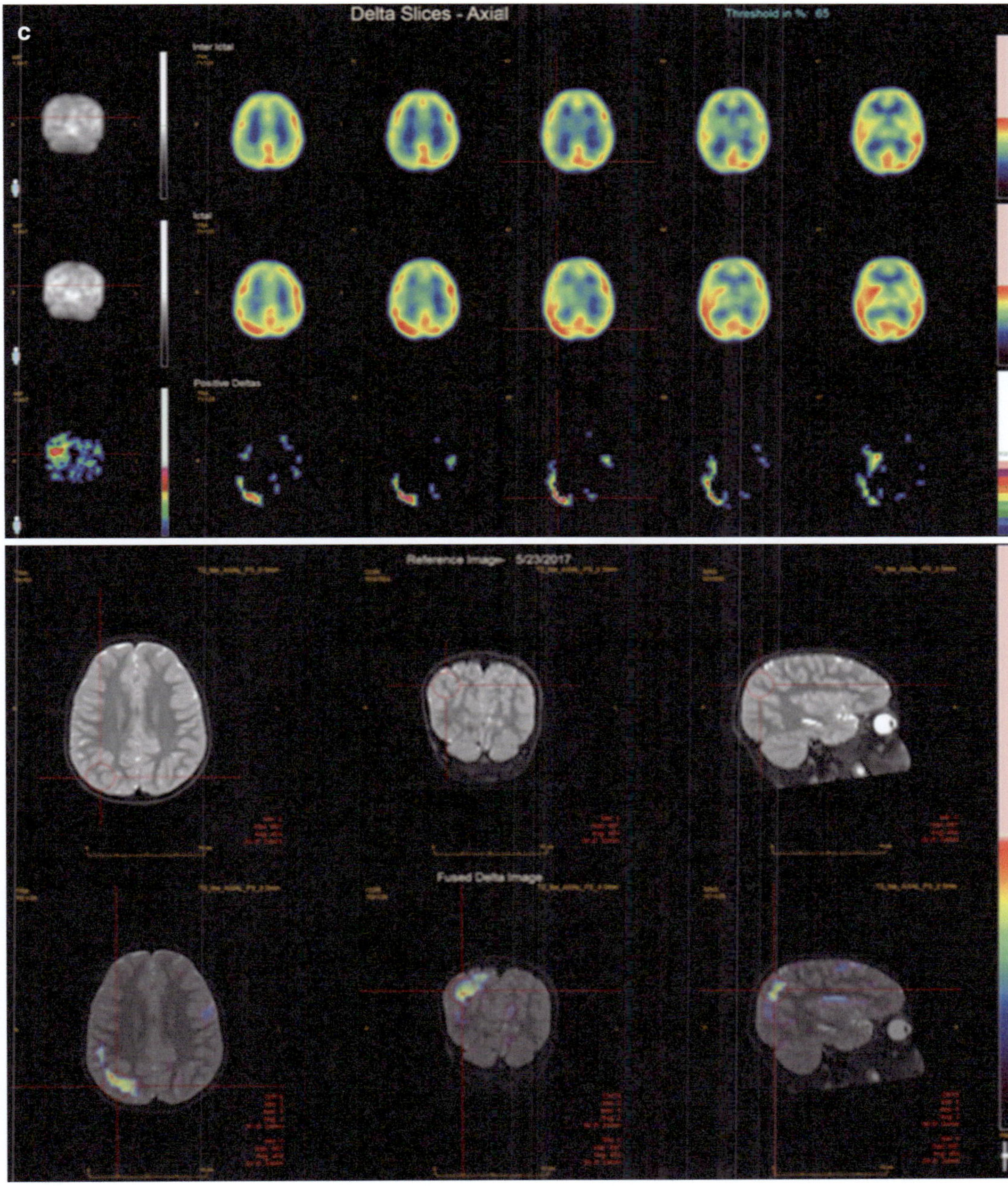

Fig. Q14 (continued)

Quiz #15

The patient is a 79-year-old right-handed female presenting with memory impairment that started about 5 years ago, getting worse over the last 1–2 years. She tried Aricept and Exelon patch, both without help. Family members noticed that she has worsening gait instability over the last 2 years. She tends to shuffle and has started to use a walker since December 2013. Brain MRI showed moderate brain atrophy, ventriculomegaly, and chronic ischemic changes of the white matter. What is the most appropriate impression for the CSF imaging study as shown in Fig. Q15?

A. Essentially normal study with transient ventricular reflux
B. Abnormal study with findings suggestive of normal pressure hydrocephalus (NPH) but without potential benefits for VP shunting
C. Abnormal study likely due to hydrocephalus *ex vacuo*
D. Abnormal study likely due to brain atrophy
E. Abnormal study with findings consistent with NPH and potential benefits for CSF shunting

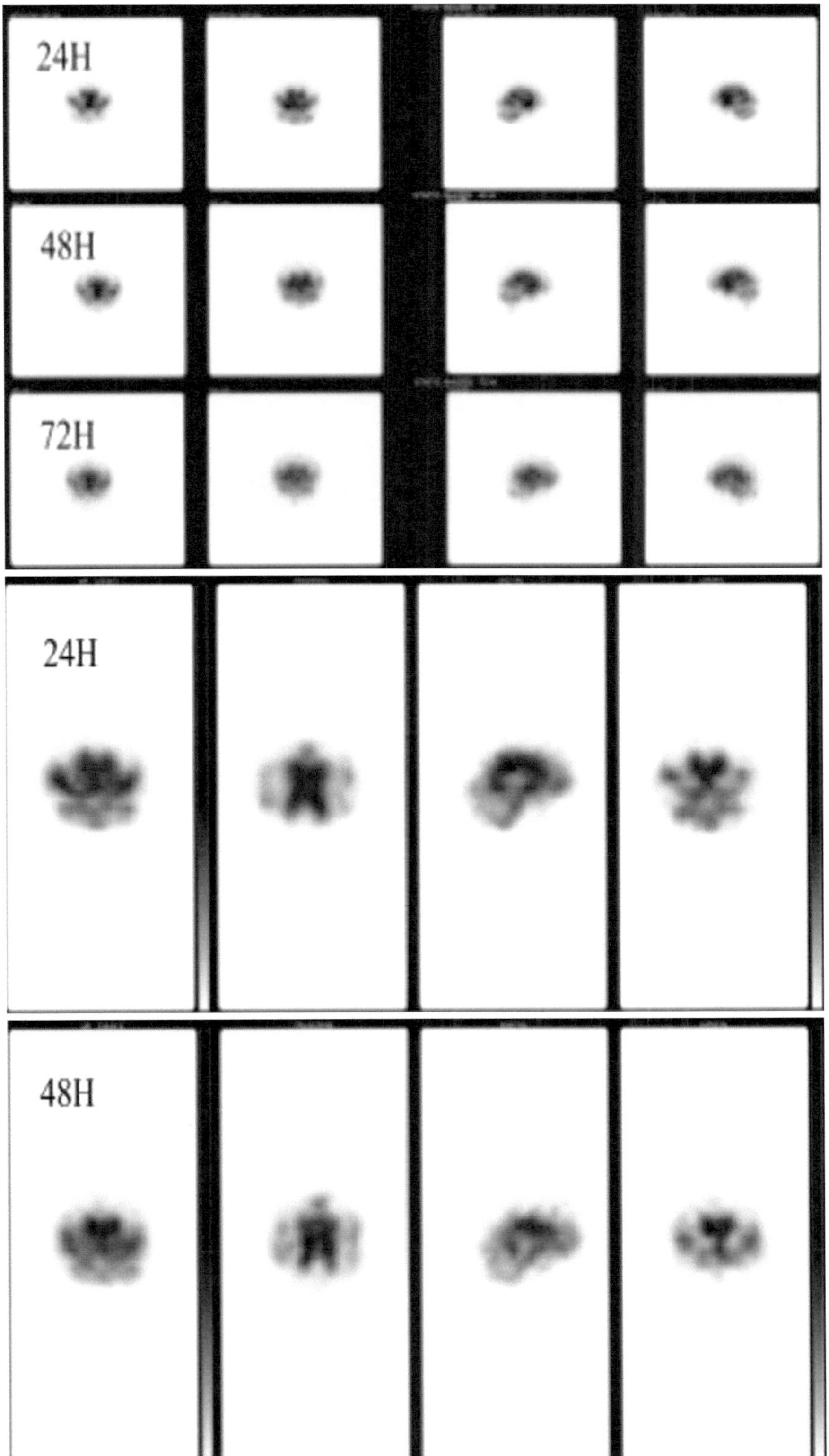

Fig. Q15

Quiz #16

The patient is a 58-year-old right-handed female presenting with progressive memory loss and severe language difficulty for 3–4 years. On neurological exam, she scored 25/30 on MMSE indicating borderline or mild dementia. In contrast, she has severely impaired verbal skills. Significant impairments were observed with more complex auditory comprehension items. Her oral expression was characterized by markedly limited language output that was vague and telegraphic and had frequent errors of repetition. Repetition, however, was intact for single words that were simple and those that were nonsense, with good repetition for simple sentences and increased difficulties as sentences increased in length and complexity. Although her speech is limited in quantity, it is qualitatively of normal volume and fluent, without evidence of halting, effortful speech, or dysarthria. A recent MR imaging of the brain was unremarkable, except for a few nonspecific hyperintense T_2 signals in subcortical white matter. Brain FDG PET images are displayed in Fig. Q16. Based on the clinical presentation and neuroimaging findings, which is the most likely neurological syndrome this patient may have?

A. Alzheimer's disease (AD)
B. Semantic variant primary progressive aphasia (svPPP)
C. Dementia with Lewy bodies (DLB)
D. Vascular disease (VD)
E. Behavioral variant FTD (bvFTD)

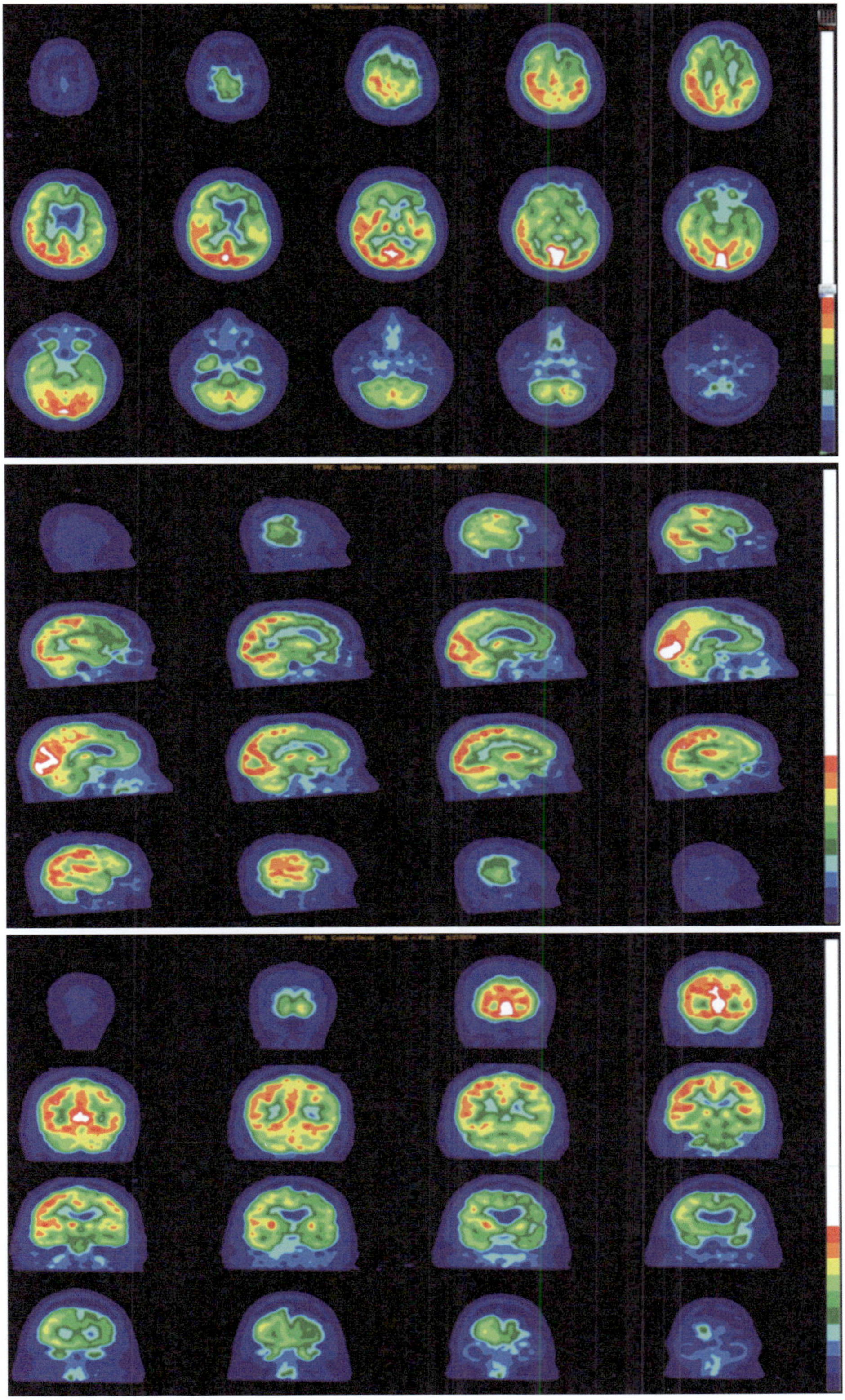

Fig. Q16

Quiz #17

The patient is a 3-year-old right-handed male with an extensive history of seizures that probably started from birth or at the early infancy according to his mother. He was treated with several antiepileptic medications, still with poor seizure control. The first type of seizure is described as staring off (with tendency to the left), nostrils' flaring, followed by either rapid or slow breathing, and often lasting a half to several minutes. The second type of seizure often occurs during sleep and manifests with tremors, stiffening, starring off with eye rolling, and slight nystagmus. Past medical history is notable for known tuberous sclerosis (TS) and polycystic kidney disease. Family history is positive for seizures in a paternal aunt. An interictal brain FDG PET was performed with images displayed in Fig. Q17. What's the most appropriate imaging impression of the FDG PET study?

A. Abnormal study showing multiple cortical infarcts with largest one in the left frontal region.
B. Findings consistent with known TS but no imaging features suggesting their epileptogenicity.
C. Findings consistent with known TS, all without epileptogenicity due to their hypometabolism on PET.
D. The larger lesions in the left frontal and anterior cingulate regions likely represent epileptogenic foci/zones.
E. Given the seizure semiology and FDG PET findings, this patient is likely to have left frontal lobe epilepsy (FLE), but no involvement of other regions.

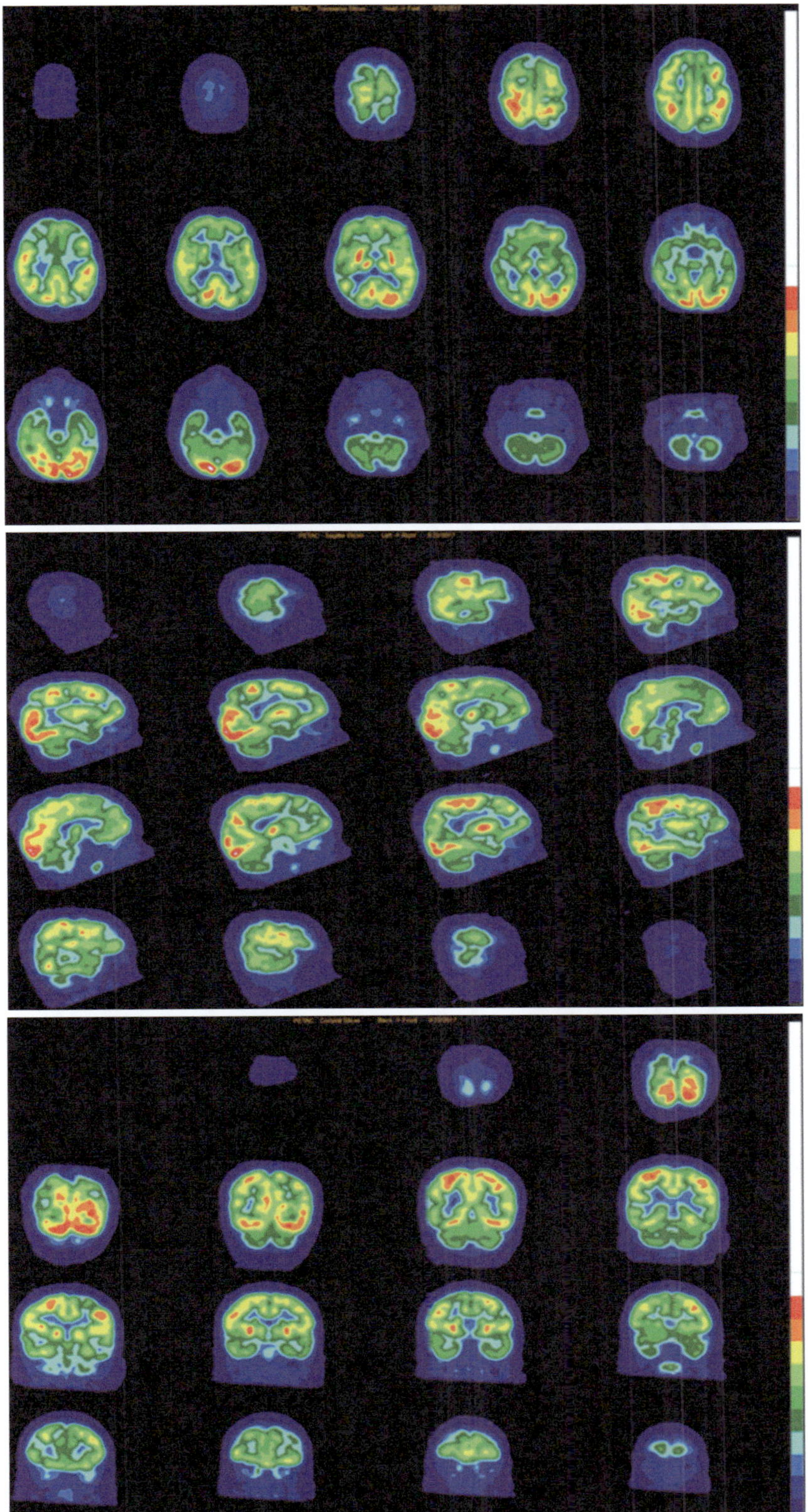

Fig. Q17

Quiz #18

The patient was a 70-year-old male with long-standing history of chronic lymphocytic leukemia (CLL) which was stable until June 2017, when transformed diffuse large B-cell lymphoma (DLBCL) was diagnosed via lymph node and bone marrow biopsies at an outside institution. He received chemotherapy with R-CHOP (rituximab, cyclophosphamide, doxorubicin hydrochloride, oncovin, and prednisolone) which was completed in December 2017 and currently on rituximab maintenance. The patient had achieved complete remission after six cycles of R-CHOP, and there was no evidence of recurrent or residual disease on multiple follow-up FDG PET CT studies from October 11, 2017, to August 28, 2018. Clinical exam and laboratory tests were also negative. The patient was asymptomatic, and he underwent another routine whole-body FDG PET CT for follow-up. The brain portion of the FDG PET CT was shown in Fig. Q18, while the rest of the whole-body PET CT was unremarkable. Maximal SUV of the cerebellar lesion was 23.8, markedly increased relative to max SUV 10.1 of the contralateral, *e.g.*, left lateral cerebellar cortex. What is the most appropriate recommendation for this patient's further workup?

A. Biopsy the right cerebellar lesion for definite diagnosis as soon as possible.
B. Do nothing, as the finding of the right cerebellar focal FDG activity may represent an imaging artifact.
C. Recommend CT of the head/brain with IV contrast.
D. Recommend brain MRI with and without contrast.
E. Recommended MRA brain with special reference to the right.

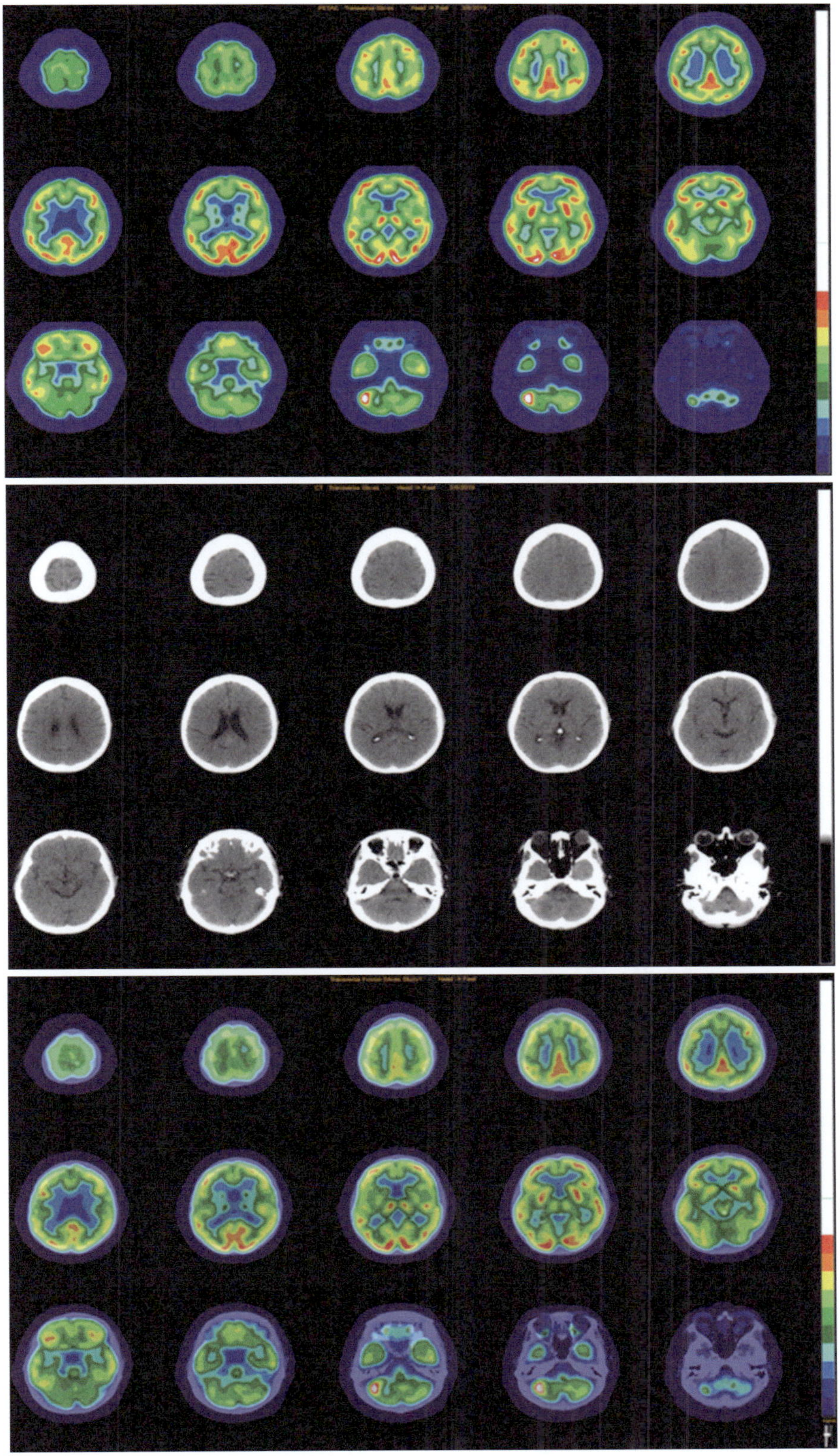

Fig. Q18

Quiz #19

The patient is a 23-year-old female presenting with positional headache for 6–7 months. CSF leak and spontaneous intracranial hypotension were suspected, for which the patient has had two empiric high-volume blood patching at an outside institution 2 months ago, still without significant symptom relief. She denies any brain or spinal procedures and no history of trauma. A recent MR imaging of the spine at an outside institution showed findings suggestive of intracranial hypotension. CSF leak study images are displayed in Fig. Q19. What's the most appropriate treatment for this patient?

A. Multiple times of epidural blood patch to cover the lower cervical spine through the lumbar spine.
B. Do nothing as spontaneous resolution of CSF leak does occur.
C. One time of high-volume epidural blood patch targeting the lumber spine.
D. Consultation for surgical repairs due to prior unsuccessful empiric epidural blood patches at an outside institution.
E. Provide pain medication and maintain well hydration.

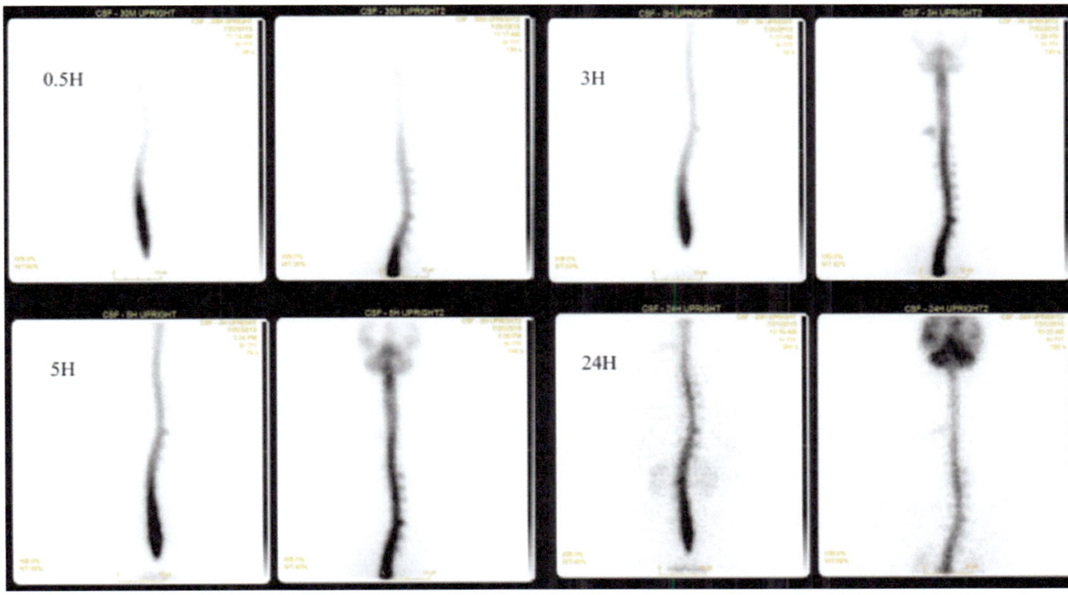

Fig. Q19

Quiz #20

The patient is an 84-year-old right-handed female presenting with worsening memory loss for several years. In addition, she has had significant mobility issues with gait shuffling and frequent falls with broken teeth and head injuries. Her daughter, who is with her, reports that her mother's memory problem and mobility issues started around the same time, with periods of confusion often worsening in the evening. Her daughter also reports that her mother sometimes had hallucination, mostly auditory. For example, a few months ago, the patient complained of hearing "crackling" noises, but other family members did not. The patient used to have significant behavioral issues and has been on risperidone for treatment for years without benefits. Neurological exam showed MMSE score of 10/30. Recent laboratory tests showed TSH, folate, and vitamin B_{12} in normal ranges. Brain perfusion SPECT images are shown in Fig. Q20. According to the clinical data and the brain perfusion SPECT findings, what is the most likely imaging impression?

A. Dementia with Lewy bodies (DLB)
B. Alzheimer's disease (AD)
C. Frontotemporal dementia (FTD)
D. Posterior cortical atrophy (PCA)
E. Vascular dementia (VD)

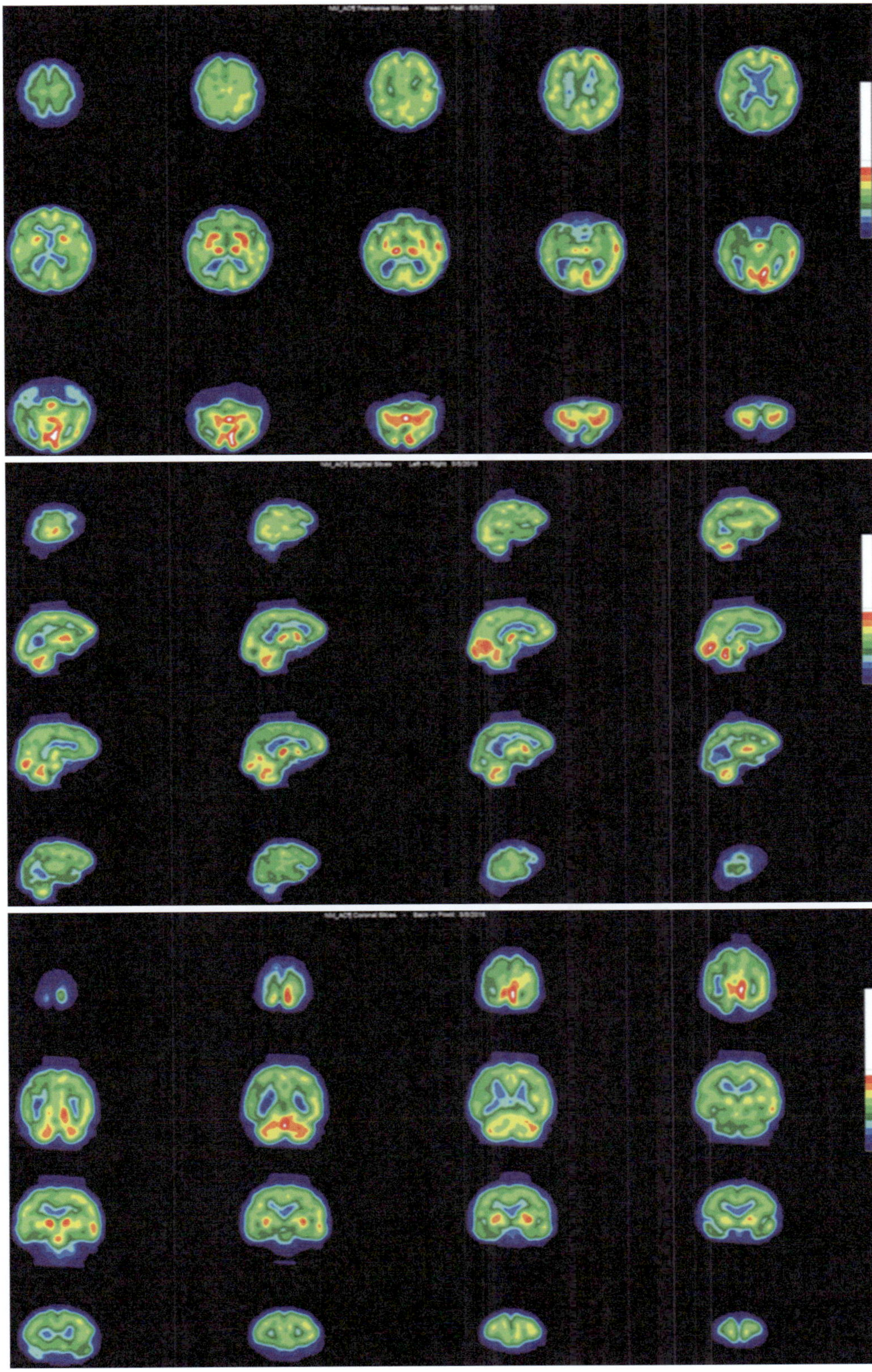

Fig. Q20

Quiz #21

The patient is a 3-year-old right-handed female presenting with medically refractory seizures that started 2 and a half years ago, per mother. During the first seizure, patient's head and eyes were deviated to the right, followed by losing muscle tone. Despite antiepileptic treatment with two medications, the seizures continue, with increasing bilateral extremity stiffness, now more in the left upper extremity at the onset. The seizures occur randomly during the day, with frequency of a few episodes a day, each lasting 30–60 seconds. Postictal sleep was noted. No aura or trigger was observed, per mother. Initial EEGs were suspicious for left hemispheric seizures, but recent EEG studies showed a possible right central (or cingulate) versus right frontotemporal/insular seizure focus. A recent CT of the head/brain was normal. Prior brain MRI was also unremarkable. Brain FDG PET images are displayed in Fig. Q21. What's the most likely epilepsy this patient may have?

A. Right frontal lobe epilepsy (FLE)
B. Right temporal lobe epilepsy (TLE)
C. Right parietal lobe epilepsy (PLE)
D. Right insular lobe epilepsy (ILE)
E. Likely multifocal epilepsy

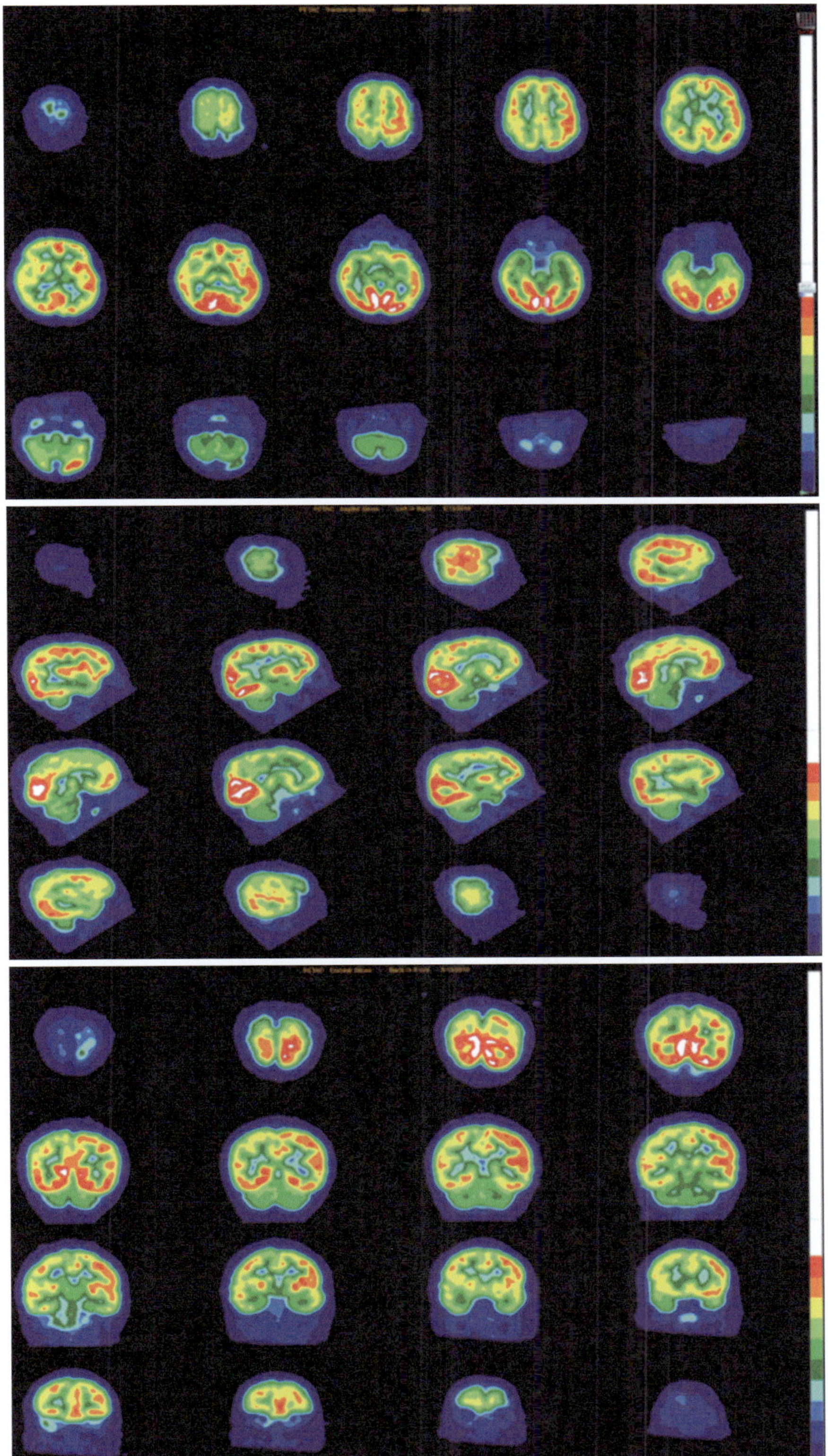

Fig. Q21

Quiz #22

The patient is a 62-year-old male complaining of right arm and hand tremor for 5 months. He has been taking Sinemet (20–325 mg, 1.5 tablets, by mouth, three times a day) for 2 months, with a good response. Past medical history is significant for hypertension, hyperlipidemia, spinal stenosis, chronic neck pain, asthma, thoracic outlet syndrome, gastroesophageal reflux disease, and obstructive sleep apnea. DaTscan images are displayed in Fig. Q22. What is the most appropriate impression of the DaTscan study?

A. Abnormal study showing dopamine transporter depletion confined to the right striatum.
B. Abnormal study showing dopamine transporter depletion of only bilateral putamen.
C. Abnormal study showing dopamine transporter depletion, right caudate nuclei > right putamen > left putamen.
D. Abnormal study suggestive of non-neurodegenerative disease (stroke, tumor, or trauma, etc.) affecting the right striatum.
E. Abnormal findings show global dopamine transporter depletion, with lateralization to the right striatum, discordant with the right-sided tremor, overall suggesting advanced PD.

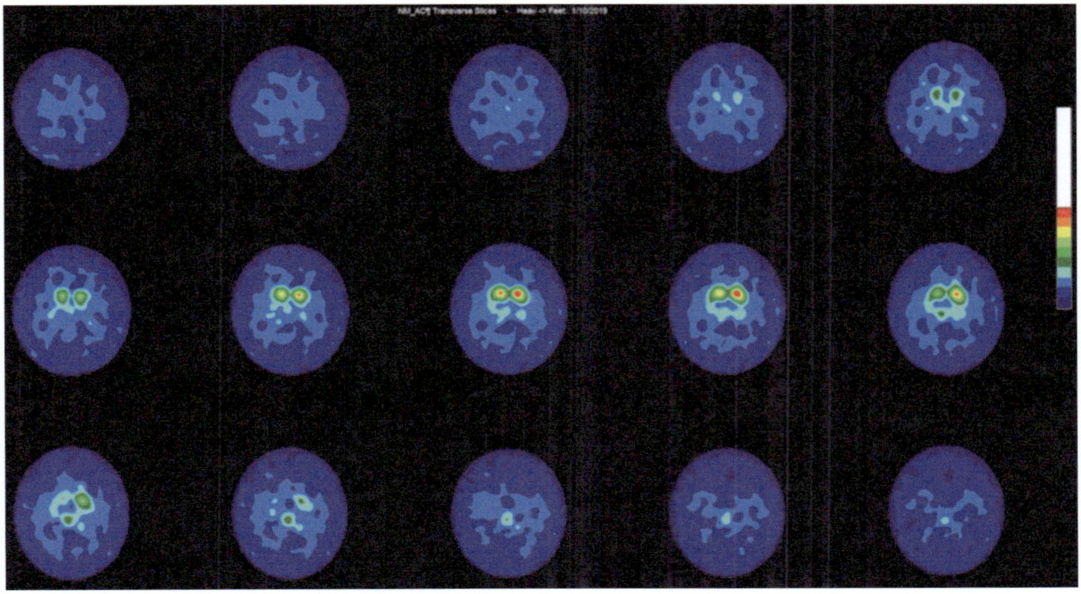

Fig. Q22

Quiz #23

The patient is a 61-year-old right-handed male presenting with worsening memory loss, behavioral problems, and speech difficulties for 2–3 years. He was brought to our emergency department by police because he was trying to steal lighters in a supermarket. He denies any hallucinations. No motor weakness or tremors were noted. There was no prior history of any psychiatric disease. During his stay in hospital, he exhibited disorganized thoughts, loss of inhibition, loss of speech, and repetitive behaviors. He refused to take medications. He had minimal interaction with peers, demonstrated increasing isolation and social withdrawal, and had difficulties attending psychiatric therapy group meetings. His judgment was poor because of disinhibition, but his sleep and appetite were good. The patient used to be a store owner, good with numbers, but has had functional decline and social withdrawal over the last few years. He has a documented history of tobacco, marijuana, and cocaine abuse. Brain MRA showed no evidence of vascular stenosis, aneurysm, or occlusion. However, brain MRI revealed generalized brain parenchymal diminution with more prominent atrophy of the temporal lobes. CT of the head/brain showed atrophy of bilateral temporal and frontal lobes and encephalomalacia in the right thalamus. Brain FDG PET images are displayed in Fig. Q23. Based on the clinical presentation and neuroimaging findings, which is the most likely neurological condition this patient may have?

A. Vascular dementia (VD)
B. Semantic variant FTD (svFTD)
C. Alzheimer's disease (AD)
D. Dementia with Lewy bodies (DLB)
E. Behavioral variant FTD (bvFTD)

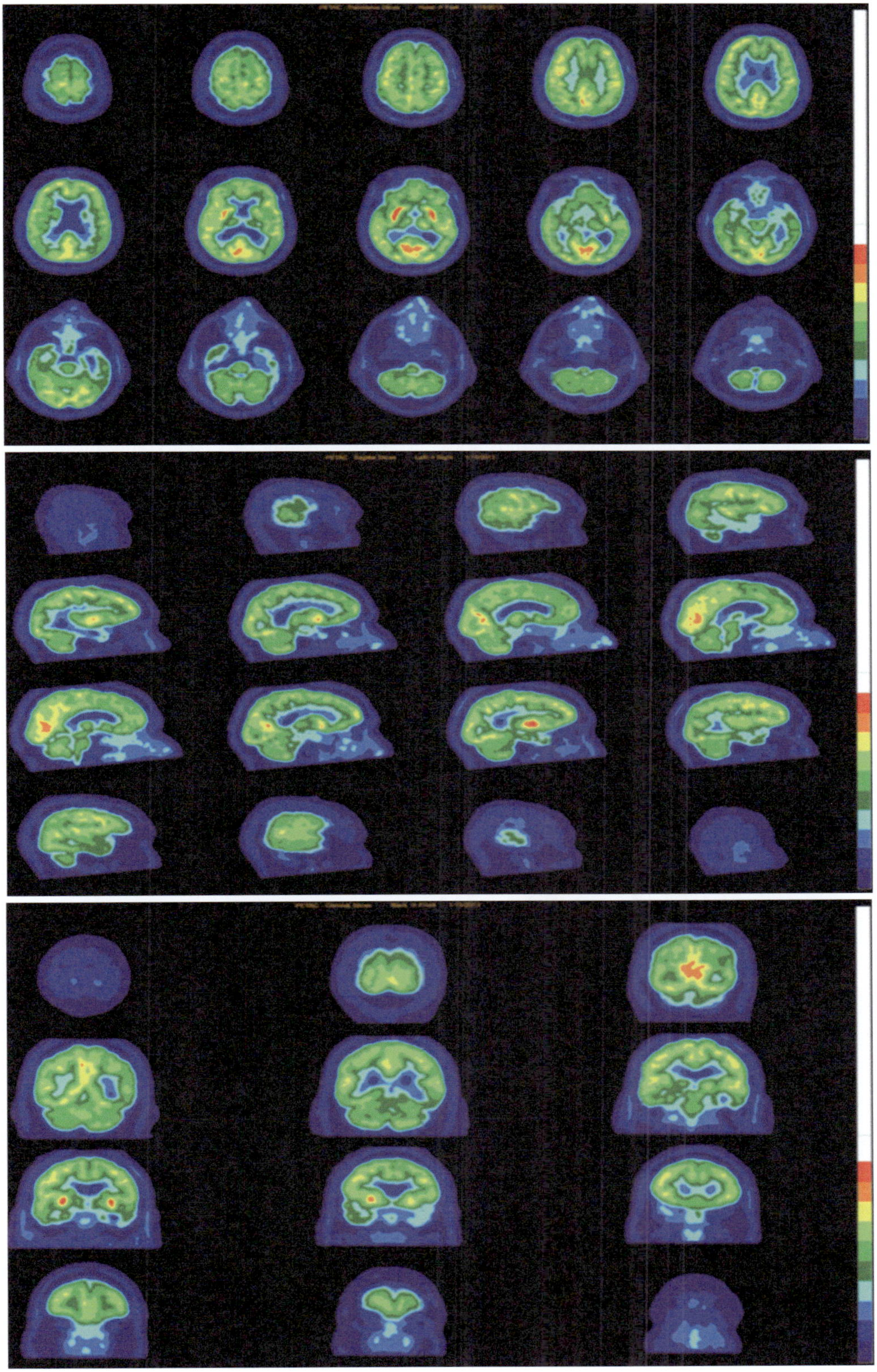

Fig. Q23

Quiz #24

The patient was a 33-year-old male with cardiac arrest 3 days ago likely due to heroin overdose per reports from police officers and EMS responders. Since admission, he was intubated and started on a cooling protocol which was discontinued due to severe hypotension despite treatment with several pressors. Past medical history was notable for polysubstance abuse (including abuse of alcohol, marijuana, and heroin), alcoholic pancreatitis, and drug abuse-related pericarditis. Neurological exam showed no purposeful movements. Pupils were fixed and dilated. There was no reaction to verbal or painful stimuli. CT of the head/brain scans showed "no acute intracranial process." In-hospital EEG revealed findings indicating severe diffuse encephalopathy. Limited images from a mobile gamma camera study (due to patient's unstable vital signs and unable to be transported to our nuclear medicine clinic) are displayed in Fig. Q24. What's the most appropriate imaging impression of the brain perfusion study?

A. Technically limited study with findings inconclusive for brain death
B. Positive study for brain death because of the "hot nose sign"
C. Negative/equivocal study due to likely perfusion to the brain stem
D. Positive study for brain death because of the early (flow) images showing no brain perfusion
E. Positive study with direct (absence of brain parenchymal perfusion) and indirect (presence of a hot nose sign) scintigraphic evidence of brain death

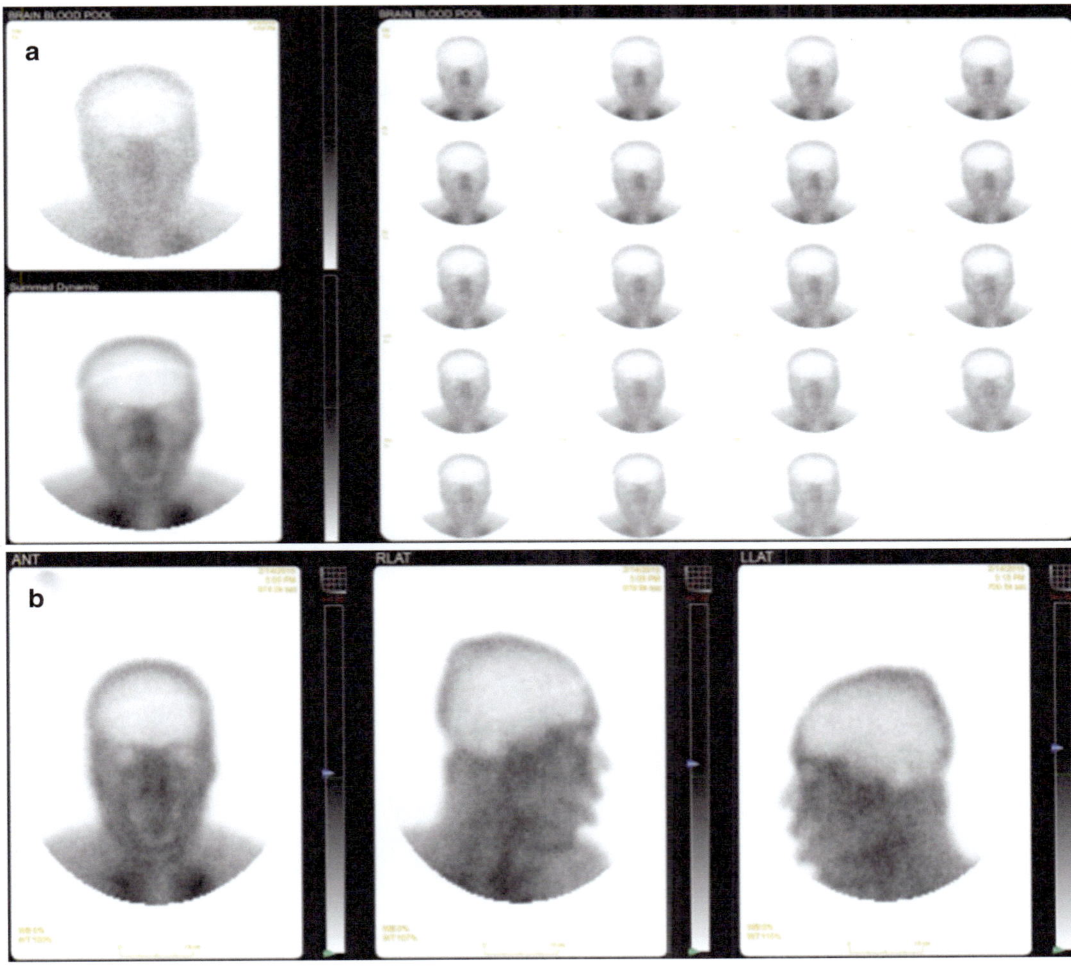
BRAIN BLOOD POOL
a
Summed Dynamic
BRAIN BLOOD POOL
ANT
b
RLAT
LLAT

Fig. Q24

Quiz #25

The patient is a 72-year-old female with progressive memory loss and difficulty in speaking for 1 year. She also reports pain and uncomfortable sensation in her legs, especially at night. She is widowed and has no history of smoking or drug/alcohol abuse. She denies history of stroke, head trauma, or seizures. Mental status exam showed no dysarthria but a nonfluent expressive aphasia, with difficulty in naming and calculating. CT of the head/brain showed mildly prominent ventricles and sulci compatible with atrophy. A recent brain MRI revealed nonspecific white matter changes. Brain FDG PET images are shown in Fig. Q25. Based on the clinical presentation and neuroimaging findings, what is the most likely neurological condition this patient may have?

A. Dementia with Lewy bodies (DLB)
B. Alzheimer's disease (AD)
C. Corticobasal degeneration (CBD)
D. Frontotemporal dementia (FTD)
E. Primary progressive aphasia (PPA)

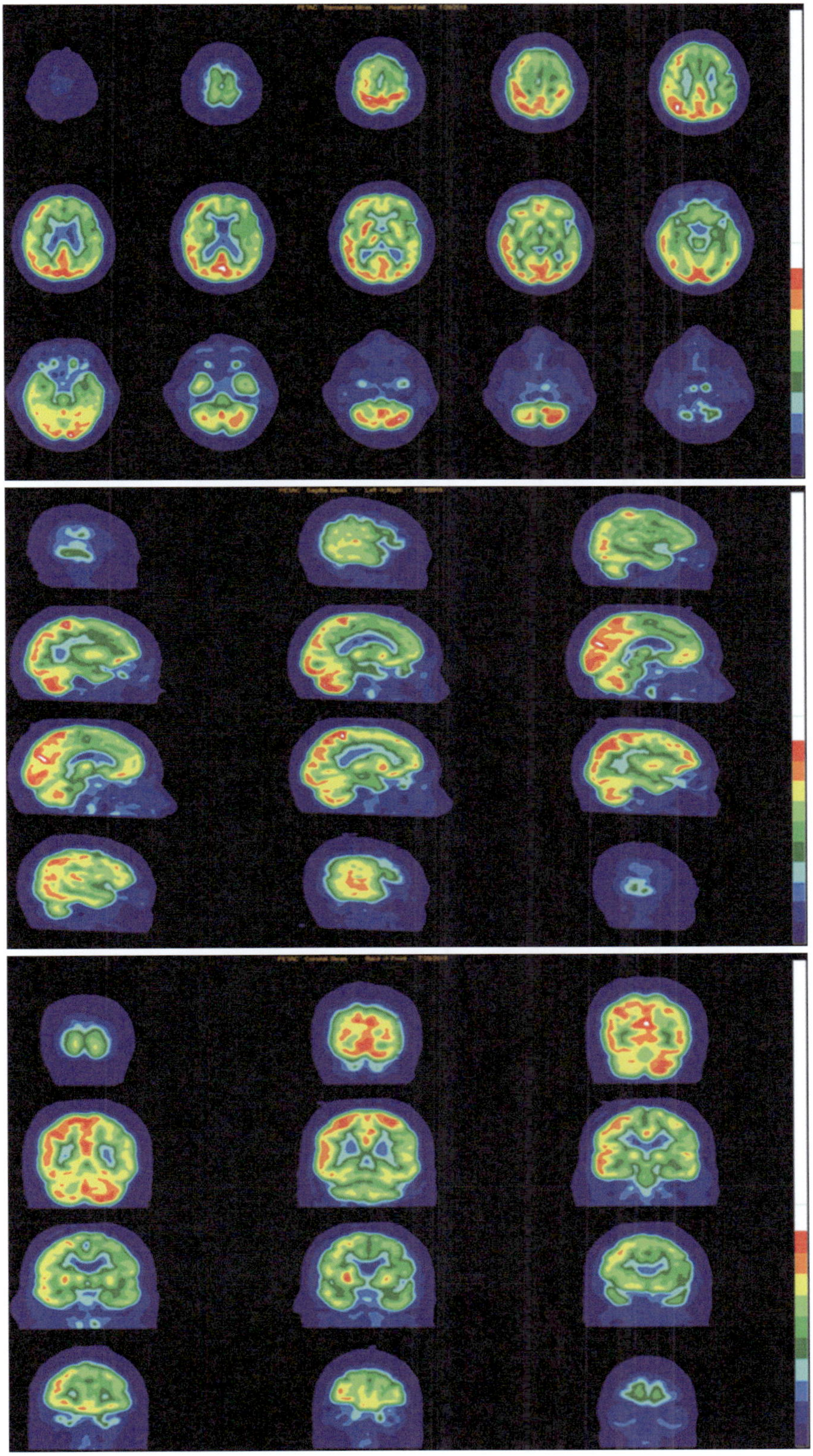

Fig. Q25

Quiz #26

The patient is a 77-year-old female presenting with rapid decline in balance and multiple falls. In addition, she has impaired memory and tremor of both hands. She denies dizziness and has no seizures. Past medical history is notable for hypertension, dyslipidemia, diabetes mellitus, and obesity. Brain MRI showed midbrain atrophy suspicious for progressive supranuclear palsy (PSP). DaTscan images and a selected MRI image showing midbrain atrophy are displayed in Fig. Q26. What is the most appropriate imaging diagnosis for this patient?

A. Abnormal DaTscan consistent with PD
B. Essentially normal DaTscan with head tilting
C. Abnormal DaTscan consistent with multiple system atrophy (MSA)
D. Abnormal DaTscan likely due to corticobasal degeneration (CBD)
E. Abnormal DaTscan likely secondary to progressive supranuclear palsy (PSP)

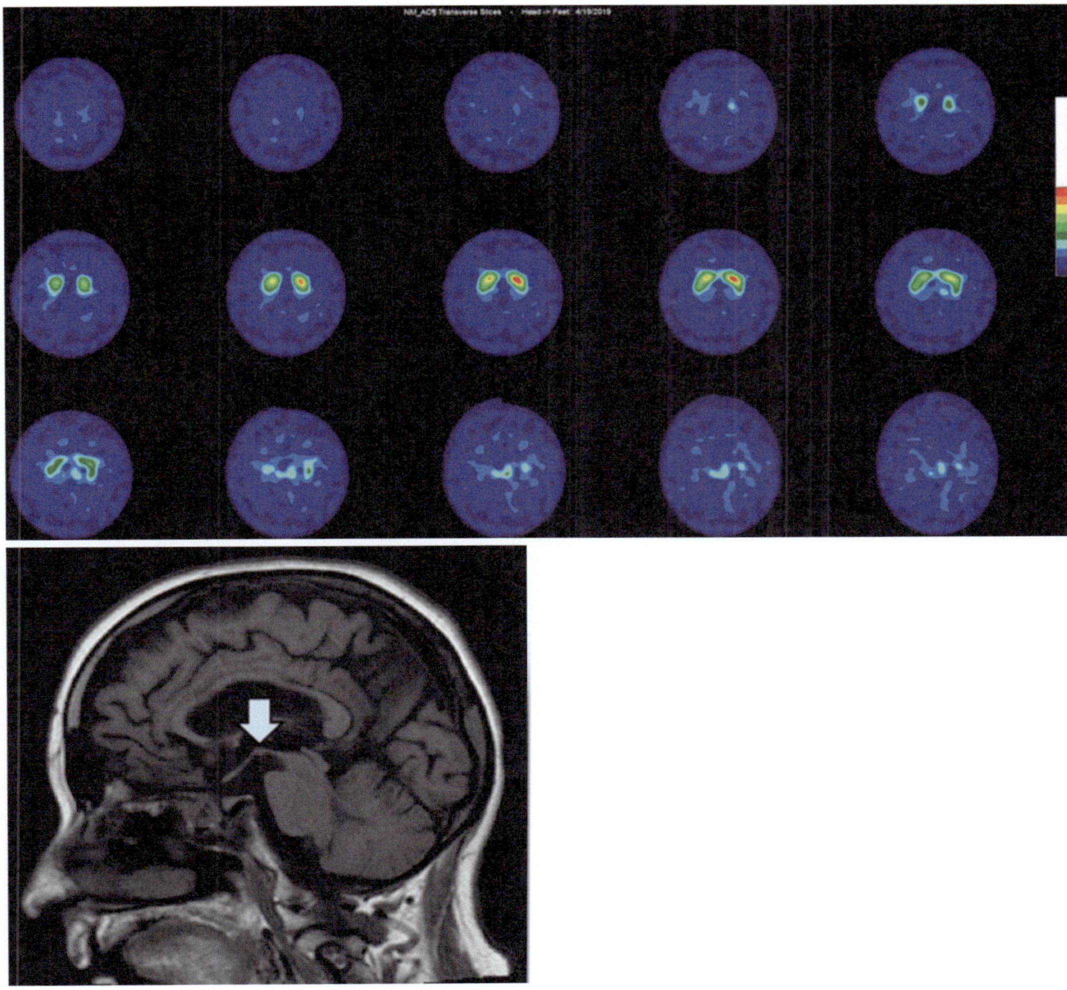

Fig. Q26

Quiz #27

The patient is a 15-year-old right-handed male presenting with intractable focal epilepsy for 4 years despite on antiepileptic medications. The seizures often occur in the afternoon from 2 to 5 pm, with frequency of once a week and usually lasting about 45 seconds to a few minutes. During the seizures, the patient reports seeing a dark curtain going down his vision and appearing scared. The seizures manifest with chewing automatism, left upper extremity flexion at the elbow with hand dystonic contracted, copious drooling, left lower extremity bicycling, and eye closed with slight left eye deviation. The seizures are often preceded by auras including feeling "weird" and lightheaded and yelling "Dad," "Mom," and "I do not feel right." EEG studies showed right temporal intermittent rhythmic delta activity (TIRDA) > occipital intermittent rhythmic delta activity (OIRDA), focal epileptiform discharges independent right posterior temporal and right anteromedial temporal, with clear propagation pathway from right posterior temporal to right anteromedial temporal region. Brain MRI with and without gadolinium was normal. FDG PET images are displayed in Fig. Q27. Based on the seizure semiology, EEG results, and FDG PET findings, what is the most likely epilepsy this patient may have?

A. Right frontal lobe epilepsy (FLE)
B. Right lateral temporal lobe epilepsy (LTLE)
C. Right mesial temporal lobe epilepsy (MTLE)
D. Right parietal lobe epilepsy (PLE)
E. Right occipital lobe epilepsy (OLE)

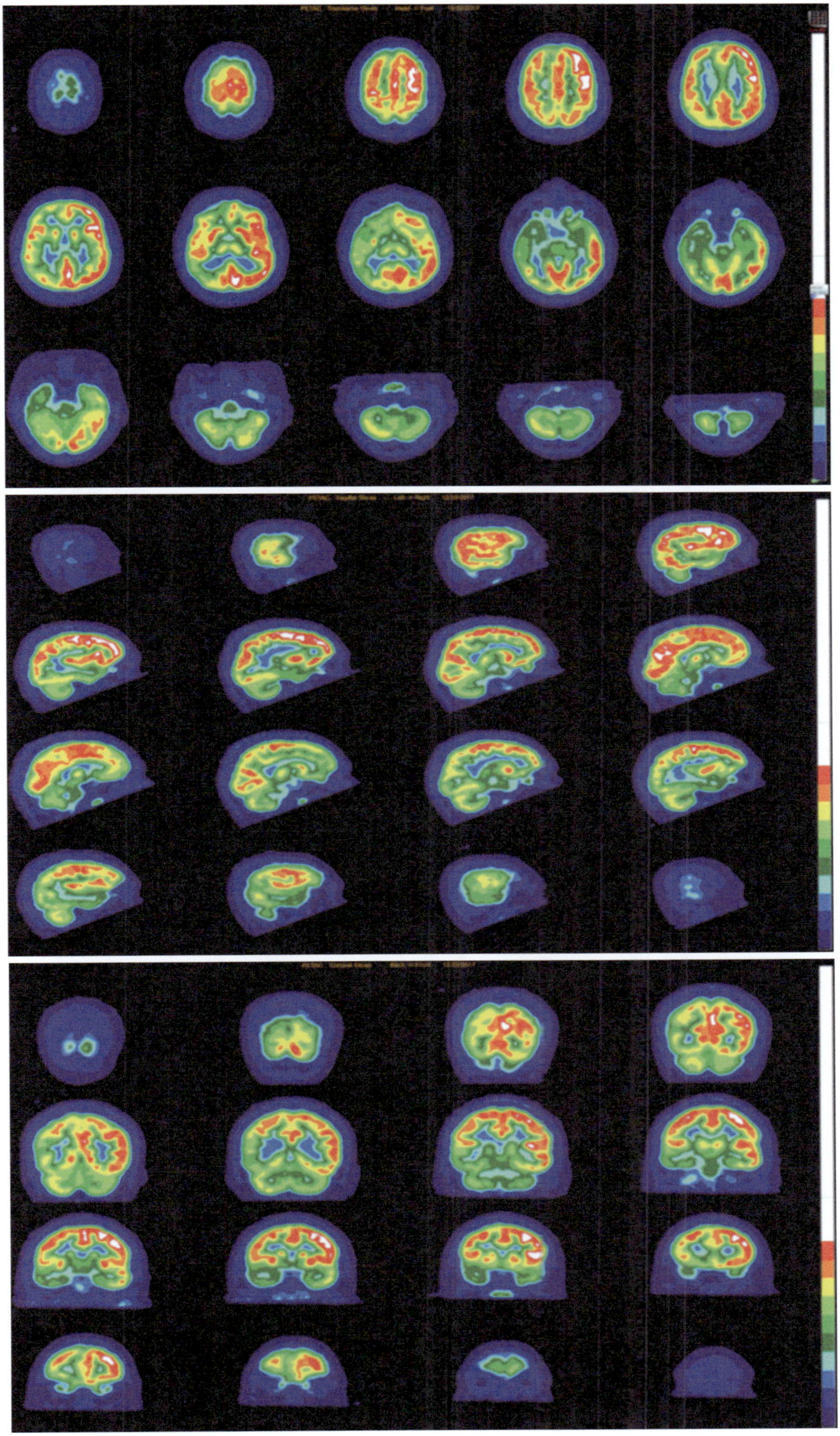

Fig. Q27

Quiz #28

The patient is a 21-year-old right-handed female with medically refractory epilepsy, and she is referred for pre-surgical evaluation. Brain MRI revealed left mesial temporal sclerosis. Brain FDG PET showed hypometabolism in left mesial temporal region, suspicious for an interictal epileptogenic focus/zone. Functional MRI (fMRI) demonstrated bilateral language representation. Magnetoencephalography (MEG) suggested right dominance but lack of visual spatial deficits, while neuropsychiatric (NP) profile was most suggestive of left dominance. Given the lack of congruence between MEG and fMRI/NP results, the Wada test was proposed to further assess functional reserve/dominance. As part of the Wada test, brain perfusion SPECT was performed, with images displayed in Fig. Q28. What is the most appropriate imaging impression of the brain perfusion SPECT study?

A. Findings consistent with expected hypoperfusion to the left brain and intact perfusion to the right brain
B. Findings highly suggestive of a poor cerebral vascular reserve (CVR) in the left MCA territory
C. Findings confirming left mesial temporal lobe epilepsy (MTLE) with seizure expansion
D. Findings confirming left mesial temporal lobe epilepsy (MTLE) with diaschisis involving the left thalamus and right cerebellum
E. Findings suggestive of right language dominance

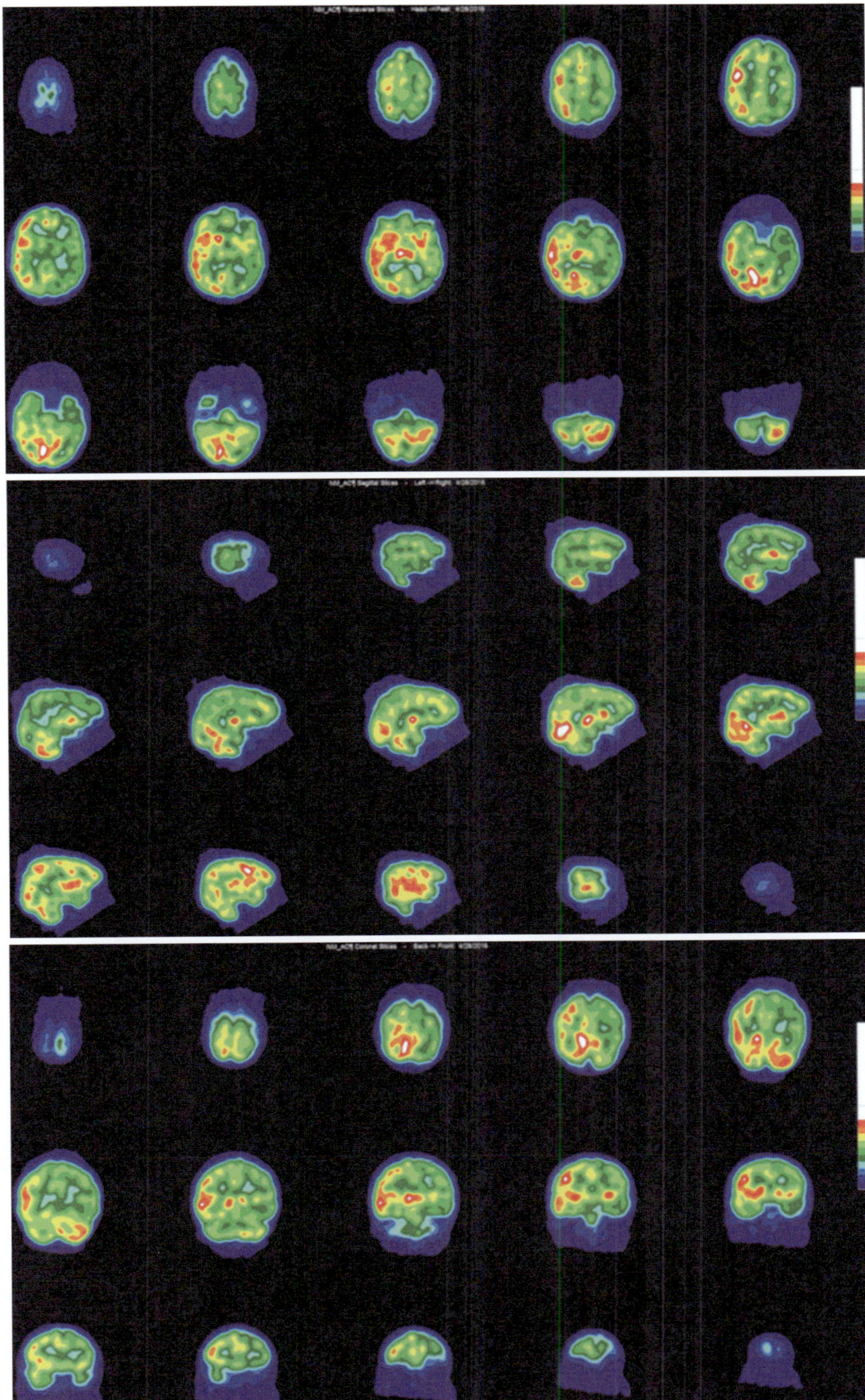

Fig. Q28

Quiz #29

The patient is a 16-year-old right-handed female presenting with an intractable seizure that started 10 years ago. The seizure was described as staring and pale, with eyes looking glassy and decreased speech. During the seizures her head and eyes deviated to the left. She has been treated with multiple antiepileptic medications, with poor seizure control. Her last seizure was 2 months ago, and it lasted about 1 minute in duration. It was described that she stared off, head and eye deviation to the left. She had left-sided twitching of the head, eyes, and mouth. The patient reported somatosensory aura (touching lip and throat/chest). After the seizure she had slurred speech and felt sleepy. Multiple EEG studies showed regional seizure activities in the right frontotemporal area. The images of ictal, interictal brain perfusion SPECTs and SISCOM analysis are displayed in Fig. Q29a–c, respectively. Based on the seizure semiology, EEG results, and scintigraphical findings, what is the most likely epilepsy this patient may have?

A. The right frontal lobe
B. The right lateral temporal lobe
C. The right parietal lobe
D. The right mesial temporal lobe
E. The right occipital lobe

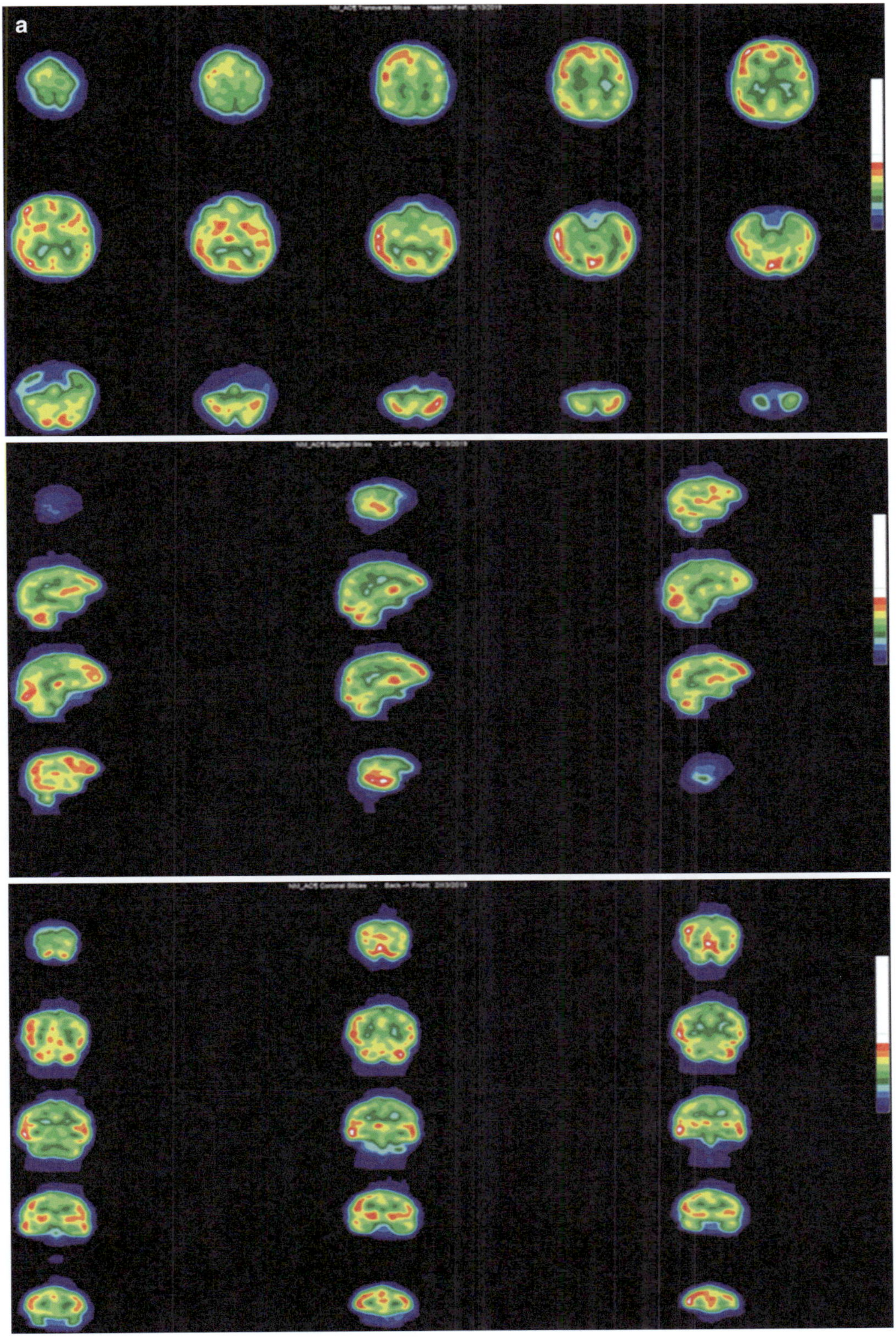

Fig. Q29 (a–c)

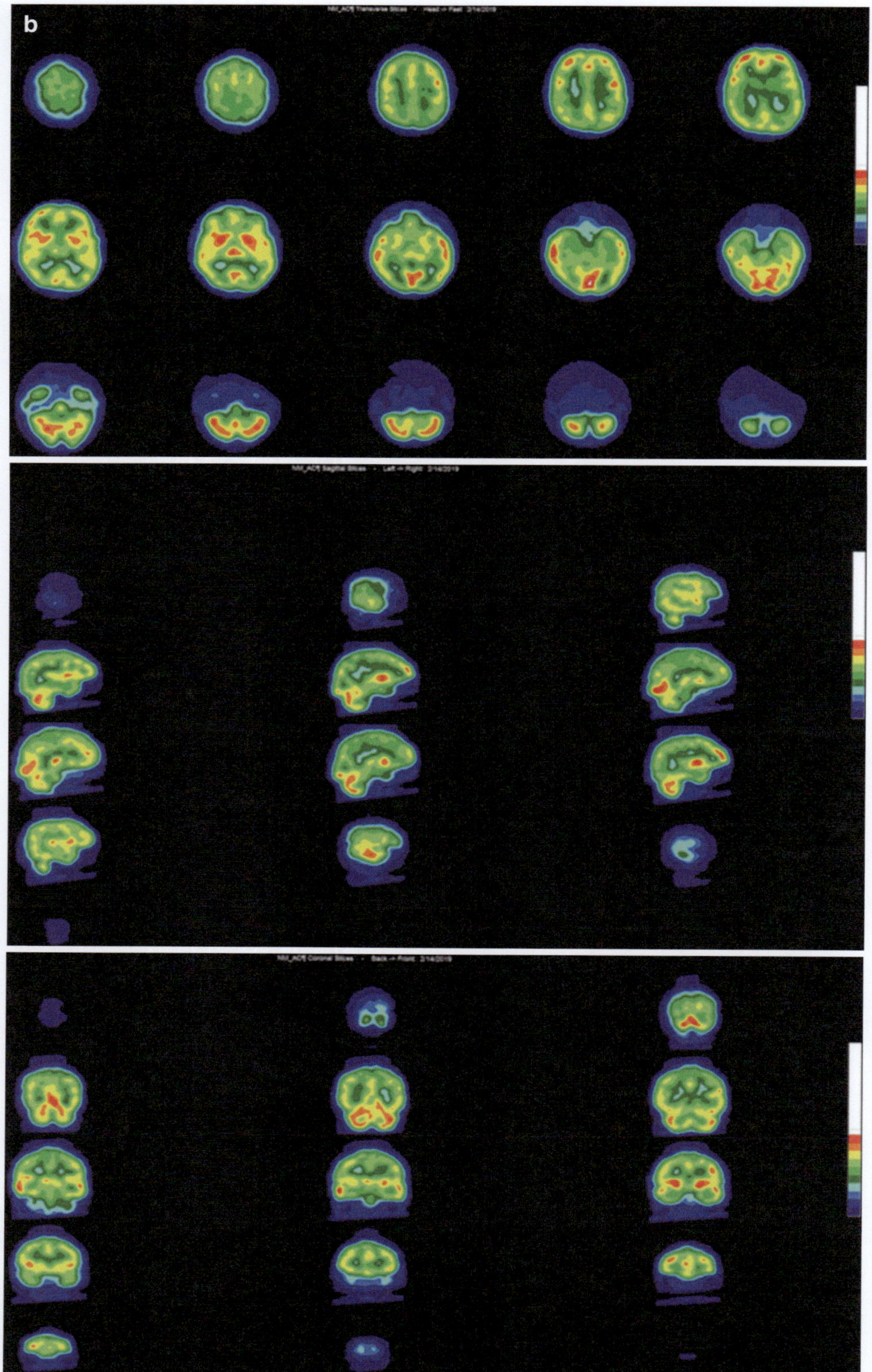

Fig. Q29 (continued)

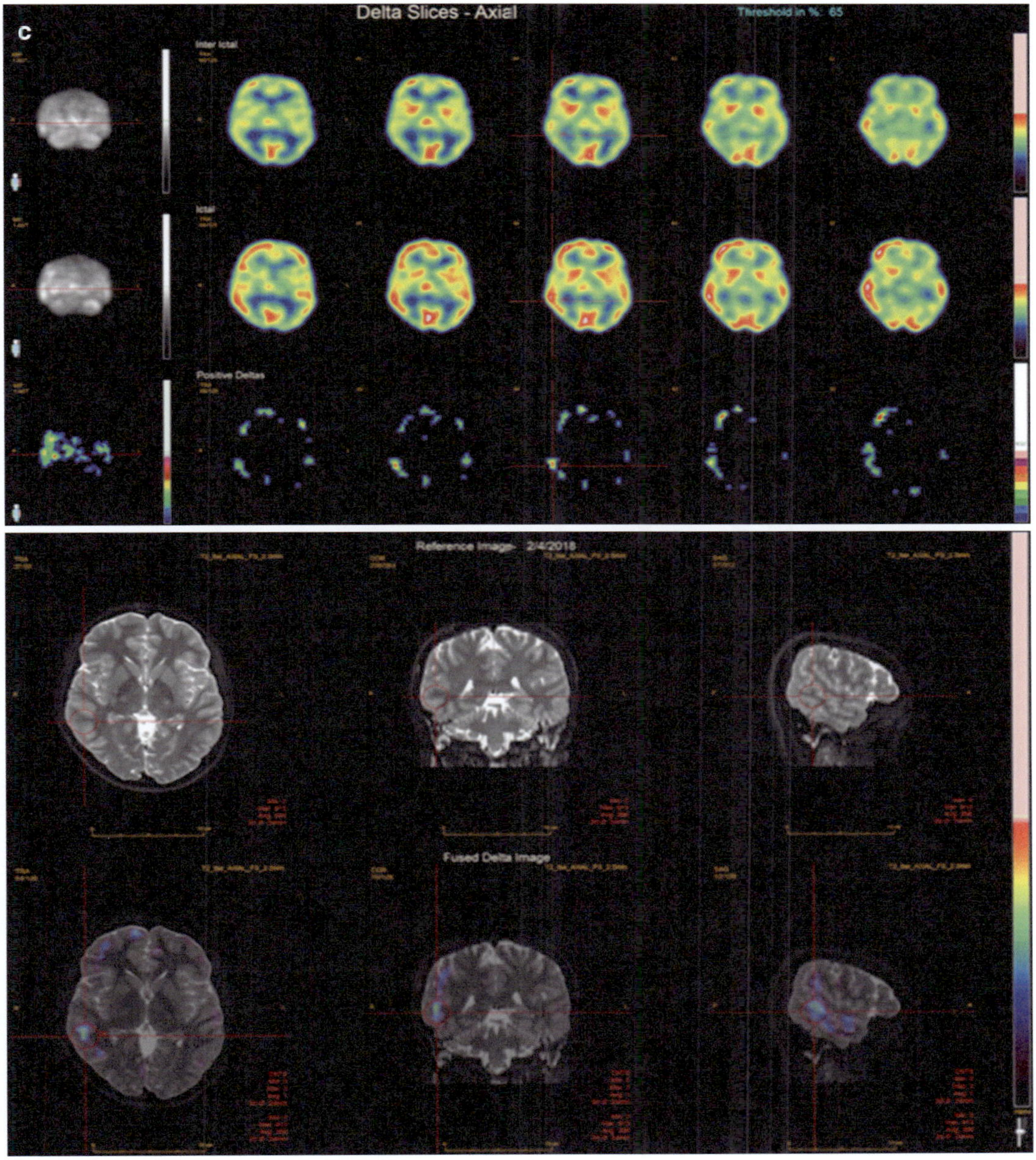

Fig. Q29 (continued)

Quiz #30

The patient is a 79-year-old male presenting with short-term memory loss, ataxia, and urinary incontinence. CT of the head/brain showed lateral ventriculomegaly, right greater than left, suspicious for normal pressure hydrocephalus (NPH), for which he underwent a high-volume CSF removal at an outside institution, which did not help. Brain MRI showed lateral ventriculomegaly, right > left. CSF images and selected MR image are displayed in Fig. Q30. What is the most likely imaging impression?

A. Findings consistent with normal pressure hydrocephalus (NPH)
B. Essentially unremarkable study except for moderately slow CSF flow
C. Findings concerning for Alzheimer's disease
D. Findings suggestive of Parkinson's disease
E. Findings consistent with hydrocephalus *ex vacuo*

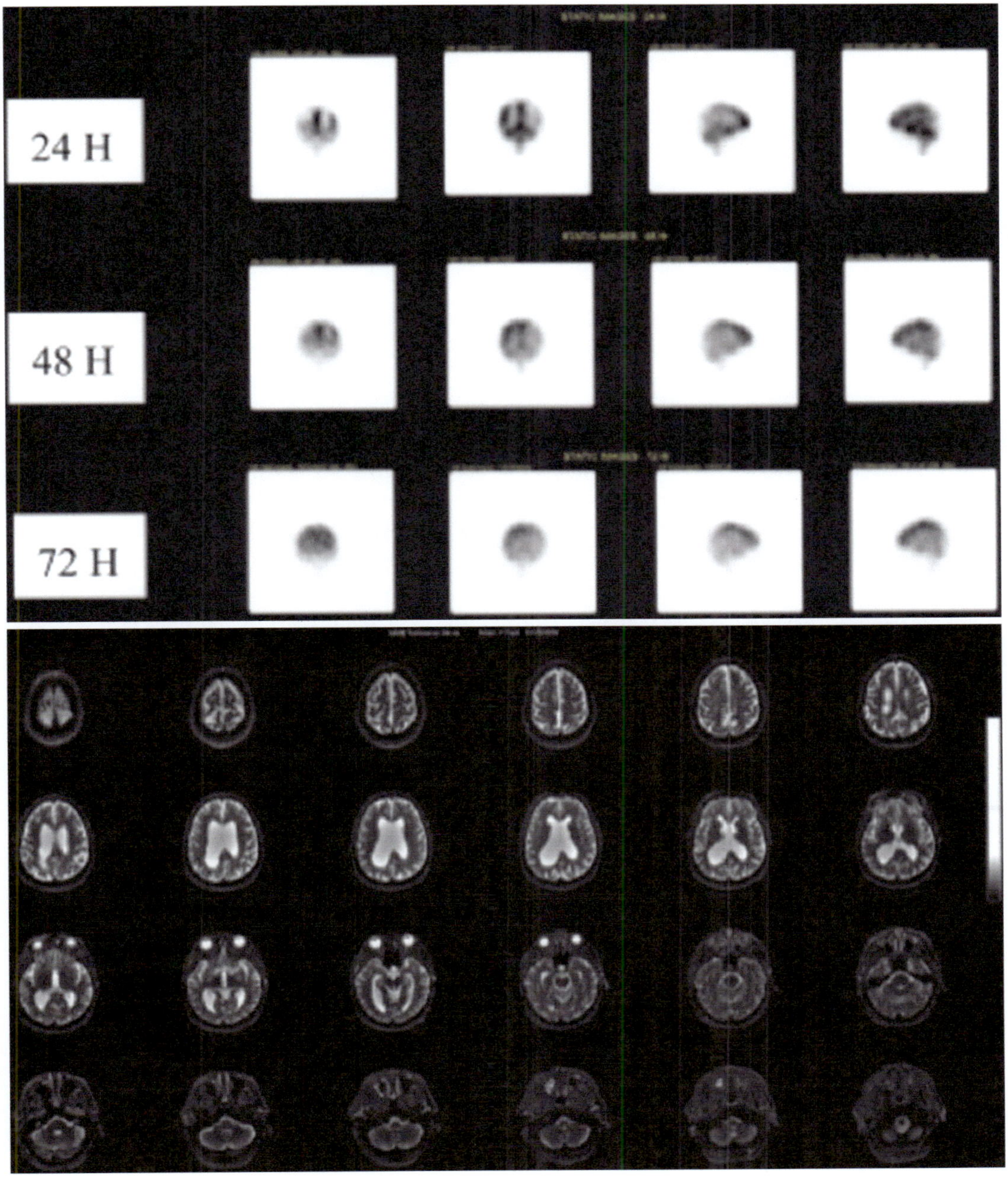

Fig. Q30

Correct Answers and Critiques

- Quiz #1 B
- Quiz #2 E
- Quiz #3 A
- Quiz #4 C

Critique: The first four quizzes are composed to cover the commonly diagnosed neurodegenerative dementias, Alzeimer's disease (AD), frontotemporal dementia (FTD), dementia with Lewy bodies (DLB), and vascular dementia (VD). In conjunction with clinical presentation and anatomic neuroimaging findings, patterns of altered glucose metabolism on FDG PET or PET CT are helpful in the diagnosis and or differential diagnosis of the four commonly diagnosed neurodegenerative conditions [1–5]. AD is the most common progressive neurodegenerative disorder. Although global/generalized cortical hypometabolism is often observed, especially in patients with advanced AD or early-onset AD (EOAD), the dominant cortical hypometabolism is located in the parietal lobe(s) including the posterior cingulate gyri and precuneus (abbreviated as PCG/PCUN), with involvement of the adjacent temporo-fronto-occipital cortices in a spread pattern. For example, within the frontal lobes, the spread hypometabolism follows the following order in terms of severity: posterior > anterior, and lateral > medial, with exception of the sensorimotor strips that may have preserved or relatively preserved metabolism; within the temporal lobes, the spread hypometabolism is more prominent in the posterior, superior, and lateral relative to the anterior, inferior, and medial; within the occipital lobes, the spread hypometabolism is superior > inferior, and lateral > medial, with preserved or relatively preserved metabolism in the primary visual cortices. In contrast, FTD, as the name implies, is characterized by dominant frontotemporal cortical hypometabolism, especially the anterior and medial portions of the frontal lobes and the anterior and inferior portions of the temporal lobes. Clinically, patients with FTD often present with behavioral changes/executive functional decline and/or impairment in language domain. DLB, however, is characterized by dominant cortical hypometabolism in the occipital lobes, and often associated with extensive involvement of other cortical regions, again in a spread pattern [6]. However, metabolism in PCG/PCUN is usually preserved; in contrast to dominant hypometabolism in the occipital regions (posterior to PCG/PCUN) and spread hypometabolism in the frontal lobes (anterior to PCG/PCUN), this unique imaging finding is referred in literature to as "cingulate island sign (CIS)," which is a highly specific neuroimaging marker for diagnosis of DLB [7]. Clinically, patients with DLB often present with complex visual hallucinations. Diagnosis of VD is often already established, based on clinical criteria with or without anatomic neuroimaging results. FDG PET or PET CT is infrequently requested for evaluation of this entity. Nevertheless, FDG PET features suggesting VD include multifocal, often severe hypometabolism, consistent with cortical and/or lacunar infarcts or both, most of the time in the middle cerebral artery territories, and lack of altered metabolic patterns suggesting other commonly diagnosed neurodegenerative dementias.

Corticobasal degeneration (CBD) is a rare neurodegenerative disorder, which is clinically characterized by asymmetric cortical dysfunction (ideomotor apraxia and alien limb phenomena) and extrapyramidal dysfunction (limb rigidity and/or dystonia) [8]. On FDG PET, CBD is featured by an imaging triad. They include (i) cortical hypometabolism in unilateral frontal lobe (posterior/middle > anterior) or frontoparietal region, (ii) hypometabolic involvement of underlying basal ganglia (ipsilateral), and (iii) crossed cerebrocerebellar diaschisis. Patients with CBD can present with memory problems, but often not dominant clinical features. None of the four cases meets the clinical and/or imaging criteria for diagnosis of CBD.

- Quiz #5 E

Critique: Glioblastoma multiforme (GBM) is the most aggressive primary brain malignant tumor often with a poor prognosis. After initial successful treatments (surgical resection, chemotherapy, and radiation), recurrence often occurs as shown in this patient in the past. Both recurrent GBM and post-radiation necrosis are contrast-enhancing on MRI [9–11]. Typical recurrent GBM on FDG PET is a focus of increased FDG activity surrounded by hypometabolism due to tumor-associated vasogenic edema and/or mass effects, whereas post-radiation necrosis is suggested by hypometabolism, e.g., decreased FDG activity. Therefore, answers A and B are incorrect. That having been said, heterogeneous and often asymmetric FDG activities secondary to prior treatments and/or coexisting conditions (*e.g.,* seizures) are often seen, making it difficult to differentiate recurrence versus nonspecific cortical activities. Nevertheless, answers C and D are also incorrect, due to the lack of MRI correlate and without surrounding hypometabolism indicating vasogenic edema and/or mass effects. In summary, FDG PET features as described, in conjunction with MRI findings, help differentiate recurrent GBM versus post-radiation necrosis.

- Quiz #6 C

Critique: Acetazolamide (Diamox) is a potent cerebral vasodilating agent. Brain perfusion SPECT study with Diamox challenge, in comparison to a baseline study (without premedication of Diamox), not only confirms cerebrovascular ischemic disease but also provides imaging evidence of cerebrovascular reserve (CVR) that is an important index for risk evaluation of cerebrovascular accidents (CVA) [12]. A good/preserved CVR is indicated by improved perfusion on Diamox study when compared to prior hypoperfusion on a baseline study, whereas decreased/worsening perfusion or persistent hypoperfusion on Diamox-challenging study is suggestive of a poor CVR. Therefore, answers A and B are incorrect. This study shows evidence of possible watershed ischemia on the baseline study, and the Diamox study reveals diffuse ischemia in the entire left MCA territories. Theoretically, vertebral artery disease can exhibit hypoperfusion in the posterior cerebral artery (PCA) territory, but clinical application of brain perfusion SPECT in the evaluation of vertebral artery ischemic disease has not yet to be established. So, answers D and E are either incomplete or inappropriate. Instead, answer C is correct, with imaging features consistent with so-called intracerebral steal phenomena (ISP) [12] in the left MCA territory.

- Quiz #7 A

Critique: Although epileptogenic foci/zones can originate from any cerebral cortical regions, majority of them are located in the temporal lobes, often referred to as TLEs. Among TLEs, majority are located in the medial (mesial) portion of the temporal lobe [13–15]. Brain FDG PET is one of the earliest approved clinical applications by the Central Medicare and Medicaid services (CMS) in the US for pre-surgical evaluation of epileptogenic foci/zones for patients with drug-resistant epilepsies. On interictal FDG PET, a typical epileptogenic focus/zone is indicated by focal cortical hypometabolism (decreased FDG activity). Although this approach has a high sensitivity, its specificity is suboptimal due to seizure propagation or expansion. Therefore, FDG PET findings need to be correlated with seizure semiology, EEG results, and other neuroimaging results. This patient's seizures proceeded with an aura (a "rush" sensation over her body), which is a typical semiologic feature indicating TLE. Her EEG results were also indicating left TLE. In addition to the clinic-electrical evidence of left TLE, MRI further showed evidence of left mesial temporal sclerosis. Consistently, FDG PET reveals dominant hypometabolism in the left medial (mesial) temporal lobe, indicating an epileptogenic focus/zone. To a lesser degree, hypometabolism is noted in the left lateral temporal lobe, likely due to seizure expansion. The right temporal hypometabolism is less prominent, with unknown etiology, although seizures started in earlier age and long-term use of multiple anti-seizure medications could contribute to the abnormality. The finding is less likely due to an additional epileptogenic focus/zone, because of lack of clinic-electrical and MRI correlate. Therefore, answers B to E are either inappropriate, incomplete, or incorrect.

• Quiz #8 D

Critique: Dopamine transporter scan (DaTscan) was approved by the FDA in 2011 to help differentiate essential tremor (ET) from tremor due to Parkinson's disease (PD), multiple system atrophy (MSA), or progressive supranuclear palsy (PSP). Normal DaTscan is in support of ET or drug-induced Parkinsonism (DIP), and it is characterized by crescent-shaped tracer activity with highest intensity in caudate nuclei tapering into putamen body and tail of both hemispheres. Since the DaTscan is abnormal and shows decreased tracer activity in the left putamen, answer A is incorrect. Rest tremor is one of the main clinical features of PD. This patient has a chief complaint of progressive weakness and ataxia, without tremor, suggesting that the pretest likelihood of PD is low. Since dopaminergic neurons in putamen are more vulnerable to neurodegenerative insults compared to those in caudate nuclei, early stage of PD often shows selectively decreased tracer activity in one or two putamens and intact tracer activity in caudate nuclei on DaTscan. This study, despite technical limitation (head tilting), shows mildly decreased tracer activity in the left putamen but preserved activity in the left caudate nuclei and entire right striatum; therefore, answers A, C and E are incorrect. Although the imaging finding is indistinguishable from early stage of PD, the lack of rest tremor and the MRI finding of marked cerebellar atrophy make answer B unlikely. MSA is originally referred to as *Shy-Drager syndrome*, also sometimes referred to as *olivopontine cerebellar degeneration* [16]. It is a rare neurodegenerative disorder, with two major variants: MSA Parkinsonian variant and MSA cerebellar variant. The DaTscan findings, in conjunction with clinical presentation and MRI results, are in support of MSA cerebellar variant, with mild involvement of the left putamen.

• Quiz #9 C

Critique: CSF scintigraphy is an imaging of choice for evaluation of Ommaya shunt patency and CSF flow/distribution for patients with leptomeningeal carcinomatosis. In clinical practice, the likelihood of Ommaya shunt obstruction is low, as most of the patients are referred for evaluation of a newly implanted Ommaya shunt for pending intrathecal chemotherapy. Once the injected tracer, via the reservoir and catheter, reaches the lateral ventricles, a normal CSF flow is indicated by tracer ascending over the top convexity and visualization of the kidneys at 24 hours, with homogenous and symmetric CSF tracer distribution in the subarachnoid spaces of both hemispheres and the spinal canal. Therefore, answers A and B are incorrect. The study shows essentially normal CSF flow in the right brain, but diffused and mildly decreased tracer activity is noted in the left hemisphere, with an area of absent tracer activity in the left parietal region. The uneven CSF flow/distribution is often suggestive of a poor treatment response and worse prognosis. So, answers D and E are incorrect.

• Quiz #10 B

Critique: DaTscan is a brain SPECT study of the striatal dopamine transporter status, with main indication to differentiate essential tremor (ET) from tremor due to dopamine neurodegenerative diseases, most of which are PD [17]. In this patient, the clinical presentation of occasional bilateral hand tremor is atypical for PD. The DaTscan finding of diffuse and severely decreased tracer activity in the entire left striatum does not follow a typical neuropathological pattern for PD, as dopaminergic neurons in putamen are more vulnerable to neurodegenerative insults in comparison to those in caudate nuclei. Therefore, answers A and C are incorrect. In contrast, tracer activity in the entire right striatum (both caudate nuclei and putamen) is normal. The abnormality in the entire left striatum is likely secondary to prior left-sided stroke, rather than a neurodegenerative process. Overall, the imaging findings are suggestive of vascular Parkinsonism, less likely due to technical or motion artifacts. So, answers D and E are incorrect or inappropriate.

- Quiz #11 C

Critique: AD is age-related and most commonly diagnosed neurodegenerative dementia. On FDG PET, AD is featured by dominant hypometabolism in the parietal lobe(s) including the PCG/PCUN, with involvement of the adjacent fronto-temporo-occipital lobes in a spread pattern, except for the sensorimotor strips and the primary visual cortices. Answers A, B, and D are incorrect, given the typical, parietal-lobe-dominant hypometabolism for AD and the lack of clinical and imaging features for FTD, VD, or DLB. Among AD patients, approximately 95% of them are diagnosed after age of 65, and they are classified as late-onset AD or LOAD. In contrast, about 5% of patients develop AD prior to age of 65 [18]. This 51-year-old male patient presents with progressive short-term memory loss for 5–6 years, well prior to the cutoff age of 65. On FDG PET, in addition to the typical pattern of altered metabolism suggestive of AD, there is evidence of generalized/global brain atrophy, and diffuse hypometabolic involvement of the frontal lobes, all indicating advanced disease, all consistent with clinical features of early-onset AD (EOAD) rather than LOAD. Therefore, answer E is incorrect.

- Quiz #12 D

Critique: Ventriculoperitoneal (VP) shunt is often placed for the treatment of normal pressure hydrocephalus (NPH). Connected to the sub-scalp implanted injection reservoir is a short catheter called proximal catheter that surgically penetrates the skull and brain cortex, with its tip ending into one of the lateral brain ventricles. A long tubing, also called distal catheter, connects with the injection reservoir and courses the neck, check, and abdomen subcutaneously, with its tip emptying into the abdominal/pelvic cavity. Although obstruction of both proximal and distal VP shunt catheters can occur, distal catheter obstruction is the most commonly diagnosed VP shunt dysfunction in clinic [19]. This study shows that the injected tracer has a free access to the ventricles and then followed by a normal CSF flow filling the spinal canal, indicating patent proximal catheter, so answer A is incorrect. The normal CSF flow within ventricles and spinal canal is further evidence of patent proximal catheter, but it does not indicate the patency of the distal catheter; therefore, answer B is also incorrect. The small amount of tracer activity seen in the urinary bladder 1 hour after tracer administration is likely due to free 111-indium in the radiopharmaceutical preparation, without clinical significance. The absent tracer activity within the entire distal catheter and the abdominal/pelvic cavity throughout the study is indicating high-grade distal catheter obstruction rather than a partial obstruction; therefore, answer E is incorrect.

- Quiz #13 B

Critique: Tremor is one of the common side effects of many antipsychotic/neuroleptic drugs, especially Risperdal (risperidone), and this is often referred to as drug-induced Parkinsonism (DIP). DIP is usually indistinguishable from PD because of their similar clinical features [17, 20]. Since antipsychotic drugs block the postsynaptic dopamine receptors, DaTscan, an imaging modality for striatal presynaptic dopamine transporters, shall be normal in patients with DIP. Despite technical limitations (head tilting and patient motion), the DaTscan shows crescent-shaped, normal tracer activity in caudate nuclei and putamen of both hemispheres. Tracer activity in the left striatum is minimally decreased when compared to the right, likely due to technical artifacts, but there is no pattern to suggest a neurodegenerative process; therefore, answer C is incorrect. Answers A and D are partially correct, but are inappropriate, and certainly not the best imaging impression. Answer E is also incorrect, as the findings of this study are consistent with DIP.

- Quiz #14 A

Critique: Parietal lobe epilepsy (PLE) can be difficult to diagnose, especially in children, due to the lack of somatosensory manifestations [13,

21, 22]. In this patient, several brain MRI studies were normal. However, EEG studies revealed focal epileptiform discharges from the right parietal/posterior temporal/centrotemporal region. Consistent with the EEG results, ictal and interictal brain perfusion SPECT studies as well as SISCOM (subtraction of ictal SPECT co-registered to MRI) analysis [23–25] reveal a robust focus, corresponding to the right parietal lobe, highly suggestive of right PLE. There is no electrical or imaging evidence of right TLE, occipital lobe epilepsy (OLE), frontal lobe epilepsy (FLE), or insular lobe epilepsy (ILE), although seizure propagation to these regions cannot be excluded. Therefore, answers B to E are incorrect.

- Quiz #15 E

Critique: One of the main indications of CSF imaging is to help diagnose normal pressure hydrocephalus (NPH), although clinical significance of this application is still under debate. NPH is clinically characterized by the triad of gait apraxia, dementia, and urinary incontinence. A well-designed and executed CSF scintigraphic study not only helps diagnose NPH but also provides imaging evidence of potential benefits for CSF shunting, especially in patients with equivocal MR imaging (ventriculomegaly) and/or recurrent/persistent symptoms. This study is abnormal with evidence of persistent ventricular reflux throughout the study, even up to 72 hours; therefore, answer A is incorrect. Although MRI showed brain atrophy and ventriculomegaly, but both were moderate, unlikely causing hydrocephalus *ex vacuo*, answers C and D are incorrect. The CSF ascending to the top convexities is very slow; however, there is moderate improvement over time, suggestive of communicating hydrocephalus, in conjunction with the persistent ventricular reflux, indicating potential benefits for CSF shunting [26, 27]. Therefore, answer B is incorrect.

- Quiz #16 B

Critique: Frontotemporal dementia (FTD) is a progressive neurodegenerative syndrome with several subtypes, mainly based on clinical presentation and neuroimaging findings. The FDG PET imaging shows dominant hypometabolism in frontotemporal regions, highly suggestive of FTD; therefore, answers A, C, and D are incorrect. In contrast to the borderline dementia (MMSE score of 25/30), there was a profound impairment in language domain. Her aphasia was without evidence of halting, effortful speech or dysarthria, consistent with fluent aphasia. However, there was no evidence of significant behavioral changes or executive functional decline, so answer E is incorrect. The FDG PET findings, in conjunction with the clinical features, meet the criteria for the newly classified semantic variant primary progressive aphasia (svPPA), one of the three variants of PPA [28]. The other two are logopenic variant PPA (lvPPA) and nonfluent/agrammatic variant PPA (navPPA). Because of substantial inconsistence across institutions, at the present time, svPPA is also referred to as "semantic dementia (SD)" or "temporal variant FTD (tvFTD)."

- Quiz #17 B

Critique: Tuberous sclerosis (TS) is a rare genetic disease, often affecting multi-system and many organs including the brain leading to drug-resistant seizures, global developmental delay, and behavioral problems. On FDG PET, TS is featured with numerous cortical tubers with decreased FDG activity, scattered in cerebral cortices of both hemispheres, even involving the cerebellar cortices. The tuberous sizes and the impaired FDG intensities vary; however, there are no FDG PET imaging features suggestive of their epileptogenicity [29]; therefore, answers A, C, and D are incorrect. Due to the multi-system involvement and seizure onset in early age, seizure semiology is often not helpful in localization or lateralization of an epileptogenic focus/zone in patients with TS, so answer E is also incorrect. Instead, brain FDG PET is often requested for a baseline study in the preparation for further workup, such as brain PET with investigational tracers [14] or ictal/interictal brain perfusion SPECTs with SISCOM analysis [23–25].

- Quiz #18 D

Critique: Relative to primary central nervous system lymphoma (PCNSL), newly developed CNS lymphoma in patients with history of peripheral lymphoma is referred to as secondary CNS lymphoma (SCNSL) [30, 31]. Because SCNSL is a rare but serious complication during lymphoma treatment and follow-up and because abnormal FDG PET findings are generally lack of high specificity, further workup with or correlation with anatomic neuroimaging is an appropriate next step. Since MRI is an imaging of choice in neurooncology, answers B, C, and E are incorrect or inappropriate. Although the FDG PET finding is highly abnormal, and a biopsy is needed ultimately for definite diagnosis, performing brain biopsy without noninvasive MR imaging is inappropriate; therefore, answer A is also incorrect.

- Quiz #19 A

Critique: Cerebrospinal fluid (CSF) leak is the most common cause of spontaneous intracerebral hypotension, in which patients often present with positional/postural and severe headache [32, 33]. The underlying causes of CSF leak are largely unknown at the present time, but the treatment of choice for CSF leak is epidural blood patching; therefore, answers B, D, and E are incorrect. Because the patient had two empiric high-volume blood patching at an outside institution without significant symptom relief, and because the CSF imaging shows severe CSF leak from the lower cervical spine through the upper lumbar spine, answer C, *e.g.*, one time of high-volume epidural blood patching only targeting the lumber spine, is inappropriate. Instead, it's anticipated that treatment with multiple rounds of high-volume epidural blood patch to cover the lower cervical spine through the lumbar spine is needed for this patient.

- Quiz #20 D

Critique: Posterior cortical atrophy (PCA) is a rare progressive neurodegenerative condition often associated with AD and is now considered as a variant of AD [34]. Brain perfusion SPECT in this patient shows dominant hypoperfusion to the occipitoparietal regions, without evidence of cortical or lacunar infarcts; therefore, answers C and E are incorrect. The relatively preserved perfusion to the PCG/PCUN, and the lack of "cingulate island sign (CIS)," makes AD and DLB less likely, so answers B and A are incorrect. In clinical services, differentiation of PCA from DLB is often difficult due to their similar clinical and neuroimaging features. Nevertheless, functional neuroimaging of PCA is characterized with marked asymmetry and less involvement of cortical lobes other than occipitoparietal [35], whereas imaging findings of DLB are less asymmetric and usually associated with global/generalized hypometabolism or hypoperfusion involving not only occipitoparietal lobes but also the frontal and temporal regions, except for preserved metabolism/perfusion in the PCG/PCUN, which is referred to as "cingulate island sign (CIS)" [6, 7].

- Quiz #21 D

Critique: Insular lobe epilepsy (ILE) is uncommon and EEG localization of insular epileptogenic activity is extremely difficult due to its deep location and rapid seizure expansion and propagation [13, 15, 21]. The seizure semiology of this patient is complex but shows a significant motor component, suggestive of possible frontal lobe epilepsy (FLE) or ILE with seizure propagation/expansion. Concordant to the EEG results suggestive of a possible right deep brain seizure focus, the FDG PET imaging shows dominant hypometabolism in the right insular lobe, to a lesser degree, in the adjacent right frontal, temporal, and parietal lobes, suggestive of right ILE with seizure expansion/propagation into the rest of the right hemisphere. Therefore, answers A, B, C, and E are incorrect or inappropriate.

- Quiz #22 E

Critique: Parkinson's disease (PD) is one of the most commonly diagnosed progressive dopaminergic neurodegenerative diseases. PD is clinically characterized by both motor and non-motor features. The motor symptoms (*e.g.*, rest tremor, rigidity, and bradykinesia) are attributed to the loss of striatal dopaminergic neurons. Since dopaminergic neurons in putamen are more vulnerable to neurodegenerative insults in comparison to those in caudate nuclei, DaTscan, depending on the PD stages, typically shows decreased or absent tracer activity, first affecting one or two putamen, later involving ipsilateral caudate nuclei, and finally bilateral caudate nuclei. Therefore, asymmetric abnormality is often seen on DaTscan. According to the recent literature, approximately 76% PD patients have clinical motor symptoms corresponding to contralateral striatal dopamine transporter depletion on DaTscan. However, discordance occurs in at least 15% patients [36]. Clinically, the patient presents with right arm and hand tremor for 5 months. His motor symptoms have improved after treatment with Sinemet, indicating a good response to L-dopa pharmacotherapy. The DaTscan shows nearly absent tracer activity in bilateral putamen, as well as both caudate nuclei, indicating advanced PD, right striatum being more affected than the left. Therefore, answers A to D are incorrect or inappropriate.

- Quiz #23 E

Critique: As aforementioned, frontotemporal dementia (FTD) is a progressive neurodegenerative syndrome with several subtypes, mainly based on clinical presentation and neuroimaging findings. In this patient, his clinical presentation is dominated by complex behavioral problems, in addition to memory loss and functional decline. Consistent with brain MRI and CT findings, FDG PET shows dominant hypometabolism in frontotemporal regions, right > left, suggestive of FTD. In contrast, metabolism in the PCG/PCUN and the occipital lobes is preserved or relatively preserved. Additionally, there is no evidence of cortical or lacunar infarcts. Therefore, answers A, C, and D are incorrect. Although the patient complains speech difficulties, the language impairment is not a dominant clinical feature, so answer B is incorrect. Instead, this patient meets the international consensus criteria for diagnosis of probable behavior variant FTD (bvFTD) [37].

- Quiz #24 E

Critique: Brain death scintigraphy is sometimes requested mainly for confirmation in patients that have met clinical criteria of brain death. The standardized imaging protocol [38] from the society of nuclear medicine practice guidelines requires acquisition of flow imaging, planar imaging, and SPECT imaging, following IV administration of radiopharmaceutical, to maintain highest accuracy. Brain perfusion study of this patient, however, was technically limited due to patient's unstable vitals. As a result, limited images were obtained using a mobile camera. Despite the technical limitation, the study showed no perfusion to the brain parenchyma including the brain stem, direct imaging evidence of brain death; instead, increased flow to the nasal region was noted, consistent with so-called "hot nose sign," indirect imaging evidence of brain death. Therefore, answers A and C are incorrect, while answers B and D are inappropriate/incomplete.

- Quiz #25 C

Critique: Corticobasal degeneration (CBD), previously referred to as cortical basal ganglia degeneration (CBGD), is a rare progressive neurodegenerative disorder, which is clinically characterized by asymmetric cortical dysfunction (ideomotor apraxia and alien limb phenomena) and extrapyramidal dysfunction (limb rigidity and/or dystonia) [8]. On FDG PET, CBD is featured by an imaging triad, including (i) cortical hypometabolism of unilateral frontal lobe (posterior/middle > anterior) or frontoparietal region, (ii) hypometabolic involvement of the underlying basal ganglia, and (iii) crossed cerebrocerebellar diaschisis. This patient presents with cortical dysfunction, such as pain and uncomfortable sensation in her legs. The FDG PET shows preserved metabolism in occipital lobes and parietal lobes including the PCG/PCUN, making DLB and AD less likely. Therefore, answers A and B are incorrect. Instead, dominant hypometabolism is noted in the left frontal lobe, more prominent in the posterior and middle portion, in conjunction with the left striatal hypometabolism and right cerebellar diaschisis, consistent with CBD rather than FTD, so answer D is incorrect. Although the patient complains of difficulty in speaking, this is not a dominant clinical feature. Also, only mild hypometabolism is noted in the left temporal lobe, likely due to disease spread from the dominantly affected left frontal lobe. There are no clinical or imaging features to suggest primary progressive aphasia (PPA). Therefore, answer E is incorrect.

- Quiz #26 E

Critique: DaTscan was approved by the FDA in 2011 for clinical use in the US to help differentiate essential tremor (ET) from tremor due to Parkinson's disease (PD), multiple system atrophy (MSA), or progressive supranuclear palsy (PSP). PSP, also referred to as *Steele-Richardson-Olszewski syndrome*, is an uncommon neurodegenerative disorder leading to progressive impairment of balance and walking, as well as eye movements [39]. This patient presented with a chief complaint of rapid decline in balance and frequent falls. Despite the lack of ophthalmological exam results, MRI showed midbrain atrophy, with a "hummingbird sign," which is an imaging hallmark of PSP. The DaTscan shows decreased tracer activity in the right striatum and possibly left putamen. Therefore, answer B is incorrect. There are no clinical or imaging features to suggest MSA or CBD, so answers C and D are also incorrect. Although the patient complains of both hand tremors, this is not a dominant clinical feature. Moreover, the DaTscan shows an essential normal left striatum and decreased tracer activity in the entire right striatum, equally affecting the caudate nuclei and putamen, in a pattern suggestive of PSP rather than PD. Therefore, answer A is incorrect.

- Quiz #27 B

Critique: Although majority of temporal lobe epilepsies (TLEs) originate from the medial (mesial) portion, approximately 20% of TLEs can arise from the lateral temporal cortex [15, 21]. Lateral temporal lobe epilepsies (LTLEs) are often difficult to diagnose due to the propensity of seizure propagation or expansion. This patient's seizures were preceded with auras, a clinical feature suggesting TLE. EEGs also showed intermittent rhythmic delta activity (TIRDA) in the right temporal region. Consistent with the clinico-electrical data, FDG PET shows dominant hypometabolism in the right temporal lobe, in conjunction with diaschisis involving the ipsilateral thalamus and contralateral cerebellum, highly suggestive of right TLE. Although mild hypometabolism is noted in the adjacent right fronto-parieto-occipital lobes, the subtle finding is likely sequelae of seizure propagation or expansion. Therefore, answers A, D, and E are incorrect. When compared to the left temporal lobe, metabolism in the right mesial temporal lobe is symmetric and is relatively preserved. In contrast, cortical metabolism in the right lateral temporal lobe is markedly decreased and, in conjunction with the normal MRI, is in support of diagnosis of LTLE rather than MTLE. Therefore, answer C is incorrect.

- Quiz #28 A

Critique: The Wada test, named after Dr. Juhn Atsuchi Wada, also referred to as "intracarotid sodium amobarbital procedure (ISAP)," is sometimes performed to help determine brain hemispheric functional dominance/reserve as part of pre-surgical evaluation [40]. Brain perfusion SPECT is occasionally requested as part of the Wada test, mainly for confirmation of expected hypoperfusion in the ipsilateral hemisphere and intact perfusion in the contralateral. The scintigraphic data predominantly reflects pharmacological effects of intracarotid sodium amobarbital, with no implication in cerebrovascular reserve (CVR), underlying disease, or hemispheric functional dominance. Therefore, answers B to E are incorrect or inappropriate.

- Quiz #29 B

Critique: As aforementioned, lateral temporal lobe epilepsies (LTLEs) are uncommon when compared to the mesial temporal lobe epilepsies

(MTLEs). But LTLEs are often difficult to diagnose due to the propensity of seizure propagation and/or expansion [41]. Although the seizure semiology in this patient is atypical for TLE, multiple EEG studies showed focal seizures with somatosensory aura and regional seizure activities in the right fronto-temporal area. The ictal/interictal SPECT studies and SISCOM analysis [23–25] reveals a delta focus co-registered to the lateral cortex of the right temporal lobe posteriorly, suggestive of right LTLE rather than MTLE. Therefore, answer D is incorrect. In contrast, there is no SISCOM data to suggest a seizure focus/zone in the adjacent right frontal, parietal, or occipital lobe, although seizure propagation/expansion cannot be excluded. Therefore, answers A, C, and E are also incorrect.

- Quiz #30 E

Critique: The underlying cause of hydrocephalus *ex vacuo* is compensatory enlargement of the CSF spaces leading to ventriculomegaly and enlargement of subarachnoid spaces, primarily secondary to marked encephalic volume loss/atrophy. This patient presented with a classic triad of ataxia, dementia, and urinary incontinence for clinical diagnosis of normal pressure hydrocephalus (NPH). CT and MRI revealed ventriculomegaly, which is indistinguishable from NPH. CSF imaging shows delayed CSF flow, more prominent in the right brain; however, there is no evidence of ventricular reflux, making NPH less likely. Therefore, answers A and B are incorrect. Although the patient complains of memory loss, there are no motor symptoms, nor MR imaging evidence, to suggest AD or PD. Answers C and D are therefore incorrect or incomplete. The diagnosis of hydrocephalus *ex vacuo* (answer E) in this patient is indirectly supported by the prior high-volume CSF removal with no symptom relief.

References

1. Brown RK, Bohnen NI, Wong KK, et al. Brain PET in suspected dementia: patterns of altered FDG metabolism. Radiographics. 2014;34:684–701.
2. Ishii K. PET approaches for diagnosis of dementia. Am J Neuroradiol. 2014;35(11):2030–8.
3. Marcus C, Mena E, Subramaniam RM. Brain PET in the diagnosis of Alzheimer's disease. Clin Nucl Med. 2014;39:e413–26.
4. Shivamurthy VKN, Tahari AK, Marcus C, et al. Brain FDG PET and the diagnosis of dementia. Am J Radiology. 2015;204:W76–85.
5. Silverman DHS. Brain F-18 FDG PET in the diagnosis of neurodegenerative dementias: comparison with perfusion SPECT and with clinical evaluation lacking nuclear imaging. J Nucl Med. 2004;45:594–607.
6. Mak E, Su L, Williams GB, O'Brien JT. Neuroimaging characteristics of dementia with Lewy bodies. Alzheimers Res Ther. 2014;6(2):18–27.
7. Lim SM, Katsifis A, Villemagne VL, et al. The 18F-FDG cingulate island sign and comparison to 123I-beta CIT SPECT for diagnosis of dementia with Lewy bodies. J Nucl Med. 2009;50(10):1638–45.
8. Armstrong MJ, Litvan I, Lang AE, et al. Criteria for the diagnosis of corticobasal degeneration. Neurology. 2013;80:496–503.
9. Chen W. Clinical applications of PET in brain tumors. J Nucl Med. 2007;48(9):1468–81.
10. Demetriades AK, Almeida AC, Bhangoo RS, et al. Application of positron emission tomography in neuro-oncology: a clinical approach. Surgeon. 2014;12(3):148–57.
11. Wang X, Hu X, Xie P, et al. Comparison of magnetic resonance spectroscopy and positron emission tomography in detection of tumor recurrence in posttreatment of glioma: a diagnostic meta-analysis. Asia Pac J Clin Oncol. 2015;11(2):97–105.
12. Vagal AS, Leach JL, Fernandez-Ulloa M, et al. The acetazolamide challenge: techniques and applications in the evaluation of chronic cerebral ischemia. AJNR. 2009;30(5):876–84.
13. Cendes F, Theodore WH, Brinkmann BH, et al. Neuroimaging of epilepsy. Handb Clin Neurol. 2016;136:985–1014.
14. Kagawa K, Chugani DC, Asano E, et al. Epilepsy surgery outcome in children with tuberous sclerosis complex evaluated with alpha-[11C]-methyl-L-tryptophan positron emission tomography (PET). J Child Neurol. 2005;20(5):429–38.
15. Rathore C, Dickson JC, Teotonio R, et al. The utility of 18F-fluorodeoxyglucose PET (FDG PET) in epilepsy surgery. Epilepsy Res. 2014;108:1306–14.
16. Massey L, Micallef C, Paviour DC, et al. Conventional magnetic resonance imaging in confirmed progressive supranuclear palsy and multiple system atrophy. Mov Disord. 2012;27:1754–62.
17. Gayed I, Joseph U, Fanous M, et al. The impact of DaTSCAN in the diagnosis of Parkinson disease. Clin Nucl Med. 2015;40(5):390–3.
18. Zhu X-C, Tan L, Wang H-F, et al. Rate of early onset of Alzheimer's disease: a systematic review and meta-analysis. Ann Transl Med. 2015;3(3):38–43.
19. Chiewvit S, Nuntaaree S, Kanchaanapiboon P, et al. Assessment of lumboperitoneal or ventriculoperitoneal shunt patency by radionuclide technique: a review experience cases. World J Nucl Med. 2014;13(2):75–84.
20. Shin H-W, Chung SJ. Drug-induced Parkinsonim. J Clin Neurol. 2012;8:15–21.
21. Kumar A, Chugani HT. The role of radionuclide imaging in epilepsy, part 1: sporadic temporal and extratemporal lobe epilepsy. J Nucl Med Technol. 2017;45(1):14–21.
22. Kumar A, Chugani HT. Application of PET and SPECT in pediatric epilepsy surgery. In: Cataltepe O, Jallo GI, editors. Pediatric epilepsy surgery: preoperative assessment and surgical treatment. New York: Thieme; 2010. p. 82–98.
23. Chen T, Guo L. The role of SISCOM in preoperative evaluation for patients with epi-

lepsy surgery: a meta-analysis. Seizure. 2016;41:43–60.
24. O'Brien T, O'Connor M, Mullan B, et al. Subtraction ictal SPECT co-registered to MRI in partial epilepsy: description and technical validation of the method with phantom and patient studies. Nucl Med Comm. 1998;19:31–45.
25. O'Brien T, So EL, Mullan B, et al. Subtraction ictal SPECT co-registered to MRI improves postictal SPECT localization of seizure foci. Neurology. 1999;52:137–46.
26. Jacobs L, Conti D, Kinkel WR, et al. "Normal-pressure" hydrocephalus. Relationship of clinical and radiographic findings to improvement following shunt surgery. JAMA. 1976;235(5):510–2.
27. Kitami K, Suzuki A, Hadeishi H, et al. Normal pressure hydrocephalus after subarachnoid hemorrhage – with regard to pathogenesis and factors influencing the efficacy of shunt surgery. No To Shinkei. 1986;38(8):781–8.
28. Gorno-Tempini ML, Hillis AE, Weintraub S, et al. Classification of primary progressive aphasia and its variants. Neurology. 2011;76:1006–14.
29. Babak N, Kalantari, Salamon N. Neuroimaging of tuberous sclerosis: spectrum of pathologic findings and frontiers in imaging. Am J Roentgenol. 2008;190:W304–9.
30. Malikova H, Burghardtova M, Koubska E, et al. Secondary central nervous system lymphoma: spectrum of morphological MRI appearances. Neuropschyiatr Dis Treat. 2018;14:733–40.
31. Tang YZ, Booth TC, Bhogal P, et al. Imaging of primary central nervous system lymphoma. Clin Radiol. 2011;66(8):768–077.
32. Ali SA, Cesani F, Zuckermann JA, et al. Spinal-cerebrospinal fluid leak demonstrated by radiopharmaceutical cisternography. Clin Nucl Med. 1998;23(3):52–15.
33. Limaye K, Samant R, Lee RW. Spontaneous intracranial hypotension: diagnosis to management. Acta Neurol Belg. 2016;116(2):119–25.
34. Meyer MA, Hudock SA. Posterior cortical atrophy: a rare variant of Alzheimer's disease. Neuro Int. 2018;10(2):51–3.
35. Gupta V, Verma R, Ranjan R, et al. Metabolic imaging patterns in posterior cortical atrophy and Lewy body dementia. Nucl Med Commun. 2019;40(12):1275–82.
36. Kuo PH, Lei HH, Avery R, et al. Evaluation of an objective striatal analysis program for determining laterality in uptake of I-123-ioflupane SPECT images: comparison to clinical symptoms and to visual reads. J Nucl Med Technol. 2014;42(2):105–8.
37. Rascovak K, Hodges JR, Knopman D, et al. Sensitivity of revised diagnosis criteria for the behavioral variant of frontotemporal dementia. Brain. 2011;134(9): 2456–77.
38. Donohoe KJ, Agrawal G, Frey KA, et al. SNM practice guideline for brain death scintigraphy 2.0. J Nucl Med Technol. 2012;40(3):198–203.
39. Ling H. Clinical approach to progressive supranuclear palsy. J Mov Disord. 2016;9(1):3–13.
40. Wada JA. A new method for the determination of the side of cerebral speech dominance. A preliminary report of the intra-carotid injection of sodium amytal in man (article in Japanese). Igaku to Seibutsugaki, Tokyo. 1949;14:221–2.
41. Vaugier L, Aubert S, McGonigal A, et al. Neural networks underlying hyperkinetic seizures of "temporal lobe" origin. Epilepsy Res. 2009;86(2):200–8.

Appendix II: Imaging Protocols

FDG PET CT Brain Imaging

Reference

Waxman AD, Herholz K, Lewis DH, et al. Society of nuclear medicine procedure guideline for FDG PET brain imaging, Version 1.0, approved February 8, 2009.

Principle

CT provides a map of the head/brain for attenuation correction and anatomic localization. Glucose is used as a dominant energy source for the brain, and FDG PET provides a distribution of glucose in the brain. Together, the attenuation-corrected PET images are useful in detection of abnormal glucose metabolism, if any, in the brain.

Indications in Our Clinic

Seizure focus/zone localization, dementia profiling/workup, differentiation of brain tumor recurrence versus post-radiation necrosis, and evaluation of traumatic brain injury.

Radiopharmaceutical and Dosage

- F-18 FDG (decay half-life:110 minutes)
- Dosage for adult patients: 10–15 mCi (370–555 MBq)
- Dosage for pediatric patients: 0.143 mCi/kg (5.29 MBq/kg), with a minimum dose of 1 mCi (37 MBq)

Patient Preparation

- NPO >4–6 hours prior to scheduled time.
- IV fluid containing dextrose or parenteral feeding should be withheld for at least 4–6 hours.
- Pregnancy and breastfeeding – See Society of Nuclear Medicine general procedure guidelines.
- For seizure patients, make sure that EEG monitoring is in place and if anesthesia is needed.

Procedure

1. Patient check-in procedure:
    (a) Check for order in chart and/or prescription.
    (b) Identify patient using two methods – verbally and by patient's identification wristband.
    (c) Explain procedure in a courteous and understandable manner.
    (d) Obtain brief but pertinent history from patient, including but not limited to current medications, drug allergies, prior neuroimaging studies (CT, MRI, PET, or SPECT), head trauma, seizures, memory issues, TIA or stroke, brain tumors and treatment history, and brain operations including shunt procedures.
    (e) Verify patient preparation conditions.

D. Wu, *Clinical Nuclear Medicine Neuroimaging*, https://doi.org/10.1007/978-3-030-40893-0

2. Patient should rest in a dimly lit, low stimulus room for at least 10 minutes prior to FDG injection. Obtain and document patient blood glucose level prior to FDG injection. Whole blood at injection site or finger stick method can be used. A blood glucose monitoring instrument called Accu-Chek Advantage is used at this institution. If blood glucose level is 150–200 mg/dL, the study will be performed or rescheduled at the discretion of on-duty physician. Once blood glucose is over 200 mg/dL, the study shall be rescheduled.
3. FDG dose is administered intravenously with insured proper radiation safety. A lead cart should be used for transporting the FDG dose to patient's prep room and lead syringe shield for the dose syringe, kept in place during injection process.
4. Total uptake time of FDG is 30–60 minutes. Patient should be relaxed and kept warm and comfortable during the uptake time.
5. After 30–60 minutes, position patient on scanning bed with head in the head holder.
   (a) Liberal use of Velcro straps is recommended to minimize motion.
   (b) Secure arms at the patient's side.
   (c) Position the knee cushion
6. Image acquisition is performed in 3D mode. Image reconstruction includes attenuation correction with typical pixel size of 2 mm. The imaging data is displayed in transaxial, sagittal, and coronal planes as well as a three-dimensional volume-rendered display.

Amyoid PET Imaging of the Brain

Reference

Minoshima S, Drzezga AE, Djekidel M, et al. SNMMI procedure standard-EANM practice guideline for Amyloid PET imaging of the brain, approved by the SNMMI Board of Directors on 01/30/2016.

Principle

CT provides a map of the brain for attenuation correction and anatomic localization. PET with either^{18}F-Florbetapir (Amyvid™, Eli Lilly) or ^{18}F-Flutemetamol (Vizamyl™, GE Healthcare) provides a distribution of amyloid plaques in the brain. Together, the attenuation-corrected PET images are useful in defining amyloid plaque status in the brain (negative versus positive). Of note, the FDA also approved the use of ^{18}F-Florbetaben (NeuraCeq™, Piramal Pharma), a third PET amyloid imaging agent in the USA; however, this radiopharmaceutical has yet to be used in our institution.

Appropriate Clinical Indications

1. Patients with persistent/progressive unexplained mild cognitive impairment (MCI)
2. Patients who meet the core clinical criteria for possible Alzheimer's disease (AD) but have an unclear clinical presentation – either an atypical clinical course or an etiologically mixed presentation
3. Patients with progressive dementia and a typically early age of onset (usually defined as 65 years or younger in age)

Radiopharmaceutical and Dosage

- ^{18}F-Florbetapir (Amyvid™, Eli Lilly) 10 mCi (370 MBq)
- ^{18}F-Flutemetamol(Vizamyl™, GE Healthcare) 5 mCi (185 MBq)

Patient Prep

No fast required

Procedure

1. Patient check-in procedure:
   (a) Check for order in chart and/or prescription.
   (b) Identify patient verbally and/or patient identification wristband.
   (c) Explain procedure in a courteous and understandable manner.
   (d) Obtain brief and pertinent history from patient, including medications and drug allergies.
   (e) Verify patient preparation conditions.
2. Injection of ^{18}F-Florbetapir or ^{18}F-Flutemetamol I.V. Insure proper radiation safety. A lead cart should be used for transporting dose to patient prep room and lead

syringe shield for the dose syringe, kept in place during injection process.

3. Total uptake time of ^{18}F-Florbetapir or ^{18}F-Flutemetamol is 45 minutes (30–50 minutes) or 60 minutes (60–120 minutes), respectively, with patient being kept warm, relaxed, and comfortable during the uptake time.
4. Patient should void urine bladder prior to scanning.
5. At the end of the uptake time, position patient on scanning bed with head in the head holder.
   (a) Liberal use of Velcro straps is recommended to minimize motion.
   (b) Secure arms at the patient's side.
   (c) Position the knee cushion.
6. Image acquisition is performed in 3D mode. Image reconstruction includes attenuation correction with typical pixel size of 2 mm. The imaging data is displayed in transaxial, sagittal, and coronal planes as well as a three-dimensional volume-rendered display.

Brain Perfusion SPECT

References

1. Juni JE, Waxman AD, Devous MD, et al. Procedure guideline for brain perfusion SPECT using ^{99m}Tc radiopharmaceuticals 3.0. Approved by SNM Board of Directors on 2/8/2009.
2. Kapucu OL, Nobili F, Varrone A, et al. EANM procedure guideline for brain perfusion SPECT using ^{99m}Tc Radiopharmaceuticals, version 2. Eur J Nucl Med Mol Imaging. Published on line: October 17, 2009.

Principle

Blood supply/perfusion to the brain is approximately 15% of the cardiac output. SPECT with appropriate radiopharmaceuticals produces tomographic images of brain perfusion in a three-dimensional distribution.

Indications in Our Clinic

1. Pre-surgical lateralization or localization of epileptogenic foci/zones
2. Evaluation of dementias and/or cerebrovascular disease
3. Evaluation of Lyme encephalopathy
4. Assessment of brain death

Radiopharmaceutical and Dosage

- Tc-99 m Neurolite (ethyl cystine dimer [ECD]): 30 mCi (1110 MBq)

Patient Prep

1. Have all the patients void urine bladder, if possible, prior to the start to the study.
2. For patients with planned premedication of Diamox (a potent cerebral vasodilator used for a challenge study), 1000 mg in 10 cc sterile water will be given IV over 2–3 minutes by a physician. For pediatric patients, Diamox dose is 14 mg/kg body weight. *Contraindications: allergy to sulfa drugs.* General caution is applied for patients with renal and hepatic insufficiency. Occasional side effects include light-headedness, vertigo, tinnitus (ringing in the ears), and flushing. These symptoms are generally transient and require no direct action beyond reassurance and keeping the patient in a supervised area until all symptoms have subsided/resolved.
3. For patients scheduled for ictal or interictal brain perfusion SPECT, Tc-99m Neurolite will be IV injected by staff members in our inpatient epilepsy monitoring unit (EMU). Make sure that the radiopharmaceutical is accurately calibrated, with clearly marked expiration in terms of date and time. For ictal studies, the seizure onset time, radioactive tracer injection time, and syringe/tube flusing time shall be clearly documented in hour/minute/second.

Procedure

1. General:
   (a) Patient check-in procedure per protocol.
   (b) Obtain pertinent history.
   (c) Start an intima insuring good IV access.
   (d) Place patient in a quiet, dimly lit room, and wait a minimum of 15 minutes before tracer dosing.
   (e) Avoid any conversation, inject the patient, and leave the room.

   (f) After tracer dosing, wait for 5 minutes before moving the patient.
   (g) Have patient return a minimum of 45 minutes and maximum of 2 hours post tracer dose for imaging.
2. For patients with scheduled premedication of Diamox, wait for a minimum of 30 minutes before tracer dosing.
3. For patients scheduled for ictal brain perfusion SPECT, clearly document the following: seizure onset time, tracer injection time, and IV flushing time in hour/minute/second, respectively.

Equipment and Setup

1. General: Using the head holder, place the patient on the table, and then hit SET. Verify the Infinia acquisition is set for the following default parameters:
   (a) LEUHR (fan beam) collimators
   (b) Step and shoot
   (c) 15 sec/frame for 120 frames (36 minutes)
   (d) 128 × 128 matrix
   (e) Zoom 1.0 pan Y: −20
   (f) Total angular range: 2 × 360
   (g) On the acquisition controller, adjust the camera heads (using hand control only) to the following parameters: bed height, 69–75; radius, 13–15 no >18 cm; and table trans (−10)–(−14).
2. For patients undergoing brain death scintigraphy, arrange with nursing staff to have respiratory therapist available for transport and during imaging, imaging in a room that has wall oxygen and suction available
   (a) Position the camera over the patient's head and acquire flow and static images.
   (b) Flow images should start before the arrival of the tracer bolus in the neck and end well after the venous phase.
   (c) Equipment and set-up with acquisition parameters in the following:
      - Dynamic phase #1: 2 sec/frame for 60 seconds (2 minutes), 128 × 128 matrix
      - Dynamic phase #2:60 sec/frame for 19 frames (19 minutes), 128 × 128 matrix
      - Static phase: acquire anterior and posterior and right lateral and left lateral images at a minimum of 20 minutes postinjection for the following parameters – 5 minutes per view, 128 × 128 matrix, and no zoom
   (d) SPECT allows better visualization of perfusion to the posterior fossa and brain stem structures and should be performed whenever possible with the following parameters:128 × 128 matrix, no zoom, and 20 seconds/stop.

Brain Dopamine Transporter Scan (DaTscan)

Reference

Djang DSW, Janssen MJR, Bohnen N, et al. SNM practice guideline for dopamine transporter imaging with ^{123}I-Ioflupane SPECT 1.0. J Nucl Med 53(1): 154–163, 2012

Principle

Brain SPECT with ^{123}I-Ioflupane that selectively binds to striatal presynaptic dopamine transporter protein in the caudate nucleus and putamen produces tomographic images indicating CNS dopamine neurons' status.

Indications

The main indication is to assist in the evaluation of adult patients with suspected Parkinsonian syndromes. DaTscan may be used to help differentiate essential tremor (ET) from tremor due to idiopathic Parkinson's disease (PD), multiple system atrophy (MSA), and progressive supranuclear palsy (PSP).

Radiopharmaceutical and Dosage

- I-123 DaTscan™
- 5 mCi via slow (15–20 seconds) intravenous injection (range 3–5 mCi)

Patient Prep

Prearrival: Review current medications to determine possible drugs that could interfere with DaTscan imaging. Potential interfering medications are listed as the following: amoxapine, amphetamine, benztropine, bupropion, buspirone, cocaine, methamphetamine, methylphenidate, mazindol, norephedrine, paroxetine, phentermine, phenylpropanolamine, selegiline, and sertraline. If the patient is on any of the medications listed on the drug interference list, consult the ordering physician to determine if the patient can be safely taken off the drug for five of its T1/2.

Pre-dosing

1. Prior to dosing patient, cross-reference with notes from radiopharmacist to ensure the potential interfering medication recommendations have been followed initially.
2. Administer a single dose thyroid-blocking agent (IOSAT tablet, 130 mg, by mouth) at least 60 minutes before the dose of I-123-DaTscan™. If patient has iodine allergy, he or she will be given a single dose of potassium perchlorate (400 mg, by mouth), 60 minutes prior to the dose of I-123-DaTscan™.
3. Advise patient to hydrate prior to and following I-23 DaTscan™ administration to permit frequent voiding.

Procedure

1. General: follow patient check-in procedure per protocol.
2. Follow pregnancy protocol for women of childbearing age.
3. Review patient history and confirm with the patient.
4. Administer one dose of thyroid blocking agent. Wait at least 60 minutes prior to dosing with I-123 DaTscan™.
5. Start the intima insuring good IV access.
6. Dose patient with I-123 DaTscan™ using a saline flush (slowly over 15–20 seconds).
7. After dosing, have patient return 3–6 hours postinjection for imaging. It is recommended to keep imaging times postinjection as consistent as possible for all patients, so a return time of 3 hours will be the standard time we always try to achieve.

Equipment Setup and Image Acquisition

1. Ensure g-level reset has been performed prior to any brain scan imaging. Using fan beam collimators (LEUHR) and the GE Infinia system, set up the patient using the I-123 DaTscan™ Brain SPECT protocol.
2. Verify that the Infinia acquisition is set for the following default parameters:
   To open patient acquisition:
   - User
   - Brain
   - SPECT fan beam (preferred)

or

   - SPECT LEHR (only if patient cannot be imaged with fan beams due to body habitus)
     (a) LEUHR fan beam collimators
     (b) 159 KEV +/− 10% window
     (c) Step and shoot
     (d) 15 sec/frame for 120 frames (36 minutes)
     (e) 128 × 128 matrix
     (f) Zoom 1.0 Pan Y: −20
     (g) Total angular range 2 × 360

3. It is important to use the head holder for all patients. A lateral head tilt may make a normal image look abnormal if transverse realignment cannot be completed successfully. Take time to make sure the patient's head is aligned properly and is straight throughout the study. Position patient with their chin down. Decrease patient motion by using head, arm, and leg straps.
4. It is vital for this study to achieve the minimal camera radius. Place the camera as close to the patient's head as physically possible without touching. The best image resolution occurs with a radius of rotation of 11–15 cm. An ideal radius for imaging successfully is 13 cm. At no time should the radius exceed 15 cm. It is more important to achieve a close radius than to include all of the lower areas of the brain. The occipital lobe of the brain should be included in the image for quantitative analysis.
5. On the acquisition controller, adjust the camera heads to the following parameters: bed height, 69–75; radius, 13–15 cm; table trans (−10)–(14); and rotate the detectors to check clearance, and then hit GO. Do not hit SET again.

6. Write down the parameters for each patient in the brain scan book and the dose sheet.
7. Process the imaging data according to the current protocol for processing DaTscan studies.

Cisternogram (CSF Scintigraphy)

Purpose

- To visualize the distribution and flow of the cerebrospinal fluid (CSF)

Indications

- To aid in the diagnosis of normal pressure hydrocephalus (NPH)
- To evaluate abnormal CSF flow patterns

Radiopharmaceutical and Dosage

- In-111 DTPA 1 mCi (37 MBq)

Patient Preparation/Scheduling

1. The referring physician should fax a completed history form, medication list, and order to our schedulers. After the schedulers have verified insurance, they will give the information to the special studies team for screening and scheduling. Any contraindication for having a lumbar puncture or a cisternogram will be determined at this time. A nuclear medicine physician needs to review history and sign.
2. The patient will be screened for anticoagulant therapy such as heparin or coumadin or new medications such as Pradaxa (dabigatran), Xarelto (rivaroxaban), and Eliquis (apixaban). If patient has had recent anticoagulant therapy, a PT, PTT clotting time should be run to determine whether a lumbar puncture can be performed. Interventional radiology department will determine the time necessary for the discontinuation of anticoagulant therapy prior to performing the lumbar puncture.

Procedure

1. General:
   (a) Follow standard check-in procedure.
   (b) Verify order and review the pertinent history that has already been completed by the special studies team.
   (c) Verify the test has been explained and all questions have been answered.
   (d) Verify patient is off all blood thinners as pre-arranged.
   (e) If patient is a female between ages 12 and 55 years, an image procedure safety assessment form regarding pregnancy should be completed.
2. Administration of radiotracer:
   (a) The lumbar puncture and subsequent dosing will be performed in interventional radiology.
   (b) When bringing the dose to interventional radiology:
      (i). Enter the dose in computer for radiopharmacy dispensing.
      (ii). Review order and explain procedure. Give patient return time for images and location of our nuclear medicine clinic.
      (iii). A final verification form must be completed.
   (c) Upon completion of the injection, the spinal needle will be removed by the radiologist. The nuclear medicine technologist will dispose of the needle and any contaminated items in the medium energy waste container in the radiopharmacy.
3. Imaging:
   (a) Patient is imaged at the following time intervals postinjection:
      (i). 24-hour static images to cover the top of the head through the pelvis including the urinary bladder and SPECT imaging the brain including the basal cisterns
      (ii). 48-hour static images and SPECT
      (iii). 72-hour static images only when requested by ordering physician
   (b) Static acquisition parameters:
      (i). Ensure current In-111 uniformity correction is in place.
      (ii). Medium energy parallel hole collimator.
      (iii). In-111 peaked on 172 KeV with a 20% window and 247 KeV with a 20% window.
      (iv). 128 × 128 matrix.

   (v). Static images are 10 minutes per projection.
   (vi). Anterior/posterior and right lateral/left lateral static views.
(c) SPECT acquisition parameters as the following:
   (i). Ensure current In-111 uniformity correction is in place.
   (ii). Medium energy parallel hole collimator.
   (iii). In-111 peaked on 172 KeV with a 20% window and 247 KeV with a 20% window.
   (iv). 64 × 64 matrix, 30 seconds/stop. 120–128 projections.
(d) SPECT image processing:
   (i). To process SPECT images on a Xeleris.
   (ii). Under "all applications", use "brain" and or "IR cisternogram SPECT Recon" as instructed to complete processing.
   (iii). Transfer SPECT raw data and transaxial oblique images (SPECT 24H_IRNC transaxial) to PACS.

CSF Leak Scintigraphy With or Without Pledgets

Purpose

- To evaluate cerebrospinal fluid (CSF) leak from the skull base or in the spine

Indications

- To aid in the diagnosis of basal skull fractures, to determine positional headache etiology, and to evaluate CSF rhinorrhea

Radiopharmaceutical and Dosage

In-111 DTPA 1 mCi (37 MBq)

Patient Preparation/Scheduling

1. The referring physician should fax a completed history form, medication list, and order to our schedulers. After the schedulers have verified insurance, they will give the information to the special studies team for screening and scheduling. Any contraindication for having a lumbar puncture or a cisternogram will be determined at this time. A nuclear medicine physician needs to review history and sign.
2. The patient will be screened for anticoagulant therapy such as heparin or coumadin or new medications such as Pradaxa (dabigatran), Xarelto (rivaroxaban), and Eliquis (apixaban). If patient has had recent anticoagulant therapy, a PT, PTT clotting time should be run to determine whether a lumbar puncture can be performed. Interventional radiology department will determine the time necessary for the discontinuation of anticoagulant therapy prior to performing the lumbar puncture.
3. Pledgets are placed by an ENT doctor, if indicated or ordered. Patients should call the ENT doctor office for a consult and or setup an appointment for a date and time for pledget placement.
4. Once date for pledget placement is arranged, make an appointment in interventional radiology for the lumber puncture to be performed. Contact the anesthesia appointment schedulers to arrange it. A script for LP will be required.
5. In-111 DTPA can be injected before or after the pledgets are placed. This will be determined prior to scheduled date and arranged by the special studies team.

Procedure

1. General:
   (a) Follow standard check-in procedure.
   (b) Verify order and review pertinent history that has already been completed by the special studies team.
   (c) Verify the test has been explained and all questions have been answered.
   (d) Verify patient is off all blood thinners as pre-arranged.
   (e) If patient is a female between ages 12 and 55 years, an image procedure safety assessment form regarding pregnancy should be completed.
2. Administration of radiotracer (intervention radiology):
   (a) The interventional radiologist will perform LP and inject In-111 DTPA intrathecally.
   (b) Prepare the patient:

1. Check order, explain procedure, and verify if patient is off all blood thinners.
2. Have patient sign the consent form.
3. Enter dose in computer for radiopharmacy dispensing.

(c) Deliver the dose to interventional radiology to be administered.

(d) A final verification form must be completed.

(e) Upon completion of the intrathecal injection, the spinal needle will be removed by the radiologist. The nuclear medicine technologist will dispose of the needle and any contaminated items in the medium energy waste container in the radiopharmacy.

3. Placement of the pledgets:

Placement of Pledgets can be done before or after injection of In-111 DTPA (always within 4 hours if injection is first). Pledgets placement will take place in an ENT doctor office. Nuclear medicine will supply the pledgets, with labeling each pledget site on the attached string. Retain the remainder of pledgets in the package to acquire the average standard dry weight.

4. Image acquisition:

(a) Patient will be imaged at these time intervals postinjection of In-111 DTPA as the following:

1. 6-hour static image
2. 24-hour static image
3. 48-hour static image (if necessary)

(b) Static acquisition parameters:

1. Ensure current In-111 uniformity correction is in place.
2. Medium energy parallel hole collimator.
3. In-111 peaked on 172 KeV with a 20% window and 247 KeV with a 20%window.
4. 128 × 128 matrix.
5. Static images are acquired for a minimum of 200 k or 10 minutes.
6. Anterior/posterior and right lateral/left lateral with the patient in the PRONE projection (if possible) to maximize leak, if any.
7. All views should be performed with a radioactive marker at the vertex skull to serve as a point of reference. If a maneuver is known by the patient to provoke leak, such as bearing down, this should be accomplished.
8. *Additionally*, obtain an anterior abdominal image at 24 hours (minimum of 10 minutes) including the stomach. This image may be acquired in supine or prone position of the patient.

5. Removal of pledgets and calculations:

(a) Remove pledgets and place in plastic bag at 24 hours.

(b) Weigh each pledget immediately using a Mettler balance to avoid any drying of the fluid on the pledgets. Always use and weigh Mettler scale liner prior to placing and weighing wet pads.

(c) Place pledgets and linear into pre-labeled tubes.

(d) Weigh a sample pledget from the lot used and record weight.

(e) e. Calculate the weight of nasal fluid: (wet pledgets weight) – (sample pledget weight and scale linear).

(f) When pledgets are removed, draw 5 ml blood in a purple top tube. Centrifuge 2000 ROM for 10 minutes.

(g) Pipette a 1 ml aliquot of plasma and transfer to a tube. 1 ml serum will be used as the blank for 1gram fluid.

(h) Count pledgets and plasma. Record values.

6. Compare cpm/ml of each pledget to cpm/mL of the 1 ml aliquot of plasma. Remember each pledget has been identified to its location. A ratio of greater than 2.5 (nasal fluid to plasma) or increased ratio of one side to the other side suggests CSF leak at the pledget site.

Radionuclide Imaging Evaluation of CSF Shunt Patency

Purposes

1. For patients with VP shunt, this procedure is useful in determining the VP shunt proximal and/or distal catheter patency and to visualize

the drained CSF distribution pattern in the abdominal and pelvic cavity.
2. For patients with Ommaya shunt, this is a procedure/imaging of choice to assess CSF communication, detect blockage of CSF pathway, evaluate CSF flow pattern, and predict distribution of chemotherapeutics.

Radiopharmaceutical and Dosage

- IN-111 DTPA 1 mCi (37 MBq)

Equipment

- SPECT Gamma camera fitted with medium energy collimator
- Aseptic materials to prepare the injection site: sterile pads, betadine prep, and sterile gloves.

Patient Prep

- None

Procedure

1. Verify order and review pertinent history that has already been completed by the special studies team.
2. Order the dose through radiopharmacy.
3. Contact neurosurgeon or neurosurgical fellow who is familiar with the shunt placement and the location of shunt injection/drug reservoir.
4. Enter dose in computer for radiopharmacy dispensing.
5. Check for order in chart and/or prescription.
6. Identify patient verbally and by patient wrist identification band.
7. Explain the procedure in a courteous and understandable manner.
8. The neurosurgeon or fellow will prepare injection site and dose patient by injecting 1 mCi

In-111 DTPA with a direct stick into the drug reservoir of the shunt device, followed by flushing the syringe with CSF or saline to assure proper administration of the dose amount.

Image Acquisition

1. Scan patient at 1–2 hours postinjection. Obtain an anterior and posterior view of the head and neck, posterior view of the spine to evaluate the extent of the radioactive tracer CSF flow, and anterior view of the abdomen and pelvis. Obtain each image for a minimum of 200 K or 10 minutes using a LFOV camera fitted with a medium energy collimator peaked at 170 KEV and 247 KEV.
2. Scan patient at 24 hours postinjection. Repeat the images obtained at 1–2 hours and include a SPECT image of the head using the same cisternogram protocol.

Image Interpretation

1. For patients with VP shunt, patent proximal catheter with normal CSF flow is indicated by radioactivity reaching basal cisterns at 1–2 hours, thoracolumbar CSF space at 2–4 hours, and parasagittal/convexities at 18–24 hours. Meanwhile, patent distal catheter is indicated by radioactivity drained into abdominal/pelvic cavity at 1–2 hours, with randomized and wide distribution and increased radioactivity over imaging time. Absent radioactivity in the ventricles and abdomen/pelvis hours after dosing is suggestive of high-grade obstruction of both proximal and distal VP shunt catheters, while selected absent radioactivity in the abdomen/pelvis is indicating high-grade distal VP shunt catheter obstruction that is the most commonly diagnosed VP shunt malfunction.
2. For patients with Ommaya shunt, patent shunt with normal CSF flow is indicated by radioactivity reaching basal cisterns at 1–2 hours, thoracolumbar CSF space at 2–4 hours, and parasagittal/convexity space at 18–24 hours. A delayed CSF flow, obstruction, or leakage is called abnormal. Distortion of anatomy of CSF space shall be reported as well.

Index

D. Wu, *Clinical Nuclear Medicine Neuroimaging*, https://doi.org/10.1007/978-3-030-40893-0

MIX
Papier aus verantwortungsvollen Quellen
Paper from responsible sources
FSC® C105338

If you have any concerns about our products,
you can contact us on
ProductSafety@springernature.com

In case Publisher is established outside the EU,
the EU authorized representative is:
Springer Nature Customer Service Center GmbH
Europaplatz 3, 69115 Heidelberg, Germany

Printed by Libri Plureos GmbH
in Hamburg, Germany